Laboratory test	Normal adult values	Variations in child
Hematology		
Hematocrit (%)	Men: 46 ± 3.1; women: 40.9 ± 3	Birth (cord blood): 52 ± 5 1 yr: 39 ± 2 5 yr: 37 ± 3 10 yr: 39 ± 3
Hemoglobin (g/dl)	Men: 15.5 ± 1.1; women: 13.7 ± 1	Birth (cord blood): 17.1 ± 1.8; 1 yr: 11.8 ± 0.5; 5 yr: 12.7 ± 1; 10 yr: 13.2 ± 1.2
Platelet count	150,000-400,000/mm^3	Newborns: 84,000-478,000/mm^3; infants: 200,000-473,000/mm^3
Red blood cell count	Men: 4.6-6.2 million/mm^3; women: 3.9-5.9 million/mm^3	3.8-5.5 million/mm^3
White blood cell count	4500-11,000/mm^3	6200-17,000/mm^3
Coagulation		
Bleeding time	Duke: 1-5 min; Ivy: 2-7 min	
Clotting time (Lee-White)	8-15 min	
Urinalysis		
Calcium (24 hr)	100-250 mg/day (diet dependent; based on average calcium intake of 600-800 mg/24 hr)	
Chloride	110-250 mEq/day	15-40 mmol/day
Creatinine	Men: 1-2 g/24 hr; women: 0.8-1.8 g/24 hr	2-3 yr: 6-22 mg/kg/24 hr; >3 yr: 12-30 mg/kg/24 hr
Cystine	Random sample negative	
Glucose	Up to 100 mg/24 hr	
Osmolality	250-900 mOsm/kg	
Oxalate	Up to 40 mg/24 hr	
Protein	30-150 mg/24 hr (method dependent)	Up to 140 mg/m^2 of body surface area is appropriate for small children
pH	4.5-8	5-7
Phosphorus	0.9-1.3 g/day (diet dependent)	
Potassium	26-123 mEq/24 hr (markedly intake dependent)	
Sodium	27-287 mEq/24 hr (diet dependent; output is lower at night)	
Specific gravity	1.003-1.029 (range in SI units)	
Urea nitrogen	6-17 g/day	
Uric acid	250-750 mg/day	
Volume	Men: 800-2000 ml/day; women: 800-1600 ml/day	500-1000 ml/day
Color	Pale to darker yellow	
Clarity	Clear	
Ketones	None	
Red blood count	0-5/high-power field	
White blood count	0-5/high-power field	
Bacteria	None/occasional in voided specimen	
Casts	0-4 hyaline casts/low-power field	
Crystals	Interpreted by physician	
Culture	Negative	
Other		
Creatinine clearance	Men: 85-125 ml/min/1.73 m^2; women: 75-115 ml/min/1.73 m^2; geriatric: 96.9 ± 2.9 ml/min/1.73 m^2	70-140 ml/min/1.73 m^2
Renal blood flow	600 ml/min/1.73 m^2; geriatric: 300 ml/min/1.73 m^2	600 ml/min/1.73 m^2
Glomerular rate	120 ml/min/1.73 m^2; geriatric: 65.3 ml/min/1.73 m^2	120 ml/min/1.73 m^2

GENITOURINARY DISORDERS

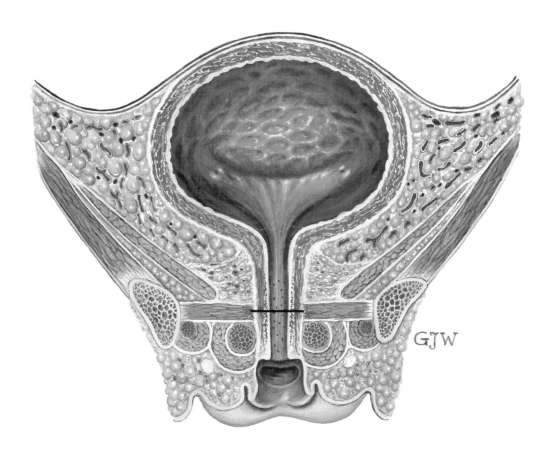

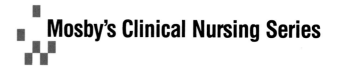

Mosby's Clinical Nursing Series

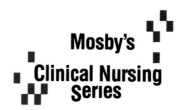

Mosby's
Clinical Nursing
Series

Cardiovascular Disorders

by Mary Canobbio

Respiratory Disorders

by Susan Wilson and June Thompson

Infectious Diseases

by Deanna Grimes

Orthopedic Disorders

by Leona Mourad

Renal Disorders

by Dorothy Brundage

Neurologic Disorders

by Esther Chipps, Norma Clanin, and Victor Campbell

Cancer Nursing

by Anne Belcher

Genitourinary Disorders

by Mikel Gray

Immunologic Disorders

by Christine Mudge-Grout

Gastrointestinal Disorders

by Dorothy Doughty and Debra Broadwell

GENITOURINARY DISORDERS

MIKEL GRAY, Ph.D., P.N.P., C.U.R.N.

Clinical Urodynamics,
Egelston Hospital for Children,
Scottish Rite Children's Medical Center,
Shepherd Spinal Center;
Clinical Professor,
Georgia State University School of Nursing,
Atlanta, Georgia

Original illustrations by
GEORGE J. WASSILCHENKO
Tulsa, Oklahoma
and
DONALD P. O'CONNOR
St. Peters, Missouri

Original photography by
PATRICK WATSON
Poughkeepsie, New York

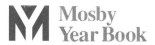
Mosby
Year Book

St. Louis Baltimore Boston Chicago London Philadelphia Sydney Toronto

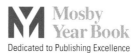
Mosby
Year Book
Dedicated to Publishing Excellence

Editor: Sally Adkisson
Project manager: Mark Spann
Production editors: Stephen C. Hetager, Christine O'Neil
Designer: Liz Fett
Layout: Doris Hallas

Acknowledgments
The author wishes to acknowledge the contributions of Ruth Gray, Office Manager for Clinical Urodynamics; Shepherd Spinal Center; Egelston Hospital Radiology Department; Life Tech, Inc., Houston, Texas; and James Lapesko, SurgiTek, Inc.

Dedication

This book is respectfully dedicated to Drs. John Woodard and Ingeborg Mauksch, whose examples of practice in urology and nursing set the standards of excellence to which I aspire.

Printed in the United States of America

Mosby–Year Book, Inc.
11830 Westline Industrial Drive
St. Louis, Missouri 63146

The authors and publisher have made a conscientious effort to ensure that the drug information and recommended dosages in this book are accurate and in accord with accepted standards at the time of publication. However, pharmacology is a rapidly changing science, so readers are advised to check the package insert provided by the manufacturer before administering any drug.

ISBN 0-8016-6876-X

92 93 94 95 96 CL/CD/VH 9 8 7 6 5 4 3 2

CONTRIBUTOR

Chapter 11, Genitourinary Drugs, contributed by

MARK BONIN, R.N., M.S.
Home Care Nurse,
St. Peters Hospice,
Albany, New York

CONSULTANTS

DOROTHY BRUNDAGE, Ph.D., R.N., F.A.A.N.
Associate Professor,
School of Nursing,
Duke University Medical Center,
Chapel Hill, North Carolina

JAMES K. BENNETT, M.D.
Shepherd Urological Associates,
Atlanta, Georgia

JANELLE FOOTE, M.D.
Shepherd Urological Associates,
Atlanta, Georgia

BRUCE G. GREEN, M.D.
Shepherd Urological Associates,
Atlanta, Georgia

THOMAS S. PARROTT, M.D.
Pediatric Urology,
Atlanta, Georgia

JOHN R. WOODARD, M.D.
Pediatric Urology,
Atlanta, Georgia

Preface

Genitourinary Disorders is the eighth volume in *Mosby's Clinical Nursing Series*, a new kind of resource for practicing nurses.

The *Series* is the result of the most elaborate market research ever undertaken by Mosby–Year Book, Inc. We first surveyed hundreds of working nurses to determine what kinds of resources practicing nurses want in order to meet their advanced information needs. We then approached clinical specialists—proven authors and experts—and asked them to develop a consistent format that would meet the needs of nurses in practice. This format was presented to nine focus groups composed of working nurses and refined between each group. In the later stages we published a 32-page full-color sample so that detailed changes could be made to improve physical layout and appearance, page by page.

Genitourinary Disorders begins with an innovative collection of highly detailed drawings that support a state-of-the-art discussion of the transport, storage, and evacuation functions of the urinary system. The chapter also provides state-of-the-art drawings and discussion of male and female reproductive anatomy and physiology.

Chapter 2 is a pictorial guide to the nursing assessment of the genitourinary system. A practical, illustrated guide to physical examination is augmented by concise, thorough examples of historical interview for the most important genitourinary system disorders.

Chapter 3 presents a review of the most current diagnostic studies, with full-color photographs of equipment and results. A consistent format for each test gives nurses information about the purpose of the examination, indications and contraindications, and associated nursing care and patient teaching.

Chapters 4 to 9 present the nursing care of patients experiencing infection or inflammation of the genitourinary system, voiding dysfunction, obstructive uropathy, urologic cancer, erectile dysfunction, or infertility, which is discussed from the perspective of the affected couple. Each disorder is presented in a format to meet advanced practice needs. Information on pathophysiology answers the most common questions nurses pose. A unique box alerts nurses to possible complications, since nurses are the health professionals in the best position to report potentially dangerous changes in patient conditions. Definitive diagnostic tests and common medical treatment options are briefly reviewed to promote collaboration among team members in designing an appropriate nursing care plan. Highlighted boxes provide detailed plans of care for specific surgical, trans-urethral, extracorporeal, and other therapeutic procedures.

The heart of the book is the nursing care, presented according to the nursing process. These pages have a color border for easy access to the nurse practicing in the acute inpatient unit, surgical/cystoscopy suite, special procedure laboratory, or ambulatory/outpatient care facility. Each nursing care plan integrates the five steps of the nursing process, including nursing diagnoses accepted by the North American Nursing Diagnosis Association (NANDA). The material can be used to develop individual care plans quickly and accurately. By facilitating the development of individualized and authoritative care plans, this book can save the nurse time for direct patient care.

In response to requests from scores of nurses participating in our research, a distinctive feature of this book is its usefulness for patient teaching. Background material allows nurses to answer common patient questions with authority. The illustrations in the book, particularly those in the anatomy and physiology, assessment, and diagnostic procedures chapters, are specifically designed to support patient teaching. Chapter 10 is a compilation of patient teaching guides that supplement specific guides for each disorder. The patient teaching guides are ideal for reproduction and distribution to patients.

The book concludes with a concise guide to commonly used genitourinary drugs. Particular emphasis is placed on antiinfective drugs and on agents used to manage voiding dysfunction and urinary stones. Highlighted boxes seen throughout the book provide information on drugs used for highly specific genitourinary disorders.

This book is intended for medical-surgical nurses, who invariably care for individuals with genitourinary disorders. The book will provide valuable information for urological nurses who practice in the inpatient unit, clinic, urodynamic laboratory, lithotripsy unit, or surgical/cystoscopy suite. It will also serve as a resource for the urological nurse preparing for specialty certification. Students will find the book an indispensable resource for learning to care for patients with genitourinary disorders, as will professional nurses who have returned to practice after a hiatus.

We hope this book contributes to the advancement of professional nursing by serving as a first step toward a body of scientific literature for nurses to call their own.

Contents

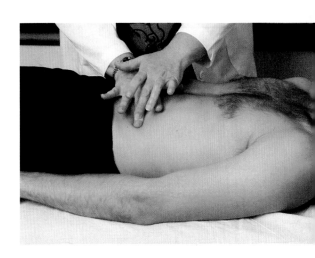

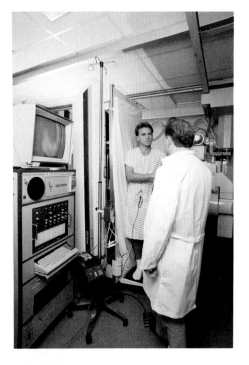

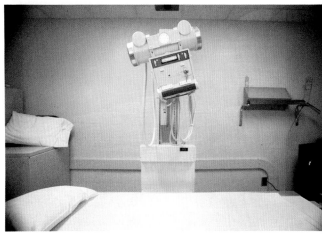

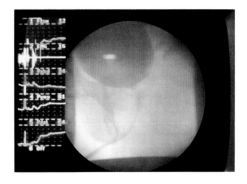

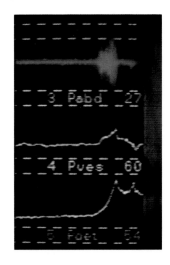

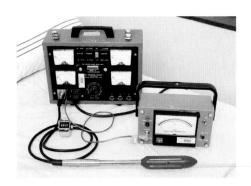

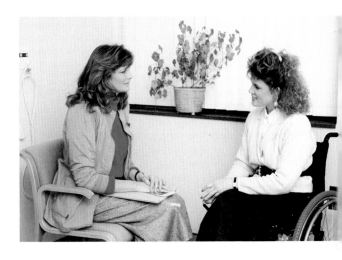

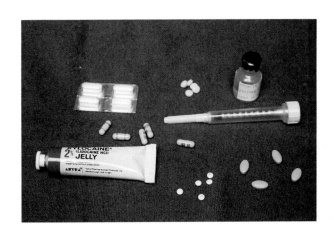

Color Plates

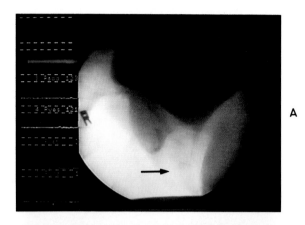

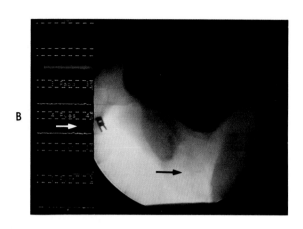

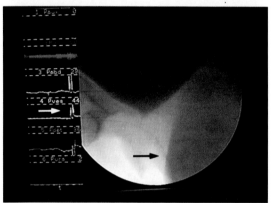

PLATE 1 **A.** Videourodynamic image shows pelvic descent with closed bladder outlet at rest. Patient is standing. Arrow indicates bladder neck below inferior aspect of symphysis pubis.

PLATE 1 **B.** Coughing causes urethral descent, transient funneling of bladder outlet with stress urinary leakage. Arrow on right indicates open urethra and arrow on left shows high intravesical pressure (121 cm H_2O) produced by cough.

PLATE 1 **C.** Following the cough the outlet rapidly closes and leakage is stopped. Arrow on left demonstrates cough occurring several seconds earlier and arrow on right shows closed bladder outlet.

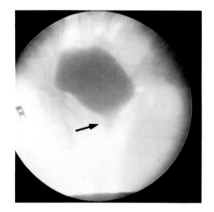

PLATE 2 Cystogram of stress incontinence caused by sphincter incompetence. Arrow indicates open bladder outlet; patient is standing without coughing or straining. Active leakage is noted.

PLATE 3 Videourodynamic image of unstable detrusor contraction producing instability (urge) incontinence. Arrow on left shows the contraction noted in intravesical and detrusor pressure channels. Arrow on right shows open bladder outlet caused by contraction.

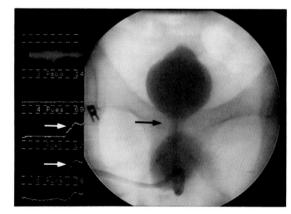

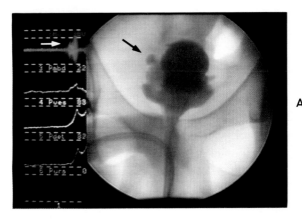
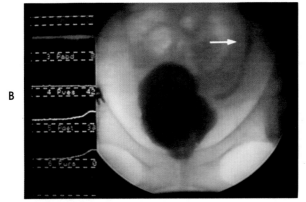

PLATE 4 A. Videourodynamic image of instability (reflex) incontinence with trabeculation caused by vesicosphincter dyssynergia. Arrow on the left indicates sphincter EMG activity of dyssynergia and the arrow on the right shows severe trabeculation with diverticula.

PLATE 4 B. Videourodynamic image of instability (reflex) incontinence with vesicoureteral reflux. Arrow indicates left reflux caused by dyssynergia.

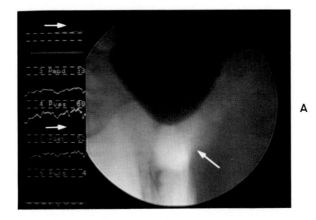
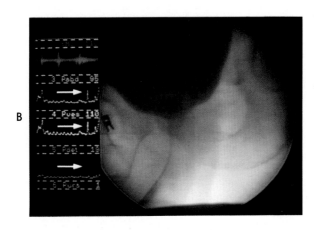

PLATE 5 A. Videourodynamic image of urinary retention caused by bladder outlet obstruction in a female. A large cystocele causes much of the bladder to lie below the outlet, producing mild mechanical obstruction. Arrow on the top left indicates poor flow and the arrow near the bottom indicates high voiding pressure (69 cm H_2O). Arrow on the right indicates large cystocele.

PLATE 5 B. Videourodynamic image of urinary retention caused by deficient detrusor contractility in a male patient. Arrows on the left indicate straining pattern noted in intravesical and abdominal pressure channels and the arrow on the bottom left shows flat detrusor pressure tracing with absent contraction.

Urinary System

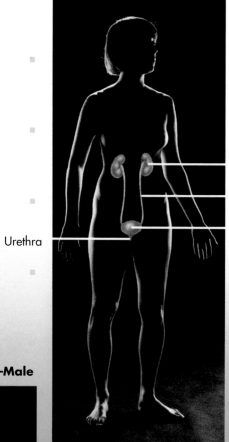

Kidney

Ureter

Bladder

Urethra

Reproductive System–Male

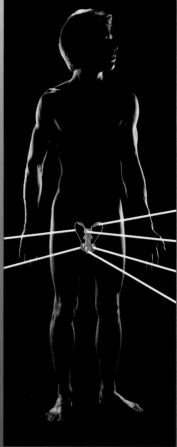

Seminal vesicle

Prostate gland

Testis

Glans penis

Ductus deferens

Epididymis

Reproductive System–Female

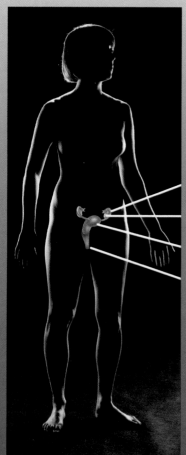

Uterine tube

Ovary

Uterus

Vagina

CHAPTER 1

Color Atlas of Genitourinary Structure and Function

The urinary system consists of the kidneys, renal pelves, ureters, urinary bladder, and urethra. Urologic nursing care focuses on changes in urine transport, storage, and elimination, in contrast to nephrologic nursing, which emphasizes care related to changes in the production of urine. Urologic nursing also addresses the male and female reproductive system, with emphasis on erectile function of the male and fertility physiology for both sexes.

KIDNEY

The kidneys are a pair of dark reddish brown organs located in the retroperitoneal space adjacent to spinal levels T12, L1, L2, and L3 (Figures 1-1 and 1-2). The convex surface of the kidneys faces away from the spine at a 90-degree angle, and the concave surface faces the spine. The concave surface contains the renal hilus and the point where the renal artery, veins, and ureter exit the organ.

The weight of an adult's kidney varies from 115 to 175 grams; women typically have slightly smaller kidneys than do men. The normal adult kidney is 11 cm long from upper to lower pole, 5 to 7 cm wide, and up to 3.5 cm thick. Normally an adult's kidneys are symmetric in shape and size, although the right kidney is situated slightly lower than the left because of the presence of the liver.

The cross-sectional anatomy of the kidney is important, because it helps explain the way urine is transported from the nephron to the renal pelvis. Two distinct sections are noted, the pelvis and the paren-

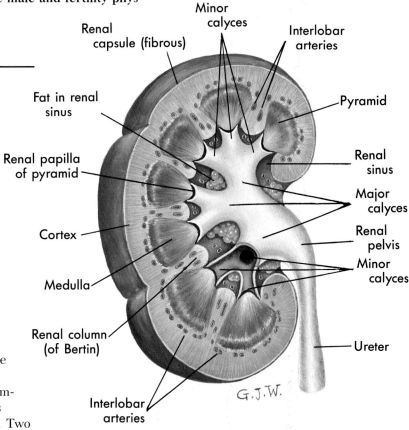

FIGURE 1-1
Cross-section of the kidney showing basic structures. (From Brundage D: *Renal disorders*, St Louis, 1992, Mosby–Year Book.)

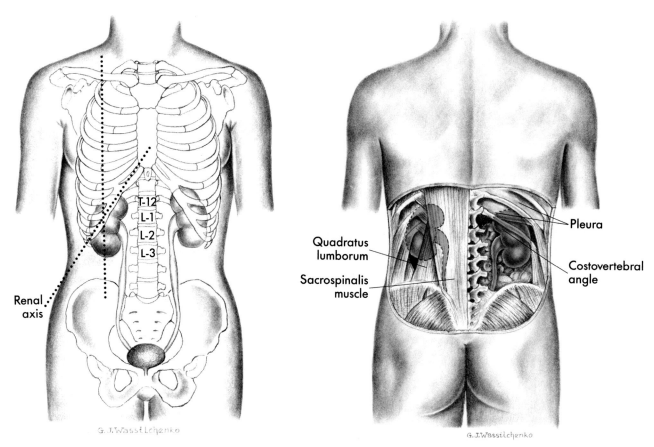

G. J. Wassilchenko

G. J. Wassilchenko

FIGURE 1-2
Anatomic relation of kidneys to spinal column. (From Thompson J et al, editors:
Mosby's manual of clinical nursing, ed 2, St Louis, 1989, Mosby—Year Book.)

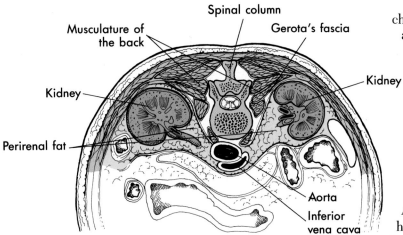

FIGURE 1-3
Protective covering of kidneys.

chyma. The **renal parenchyma** comprises a cortex and medulla that are visible to the unaided eye. The **renal medulla** contains the pyramids, conical-shaped structures with bases oriented toward the lateral border of the kidney and apices approaching the renal hilus. The **renal cortex** surrounds the medulla, forming columns and lobules that surround and fill the space between pyramids.

The coverings of the kidney are also important, because they support the kidney and protect it from physical stress or trauma (Figure 1-3). A capsule of dense connective tissue loosely adheres to the renal cortex. It is surrounded by a layer of perirenal fascia and enclosed within a layer of perinephric fat. The entire kidney and the superiorly located adrenal gland are covered in another layer of dense connective tissue, called Gerota's fascia. The kidneys are further protected by the diaphragm, abdominal muscles, quadratus lumborum muscles, and overlying ribs. Collectively, these structures form a shock absorber and protective shields that guard against damage to the urinary system from blunt or penetrating trauma.

The blood supply of the kidneys arises from the renal arteries that branch directly from the abdominal aorta (Figure 1-4). Normally an adult has one or more renal arteries. Renal veins are paired with the arteries and empty into the inferior vena cava. Lymphatic channels drain into paraaortic and para vena caval node chains.

The most important function of the kidneys is producing urine. The kidneys filter water and solutes from the bloodstream and then selectively reabsorb or excrete fluids and solutes. Renal function requires a low-pressure, obstruction-free transport and storage system from the renal pelvis to the urethral meatus. Disorders of the urinary system transport, storage, or expulsive functions endanger the urine formation function when they lead to obstruction, elevated urinary system pressure, and stasis.

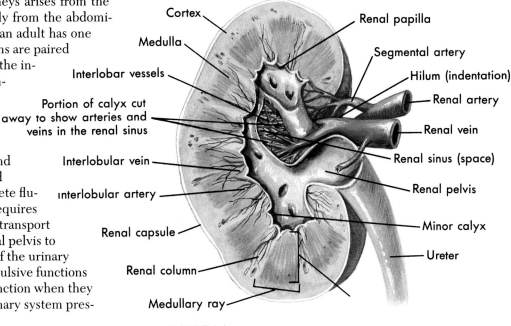

FIGURE 1-4
Blood supply of kidneys. (From Seeley.[15])

RENAL PELVIS AND URETERS

Each kidney drains urine into the bladder via a renal pelvis and ureter (Figure 1-5). The renal pelvis and ureter form a continuous tube extending from the renal hilus to the base of the bladder. The pelvis is a funnel-shaped structure that originates at the major calyces and tapers into the ureter at the ureteropelvic junction (UPJ). The tube-shaped ureter is approximately 24 to 30 cm long; the left ureter is slightly longer than the right one because of the difference in the kidneys' location. The ureter follows a course from the renal pelvis to the bladder that resembles an inverted **S**. The ureter travels medially from the ureteropelvic junction to pass over the psoas muscle to the sacroiliac joint of the bony pelvis. It then turns laterally toward the ischial spine of the pelvis and curves back toward the base of the bladder, where it inserts into the trigone muscle.

The lumen (interior) of the ureter varies in diameter from 0.2 to 1 cm. Three areas of the lumen are particularly narrow and susceptible to obstruction by calculi (urinary stones): the ureteropelvic junction, the point where the ureter crosses the iliac arteries, and the ureterovesical junction.

The microscopic anatomy of the ureters is defined by three layers. The innermost layer is an epithelial mucosa consisting of transitional-cell epithelium that is resistant to secretion or reabsorption of urine contents.

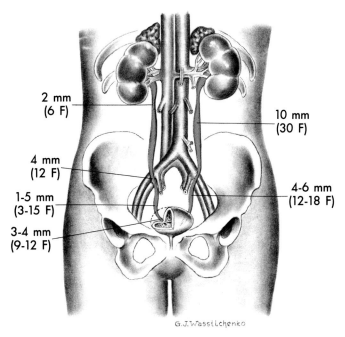

FIGURE 1-5
Course of ureter with its varying internal luminal sizes. (From Thompson J et al, editors: *Mosby's manual of clinical nursing*, ed 2, St Louis, 1989, Mosby–Year Book.)

A submucosal lamina propria, containing nerves and vascular elements, lies just outside the epithelium. It is bounded by a layer of smooth muscle. These smooth muscle bundles are arranged into a complex meshwork of interconnecting bundles. The purpose of the ure-

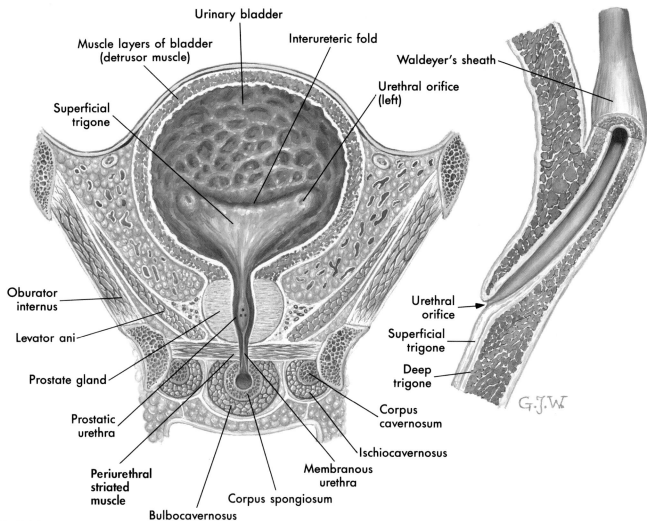

Labels on figure:

Urinary bladder
Muscle layers of bladder (detrusor muscle)
Interureteric fold
Waldeyer's sheath
Urethral orifice (left)
Superficial trigone
Oburator internus
Levator ani
Prostate gland
Prostatic urethra
Periurethral striated muscle
Bulbocavernosus
Corpus spongiosum
Membranous urethra
Ischiocavernosus
Corpus cavernosum
Urethral orifice
Superficial trigone
Deep trigone
G.J.W

FIGURE 1-6
Ureterovesical junction.

teral smooth muscle is to transport urine from the kidneys to the bladder in response to neural, chemical, or mechanical influences.

The arterial blood supply of the ureters varies among individuals. Upper ureteral segments may receive blood from branches of the renal, gonadal, or adrenal arteries, and lower (pelvic) segments may receive blood from branches of the obturator artery, deferential artery (men), or uterine artery (women). Venous blood drains into a venous plexus and leaves the ureter via vessels that parallel the arterial supply. Lymphatic drainage is provided by paraaortic or renal node chains and common or external iliacs.

URETERAL FUNCTION

The renal pelvis and ureter transport urine from the kidney to bladder in an antegrade fashion, a process called efflux. The ureters transport urine by means of muscle contraction or peristalsis. Urine transport in the ureter may be compared to peristalsis of the bowel. The renal pelvis stores only a small amount of urine (15 to 20 ml) before distention propagates a peristaltic wave thought to originate from pacemaker cells in the calyces. This causes a propulsive contraction

that forces a bolus of urine from the renal pelvis to the ureter. The smooth muscle of the ureter contains gap junctions that act as a single unit. Thus a single peristaltic wave causes a chain of contraction that pushes the urine through the entire ureteral course and into the bladder.

Besides mechanical distention, neural, endocrine, and pharmacologic factors also modulate ureteral smooth muscle contractions. Stimulation of alpha-adrenergic receptors in the ureteral wall increases the number and amplitude (strength) of contractions, whereas stimulation of beta-adrenergic receptors causes ureteral relaxation. Stimulation of cholinergic receptors in the ureters is thought to cause more vigorous peristalsis through the release of catecholamines. Administration of epinephrine or catecholamines enhances peristalsis. Hormonal changes related to pregnancy only indirectly influence ureteral dilation and the organ's ability to propagate peristaltic waves.

URETEROVESICAL JUNCTION

The ureterovesical junction has three components: the lower portion of the ureter, the trigone muscle, and the adjacent bladder wall (Figure 1-6). The lower segment of the ureter enters the bladder at the lateral aspect of the trigone muscle, near the urethrovesical outlet. The portion of the ureter that travels through the bladder wall is unique from upper ureteral segments and is called the intravesical ureter. It is approximately 1.5 cm long and is divided into an intramural segment, which is surrounded by the detrusor muscle, and a submucosal segment, which courses under the bladder mucosa. The intravesical ureter terminates as the ureterovesical valve, which opens into the bladder vesicle.

The lower segment of the ureter is anchored to the bladder by an adventitia of dense connective tissue. The superficial layer of the adventitia is an extension of the connective tissue of the bladder wall, and the deep layer is an extension of ureteral adventitia. Between these layers is Waldeyer's sheath, a plane of loose connective tissue that gives the intravesical ureter mobility, needed to accommodate changes in bladder structure as the bladder fills with urine.

The intravesical ureter also differs from upper ureteral segments in the arrangement of smooth muscle bundles. Whereas the upper ureteral segments form a complex meshwork, the intravesical ureteral bundles are more simply arranged in a longitudinal fashion, promoting closure of the lumen. These muscle bundles fan out and terminate in the trigone muscle of the bladder base.

The trigone is divided into two parts, superficial muscle and deep muscle. The deep trigone is made up of flat, tightly bound smooth muscle bundles; it is a continuation of Waldeyer's sheath. It terminates at the bladder neck in a layer of circular smooth muscle bundles that contribute to continence. The superficial trigone is an extension of the muscle bundles of the intravesical ureter. The longitudinal muscle bundles extend to the bladder neck in women and into the proximal urethra in men.

The part of the bladder wall adjacent to the ureterovesical ureter also is unique. It contains circular and longitudinally arranged smooth muscle bundles that help secure the intravesical ureter as it enters the bladder. The detrusor muscle bundles near the ureterovesical junction are the strongest, most resilient muscles of the bladder. This strength is important in protecting the continuity of the ureterovesical junction against physical stress or trauma.

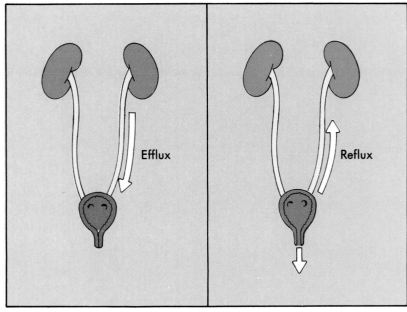

FIGURE 1-7
Function of ureterovesical junction.

Function of the Ureterovesical Junction

The ureterovesical junction allows urine to pass from the upper urinary tract (kidneys and ureters) to the lower urinary tract (bladder and urethra) and prevents regurgitation of urine in the opposite direction. The antegrade movement of urine from the upper to the lower urinary tract is called *efflux*, and retrograde movement from the bladder to the ureters or kidneys is called *reflux* (Figure 1-7). During bladder filling, intravesical pressure remains relatively low, and the detrusor muscle remains relaxed. Thus the pressure produced by peristaltic waves in the ureters propels spurts of urine through the ureterovesical junction into the bladder. During micturition, however, intravesical pressure is elevated for some time, favoring reflux of urine from the bladder to the upper urinary tract; this unfavorable condition is prevented by active and passive adaptation of the ureterovesical junction. Immediately before the detrusor muscle contracts, the muscles of the intravesical ureter and trigone contract, preventing any urine from moving through the junction. This tone is maintained for approximately 20 seconds after micturition has been completed. In addition, contraction of the detrusor muscle closes the ureterovesical junction, further reducing the possibility of reflux. This mechanism also protects the bladder from reflux during the precipitous rise in pressure noted during physical exercise or stress. After the intravesical ureter and trigone muscles relax, efflux of urine resumes and the bladder begins to refill with urine.

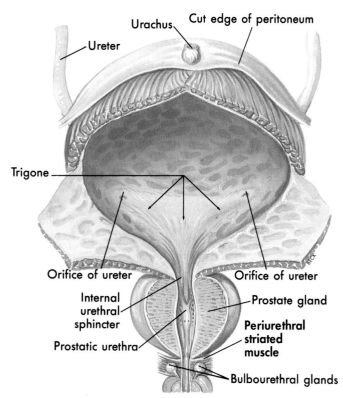

FIGURE 1-8
Anteroposterior view of bladder. (From Thibodeau GA: *Anatomy and physiology*, St Louis, 1989, Mosby–Year Book.)

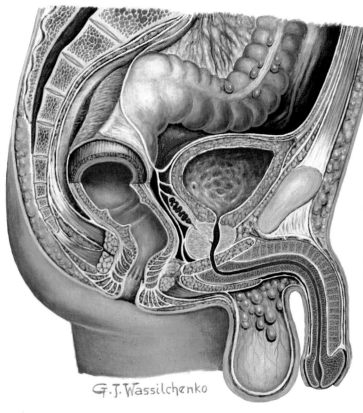

FIGURE 1-9
Lateral view of bladder showing relation to surrounding perineopelvic structures.

URETHROVESICAL UNIT (LOWER URINARY TRACT)

The urethrovesical unit consists of the urinary bladder, urethra, and pelvic floor muscles. Together these organs form a functional system that allows the bladder to fill with and store urine until the individual empties the system through voluntary expulsion, called micturition.

URINARY BLADDER

The urinary bladder is a hollow, muscle-lined organ located in the true pelvis of the adult (Figures 1-8 and 1-9). Its shape varies with the amount of urine it contains. An empty bladder lies entirely in the pelvis in approximately the shape of a tetrahedron. As it fills, the bladder assumes a more spherical shape as its dome and upper aspect enter the abdomen, approaching the level of the umbilicus.

The central opening (vesicle) of the bladder is interrupted by three openings. The ureterovesical valves mark the termination of the intravesical ureters in the base of the bladder. At its most inferior aspect, a single outlet, the bladder neck, connects the bladder to the urethra. The bladder neck and base are configured in a triangular fashion, and their shape remains fixed, regardless of how much urine the bladder contains.

In contrast, the upper parts of the bladder can change shape considerably in response to varying urine volumes. Above the base of the bladder, the apex and lateral aspects of the detrusor muscle are visible. The bladder is anchored to the abdominal wall by the urachus, and the organ approaches the umbilicus in the abdomen as it fills to 300 milliliters or more.

The microscopic anatomy of the bladder is characterized by four layers (Figure 1-10): the urothelium, the vascular submucosa, the smooth muscle bundles of the detrusor, and the protective adventitia. The urothelium is made up of transitional epithelial cells that are six to eight cells deep in the empty organ. As the bladder fills, the urothelium increases its surface area to accommodate the increasing volume of urine by stretching to a structure only two or three cells thick. This process occurs by smoothing of redundant macroscopic and microscopic wrinkles and by changes in the configuration of specialized protein structures in the urothelium. The urothelium is remarkable for its impermeability to excretion or reabsorption of water or solutes, a characteristic necessary to prevent reaccumulation of urinary waste products before expulsion.

The submucosa of the urinary bladder lies immediately beneath the urothelium. It consists of connective tissue, arteries, veins, lymphatic channels, and nerves.

Adventitia Smooth muscle of detrusor Vascular submucosa

Urothelium

Urothelium — transitional epithelium

Filled (stretched) bladder   Empty bladder

FIGURE 1-10
Microscopic anatomy of the bladder.

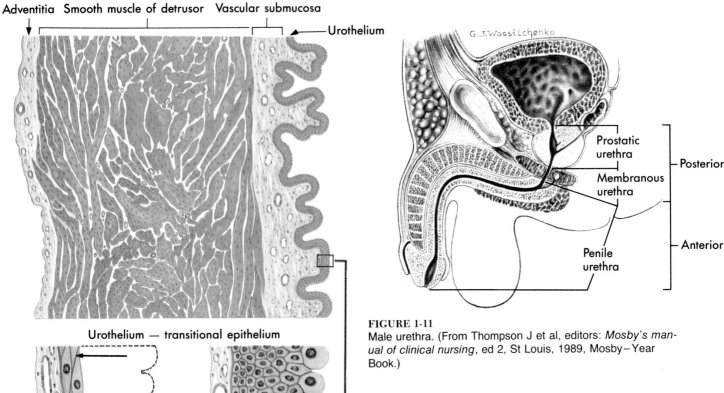

FIGURE 1-11
Male urethra. (From Thompson J et al, editors: *Mosby's manual of clinical nursing*, ed 2, St Louis, 1989, Mosby–Year Book.)

URETHRA

The urethra extends from the bladder neck to an external meatus. It has a sphincter mechanism that serves the dual purpose of preventing leakage between episodes of micturition and serving as a nonobstructing conduit during urination.

Male Urethra

The male urethra extends from the bladder neck through the prostate and the penile shaft to its meatus at the glans penis (Figure 1-11). It is divided into two segments, the proximal, or sphincteric, urethra and the distal, or conduit, urethra. After exiting the bladder at the bladder neck, the proximal urethra extends approximately 3 cm through the vertical axis of the prostate, near its anterior border. The posterior segment of the prostatic urethra is raised by the verumontanum. The verumontanum tapers at its inferior and superior aspects to form the cristae, small pores that secrete prostatic fluid during ejaculation.

The membranous urethra is approximately 2.5 cm long and lies just below the prostate. It pierces the pelvic floor muscles at a point called the pelvic diaphragm. Immediately adjacent to the membranous urethra are the periurethral muscles; intrinsic to the membranous urethra are the C-shaped fibers of the rhabdosphincter. The membranous urethra is the least distensible segment of the male urethra and is particularly susceptible to urethral stricture.

The distal (conduit) urethra tunnels from the membranous segment through the penis to its termination at the fossa navicularis. It is divided into the bulbous, pendulous, and glandular urethras. The bulbous and pendulous urethras together are approximately 15 cm

The smooth muscle bundles of the bladder wall are collectively referred to as the detrusor muscle. The muscle bundles are interspersed with collagenous supporting tissue in a complex meshwork that is not readily definable in specific layers. An autonomic plexus occupies the detrusor muscle bundles in a nearly 1:1 ratio.

The adventitial layer of the bladder is composed of connective tissue. It is loosely connected to the peritoneal fascia of the pelvis and anchored to the abdominal wall by the urachus.

Arterial blood to the bladder is derived from branches of the inferior hypogastric or internal iliac artery. In women, small branches from the uterine, vaginal, or obturator artery may feed the bladder. Inferior and superior vascular pedicles are noted. Unlike other structures of the urinary system, venous blood from the bladder does not follow arterial routes. Venous blood leaves the bladder via the anterior plexus of Santorini and flows laterally into a neurovascular sheath surrounded by lateral vesicle ligaments. Lymphatic drainage from the bladder enters the vesical, internal, and common iliac arteries and hypogastric chains.

long and extend from the membranous segment to the base of the penis. The penile urethra is encased in the corpus spongiosum under the cavernosal bodies. It terminates in the fossa navicularis, a dilated chamber 2.5 cm long that lies near the corona of the glans penis.

The microscopic anatomy of the male urethra comprises an inner urothelium lined by transitional epithelium and abundant secretory cells. Immediately underneath is a submucosal layer with vascular elements, lymphatic channels, and nerves. The proximal (sphincteric) urethra contains smooth muscle bundles and specialized skeletal muscle fibers of the rhabdosphincter.

The arterial blood supply of the male urethra arises from branches of the internal pudendal artery. Venous blood drains from the deep penile vein and pudendal plexus. Lymphatic channels empty into the subinguinal node chain.

Female Urethra

Compared to the male system, the female urethra traces a relatively short, straight course from the bladder neck to the external meatus (Figure 1-12). (Also refer to Figure 1-23 on p. 17.) It is made up of a single segment comparable to the proximal (sphincteric) urethra in men. In nulliparous women, the urethra is approximately 3 to 5 cm long. It exits the bladder neck at a 16-degree angle, travels parallel to the vagina, and terminates just superior to the vestibule. The distal (conduit) urethra is fused to the anterior vaginal wall. The proximal urethra contains smooth muscle bundles, and its middle third is lined by specialized C-shaped skeletal muscle fibers that form the rhabdosphincter.[5] Pelvic floor muscles also approach the distal segment of the female urethra, forming the periurethral musculature.

The microscopic anatomy of the female urethra is characterized by three layers. An inner urothelium comprises transitional epithelium with abundant mucus-producing cells. The submucosa contains nerves, lymphatic channels, and a particularly rich vascular network. Smooth muscle bundles are noted at the bladder neck in women; their contribution to continence remains unclear. The intrinsic skeletal muscle fibers that form the rhabdosphincter are abundant in the middle third of the female urethra. In addition, the periurethral muscles of the pelvic floor, noted in the distal portion of the female urethra, contribute to the urethral sphincter mechanism.

PELVIC FLOOR MUSCLES

The pelvic floor muscles form the final component of the urethrovesical unit (Figure 1-13). The pelvic floor muscles are a group of muscles made up predominantly of slow-twitch fibers that support the viscera of the pelvis. However, unlike with the rhabdosphincter, fast-twitch fibers that respond rapidly to sudden pres-

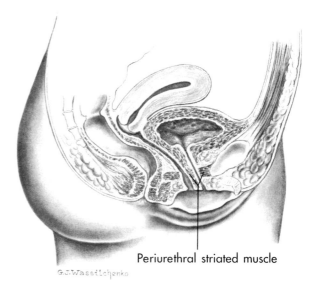

Periurethral striated muscle

G.J.Wassilchenko

FIGURE 1-12
Anatomic relations of female urethra. (From Thompson J et al, editors: *Mosby's Manual of Clinical Nursing*, ed 2, St Louis, 1989, Mosby–Year Book.)

sure changes caused by exercise, coughing, sneezing, or other forms of physical exertion are also seen in the pelvic floor muscles.[6]

The pelvic floor muscles extend from the anterior to the posterior aspects of the bony pelvis, forming a sling that supports the urethrovesical unit, rectum, and certain reproductive organs. In men, the pelvic floor muscles are divided into superior and inferior divisions. The superior portion forms part of the rectal sphincter and the periurethral muscles that contribute to the urethral sphincter mechanism. The inferior portion of the pelvic floor muscles contributes primarily to the rectal gutter. In women, the superior part of the pelvic musculature also forms the periurethral muscles and part of the anal sphincter, whereas the inferior division contributes only indirectly to urethrovesical functioning.

PHYSIOLOGY OF URETHROVESICAL UNIT

The function of the urethrovesical unit is to serve as a filling and storage compartment for urine. At controlled intervals, the urethrovesical unit also expels the bladder's contents through micturition. In adults, voluntary control over the functioning of the urethrovesical unit is called urinary continence. (See box on page 9.)

ANATOMIC INTEGRITY OF URETHROVESICAL UNIT

An intact urinary system transports urine from the kidneys to the ureters to the bladder for expulsion via the urethra. Any interruption in the structural integrity of the system will bypass the normal transport, storage, and expulsive tract, resulting in extraurethral urine loss. Ectopia and fistulous tracts are examples of interruption of structural integrity that may cause loss of continence.

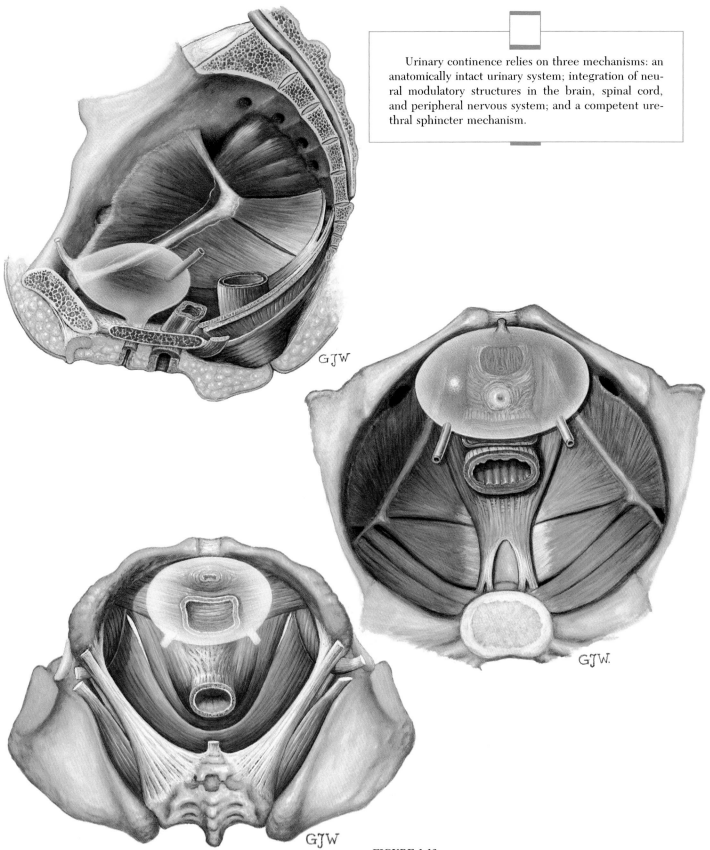

Urinary continence relies on three mechanisms: an anatomically intact urinary system; integration of neural modulatory structures in the brain, spinal cord, and peripheral nervous system; and a competent urethral sphincter mechanism.

FIGURE 1-13
Bladder relationship with pelvic floor muscles.

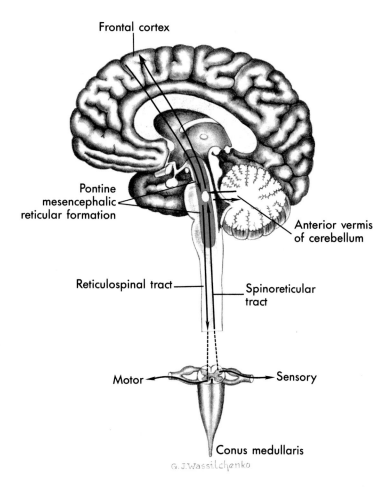

FIGURE 1-14
Central nervous system innervation of the bladder including
the pons. (From Thompson J et al, editors: *Mosby's manual of
clinical nursing*, ed 2, St Louis, 1989, Mosby–Year Book.)

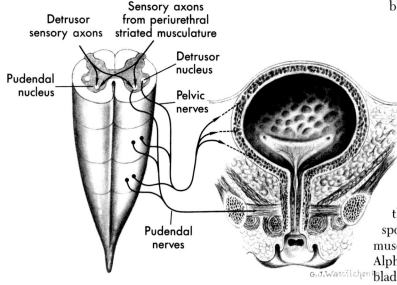

FIGURE 1-15
Sacral micturition center and peripheral bladder innervations.
(From Thompson J et al, editors: *Mosby's manual of clinical
nursing*, ed 2, St Louis, 1989, Mosby–Year Book.)

NEUROLOGIC MODULATION OF URETHROVESICAL UNIT

The second mechanism necessary for continence comprises neural modulatory centers in the brain, spinal cord, and peripheral nervous system. Several brain structures influence bladder function (Figure 1-14). A detrusor motor area is located in the cerebral cortex, and bladder function is also influenced by the thalamus, hypothalamus, basal ganglia, and possibly by the limbic system. The net effect of the brain on the urethrovesical unit is to suppress detrusor contractions until the individual wishes to urinate. The term *stable bladder* is used to describe volitional control over the timing of bladder emptying.

The brainstem also plays an important role in controlling the detrusor reflex. Two centers, located in the pons, directly modulate the act of micturition. An "M" center instigates the detrusor reflex, and an "L" center coordinates pelvic floor tone with the resulting bladder contraction.[8,9] In infants, the pontine micturition center acts without input from higher centers in the brain. Thus the infantile pons responds to stretch receptors in the bladder, producing a voiding response coordinated to filling with urine. In a continent adult, the pons responds to messages from the brain, and voiding occurs only when "permission" has been given by higher brain centers. The response is a contraction of the bladder and coordinated relaxation of pelvic floor muscles, allowing efficient emptying.

The spinal cord acts as mediator of messages from higher nervous centers in the brain and pons (Figure 1-15). The sympathetic nervous system sends signals from nerve roots at spinal levels T10 to L2 to the bladder and sphincter mechanism. These signals promote bladder filling and storage, causing the detrusor to relax and the sphincter to close. Parasympathetic signals arise from nerve roots at sacral levels 2 through 4. These signals promote voiding, causing the detrusor muscle to contract and the sphincter mechanism to relax. Somatic input to the pelvic floor muscles arises from sacral roots 1 through 3. These nerves control the pelvic floor muscles.

Three peripheral nerves transmit messages from the central nervous system to the bladder (see Figure 1-16). The hypogastric plexus primarily transmits sympathetic input to the bladder. Beta-adrenergic nerve endings respond to sympathetic input, causing the detrusor muscle to relax, thus favoring filling and storage. Alpha-adrenergics (excitatory nerve endings at the bladder neck, proximal urethra, and rhabdosphincter) also receive sympathetic signals. They respond by increasing the sphincter closure tension, promoting the filling and storage functions of the urethrovesical unit.

The pelvic plexus transmits parasympathetic signals to the detrusor muscle bundles. Cholinergic (muscarinic) receptors in the bladder wall respond by contracting the detrusor muscle, promoting voiding. In addition, cholinergic receptors in the rhabdosphincter may promote relaxation of the sphincter mechanism, further promoting micturition just as the pons produces reflex relaxation of the periurethral striated muscles.

The pudendal nerve transmits signals from the brain and pons to the pelvic floor skeletal muscles, including the periurethral muscles. During bladder filling these muscles provide tone that helps close the urethral sphincter while they reflexively relax (under pontine control) during micturition. Nonetheless, the pelvic floor muscles remain under voluntary control. Thus they can be used to willfully interrupt the urinary stream should the individual desire to stop micturition before the bladder is empty. The pelvic floor muscles add to sphincter closure by contracting rapidly during periods of physical stress.

Control of the detrusor reflex requires coordination of these elements of the nervous system (Figure 1-16). During bladder filling, the bladder transmits messages to the brain and pons when the volume of urine stimulates the stretch receptors in the bladder wall. The brain inhibits the detrusor reflex until the individual wishes to urinate. As a result, sympathetic signals to the bladder predominate, and the detrusor remains relaxed while the sphincter mechanism remains closed. At an appropriate time and place, micturition ensues. The brain releases its inhibitory control over the pons, and parasympathetic input to the bladder predominates, causing the detrusor to contract and the sphincter mechanism to relax. When the bladder is empty, the detrusor contractions stop, the sphincter closes, and filling and storage resume.

SPHINCTER MECHANISM

The third crucial element of continence is a competent urethral sphincter mechanism. The urethral sphincter mechanism consists of two principal components, the elements of compression and the elements of active tone (Figure 1-17). The coaptation (closure) of the urethral lumen is the first crucial element of forming a watertight seal to prevent leakage between episodes of micturition. The softness of the urethral wall is necessary for the sphincter to close in response to active tension. In contrast to the stiff walls of a rigid pipe, which do not close when the pipe is empty, the soft

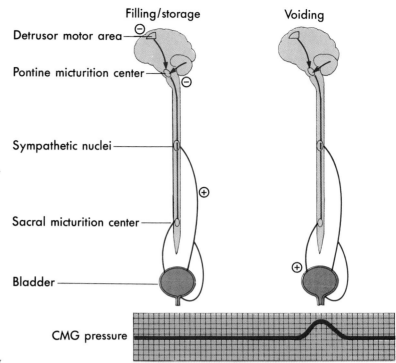

FIGURE 1-16
Filling/storage and voiding with cystometrogram (CMG) pressure.

mucosae of the urethra close passively unless intraurethral pressure forces them open. However, even with this passive closure, microscopic grooves that can allow urine to leak persist. These openings are sealed by the mucus produced by the urethral epithelium. This closure is further assisted by the rich vascular cushion in the submucosal layer of the urethral sphincter. This vascular cushion contains numerous arteries and veins that promote urethral closure by transmitting pressure from surrounding muscular elements and by adding closure pressure via their intramural pressure.

Active tension needed to maintain urethral closure in instances of physical stress is provided by muscles inside and adjacent to the urethral wall. Smooth muscle bundles in the proximal urethra and bladder neck are oriented in longitudinal and circular fashion, providing active tension designed to close the urethral lumen. In addition, specialized skeletal muscle fibers form the triple-innervated rhabdosphincter, which is especially designed to provide the prolonged tension needed to prevent leakage during long periods between voiding episodes. Muscular fibers from the pelvic floor muscles that surround the urethra also contribute to closure, particularly during periods of intense physical stress. The muscular components of the

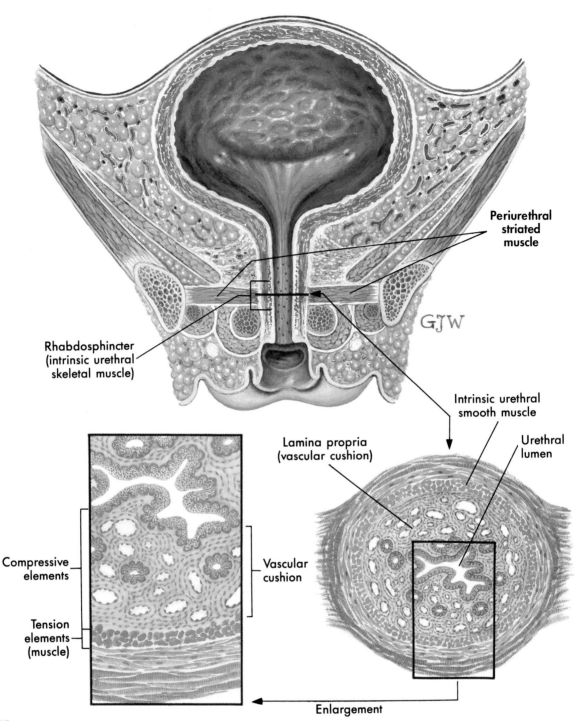

Periurethral striated muscle

Rhabdosphincter (intrinsic urethral skeletal muscle)

GJW

Intrinsic urethral smooth muscle

Lamina propria (vascular cushion)

Urethral lumen

Compressive elements

Tension elements (muscle)

Vascular cushion

Enlargement

FIGURE 1-17
Sphincter mechanism.

sphincter mechanism are aided by supportive structures (pelvic floor muscles, endopelvic fascia, tendons, and the pelvic bone) that provide the best anatomic position for effective closure of the urethral lumen.

The competence of the urethra is illustrated by its response to foreign objects and to a precipitous rise in pressure in the abdomen. The elements of urethral compression keep a normal sphincter mechanism closed even when a stiff tube such as a catheter is inserted. The effectiveness of the active tension elements of the urethra is illustrated by the tremendous rise in abdominal pressure during exercise that favors leakage. Although intraabdominal pressure may increase by 120 cm H_2O or more during running, jogging, weight lifting, or high-impact aerobics, the sphincter remains closed because the various pressures are effectively transmitted to the urethra and active tone is maintained by the muscular elements of the mechanism.

MALE REPRODUCTIVE SYSTEM

The male reproductive system has six components: the scrotum, the paired testes, the epididymides and vasa deferentia, the seminal vesicles, the prostate, and the penis (Figure 1-18). The two functions of the male reproductive system are to effect an erection of sufficient rigidity and duration to penetrate the vagina and to produce spermatozoa and semen capable of fertilizing the female's ovum.

SCROTUM

The scrotum is a cutaneous sac that lies below the pubic bone. It houses the lower portion of the spermatic cord, the testes, and the epididymides. The scrotum is made up of a deeply pigmented or reddish skin with underlying muscle and fibrous projections that cover its internal elements. The skin of the scrotum is rugated (wrinkled) and has a median raphe that marks the separation of the two hemiscrotums, each containing a testis, epididymis, and spermatic cord. Immediately beneath the skin is the dartos muscle, composed of smooth muscle bundles and elastic tissue. The dartos is a continuation of the suspensory ligament of the penis and superficial fascia of the abdomen and pelvis. The testes lie under a reflection (extension) of the abdominopelvic fascia that has an incomplete septum, further dividing the hemiscrotal compartments.

TESTES

The testes are a pair of oval organs that lie in the scrotum (Figure 1-19). Each testis is approximately 4 to 5 cm long and 2.5 cm wide. The left testis typically is lower than the right. Arterial blood reaches the testis via branches of the spermatic artery, and venous blood drains through branches of the spermatic vein. The dependent position of the testes is important, because it allows the arterial blood to cool by approximately 2 degrees Celsius, thus promoting effective sperm production. Lymphatic drainage exits the testes via the spermatic cord before emptying into the lumbar and mediastinal nodes.

The microscopic anatomy of a testis centers around the seminiferous tubules, which form the functional unit of the organ. The tubules have four to eight layers of stratified epithelial cells surrounding a central lumen. The cells are either spermatogenic (capable of forming spermatids) or supportive (nutritive). The seminiferous tubules account for 75% of the testicular

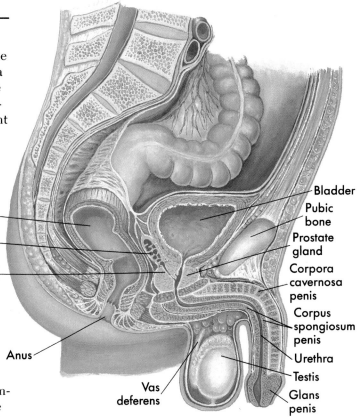

FIGURE 1-18
Male pelvic organs. (From Seidel.[23])

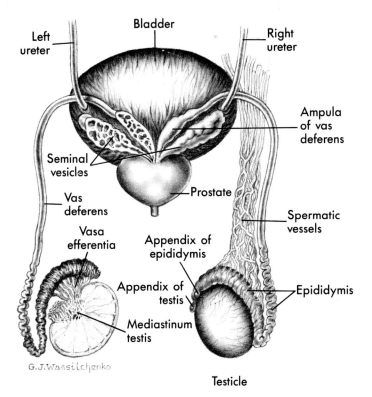

FIGURE 1-19
Testes. (From Thompson J et al, editors: *Mosby's manual of clinical nursing*, ed 2, St Louis, 1989, Mosby–Year Book.)

mass; their collective length approaches 1 mile. The remainder of the testis is composed of interstitial cells, including Leydig's cells, which produce testosterone and vascular, neural, and lymphatic elements.

The testis has three protective coverings, the tunica vaginalis, the tunica albuginea, and the tunica vasculosa. The tunica vaginalis, an extension of the peritoneum, encases the testis. The tunica albuginea penetrates the organ and divides the seminiferous tubules into lobules. The tunica vasculosa is a system of blood vessels that provides nourishment to the seminiferous tubules and interstitial cells.

EPIDIDYMIS AND VAS DEFERENS

The epididymis and vas deferens constitute a system of tubes designed to provide maturation, storage, and transport of sperm cells (see Figure 1-20). The epididymis is a sausage-shaped structure situated on the posterolateral surface of the testis. Inside the epididymis is a long, tortuous tubular structure with abundant ciliary projections; it is designed to transport spermatids. Because the epididymis has little muscle in its walls, it relies on ciliary action for sperm transport. The head of the epididymis connects to the testis, and its tail opens into the vas deferens.

The vas deferens is the more muscular tubule that originates at the tail of the epididymis and terminates into the seminal vesicles. The vas deferens begins as a tortuous tubule, descending along the posterior aspect of the testis. It then straightens and turns upward, along the spermatic cord, leaving the scrotum and ascending to the level of the deep inguinal ring. From there the vas deferens exits the spermatic cord, crosses the ureter, and traverses the prostate to its termination in the ejaculatory duct. The terminal portion of the vas deferens, called the ampulla, consists of a 10-cm-long dilated segment with several pouches, or diverticula.

SEMINAL VESICLES, EJACULATORY DUCTS, AND PROSTATE

The seminal vesicles are a pair of hollow muscular organs that lie between the posterior wall of the bladder and the rectum. They interact with the ejaculatory ducts to transport and propel sperm into the urethra during ejaculation (see Figure 1-19). The blood supply of the seminal vesicles is similar to that of the prostate.

The prostate is located at the base of the bladder and is pierced through its vertical aspect by the proximal urethra (Figure 1-20). The prostate contains both fibromuscular and glandular elements. Clinicians divide the prostate into the intraurethral lobe (anterior and right and left lateral) and the extraurethral lobe (posterior and median). The right and left lateral intraurethral lobes form the walls of the prostatic urethra and may produce a compressive obstruction during late adulthood. The posterior lobe also bears clinical significance because of its susceptibility to neoplasia during later life. The apex of the prostate is situated inferiorly, away from the bladder and near the rectal sphincter, whereas its base is situated nearest to the base of the bladder.

The microscopic anatomy of the prostate comprises glandular and fibromuscular elements. The fibromuscular tissue consists of smooth muscle bundles with abundant alpha excitatory, sympathetic receptors. The glandular tissue of the prostate is made up of follicles that drain into 12 to 20 excretory ducts, which in turn drain into the proximal urethra.

Arterial blood for the prostate arises from branches of the internal pudendal, rectal, and vesical arteries. Venous blood leaves the prostate and drains into the deep penile or internal iliac veins. Lymphatic drainage reaches the external iliac or sacral nodes.

PENIS

The penis is a cylindrical organ that extends from a root in the perineum and ends at the glans or termination of the foreskin (Figure 1-21). It is attached to the pelvic floor by the suspensory ligament, the corpora cavernosa, and an extension of Buck's fascia. The skin of the penis is characterized by its thin, distensible nature and relatively dark pigmentation. At its distal aspect, the penile skin is folded over onto itself, forming the foreskin that covers the glans penis.

The microscopic anatomy of the penis is characterized by the vascular sinusoids of the corpora cavernosa bounded by the fibrous, noncompliant tunica albuginea (see Figure 1-21). Inferior to the cavernosal bodies is the corpus spongiosum, which contains the pendulous urethra.

The arterial blood supply of the penis is provided by the internal pudendal artery, which branches into the dorsal and deep arteries that provide the blood volume needed for tumescence (Figure 1-22). Nutritive needs for the penis and urethra are met by branches of the external pudendal and femoral arteries. The venous drainage of the corporal bodies is provided by the crural (deep) and dorsal veins, which empty into the hypogastric vein. Lymphatic channels drain into subinguinal and superficial iliac nodes.

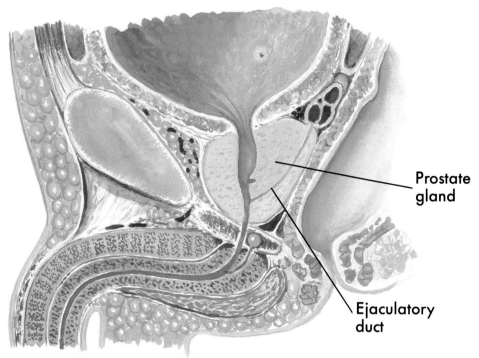

Prostate gland

Ejaculatory duct

FIGURE 1-20
Anatomy of the prostate gland. (From Seidel.[23])

SPERMATOGENESIS AND SPERM TRANSPORT

The testes, epididymides, vasa deferentia, seminal vesicles, ejaculatory ducts, and prostate function as a system to produce viable sperm cells, which are contained in a supportive semen designed for reproduction. The function of the reproductive system is regulated by a hormonal axis, and the act of ejaculation is regulated by neuromuscular activity modulated by endocrine influences.

The central hormonal axis regulating spermatogenesis originates in the hypothalamus, where luteinizing hormone–releasing hormone (LHRH) is released. It travels to the pituitary gland, causing production of luteinizing hormone (LH) and follicle-stimulating hormone (FSH). Both FSH and LH act at receptor sites in the testes to stimulate production of the male androgens, primarily testosterone and dihydrotestosterone. These hormones, in turn, stimulate the production of spermatozoa. As with all hormonal systems, the FSH-LH-testosterone axis is subject to negative feedback, which protects the body from overproduction of any hormonal elements.

The gonadal androgens are crucial to the production of mature, viable sperm cells. Spermatogenesis begins within the seminiferous tubule; during the first phase, primitive spermatogonia undergo mitotic division to form primary spermatocytes, which have 92 chromosomes. During the second phase of spermatogenesis, two meiotic divisions occur, producing four secondary spermatogonia with the haploid number of chromosomes (23) necessary for fertilization. The third phase of spermatogenesis, spermiogenesis, is the maturation of spermatids into viable spermatozoa capable of moving independently and fertilizing the ovum.

The process of spermiogenesis requires approximately 74 days and is divided into four phases. In phase 1 the small granules of hyaluronidase, protease, and other substances form a vesicle at the head of the sperm that can penetrate the membrane of the ovum. During the second phase a cap appears around this acrosomal vesicle. The centrioles of the spermatid begin to move, in preparation for formation of the tail, which is necessary for forward motility. During the fourth phase, the spermatid undergoes the final metamorphosis into the structure of a mature spermatozoon. Maturation begins within the seminiferous tubule and is completed in the epididymis.

Transport and maturation of spermatids

The vasa deferentia, seminal vesicles, and ejaculatory ducts assist reproductive function primarily by transporting mature sperm cells. The vasa deferentia and prostate also contribute needed nutrients to the semen that accompany spermatozoa during ejaculation.

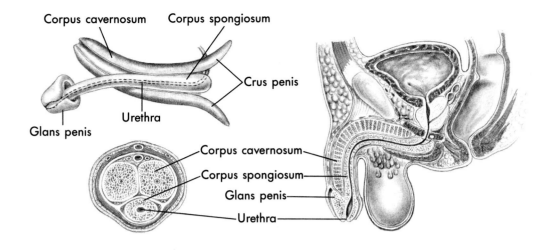

FIGURE 1-21
Anatomy of the penis. (From Seidel.[23])

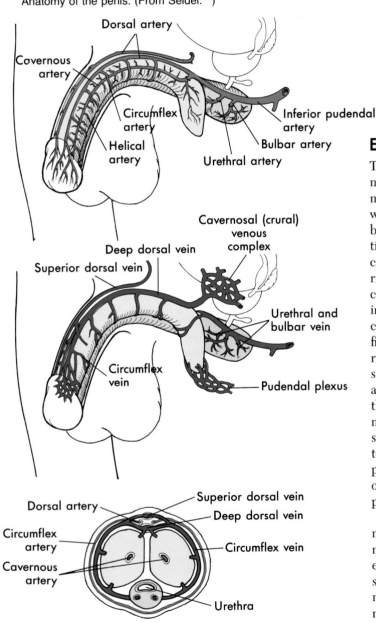

FIGURE 1-22
Vascular supply to penis.

ERECTILE FUNCTION IN THE MALE

The physiology of erectile function in men is determined by neurovascular events and modulated by hormonal influences. An erection of the penis is attained when the corporal bodies become engorged with blood, producing sufficient rigidity for vaginal penetration. The neurovascular events that produce tumescence begin with smooth muscle relaxation at the arteriolar level. This increases arterial blood flow to the corporal bodies. Initially the increased volume only increases the volume and length of the penis, as the compliant sinusoid spaces in the corporal bodies are filled. However, after the sinusoidal spaces fill, penile rigidity and cavernosal pressure increase rapidly as the sinusoids press against the relatively stiff, noncompliant, fibrous coverings of the penis. Engorgement of the cavernosal bodies by blood is maintained by venous occlusion. Three mechanisms for venous occlusion have been proposed: increased smooth muscle tone may occlude drainage; valves in the veins may prevent excessive drainage; or mechanical compression of the penile veins may occur as the corporal sinusoids press against the fibrous tunica albuginea.

The neurotransmitter that produces the smooth muscle relaxation needed for penile engorgement remains unclear; it may be a nonadrenergic, noncholinergic compound such as substance P. Paracrine substances, including prostaglandin E_1, clearly exert a modulatory effect. The male androgens also exert a modulatory effect that affects libido rather than the immediate neurovascular events of a penile erection.

FEMALE REPRODUCTIVE SYSTEM

The female reproductive system consists of four parts: the external genitalia, or vulva; the vagina; the fallopian tubes; and the ovaries (Figure 1-23). Collectively the organs of the female reproductive system act to produce an ovum capable of fertilization by a spermatozoon and to sustain a pregnancy and deliver a living offspring. This discussion focuses on the physiology related to the clinical aspects of fertility.

EXTERNAL GENITALIA

The external genitalia include all visible structures from the pubis to the perineum (Figure 1-24). The mons pubis is a slightly elevated area of hair-bearing skin over a layer of fat and the symphysis pubis bone. Immediately inferior to the mons pubis are the labia majora. The labia are two rounded folds of skin that originate at the mons pubis, surround the vestibule, and merge into the perineum. The outer aspects are hair-bearing skin, whereas the inner surfaces are hairless and have abundant sebaceous follicles, giving them a smooth, moist appearance. Medial to the labia majora are the labia minora. These thin folds of moist skin that merge superiorly at the frenulum of the clitoris and inferiorly at the frenulum of the labia majora.

The clitoris consists of two cavernosal bodies encased in a dense fibrous membrane. It is 2 cm or less in length, even when the cavernosal bodies are fully engorged. The vestibule is the area between the labia minora. It contains the urethral meatus, the ducts of Bartholin's glands, Skene's ducts, and the vaginal opening. The vaginal opening may be covered by the hymen, a mucous membrane fold with a rich vascularity and relatively few neural elements.

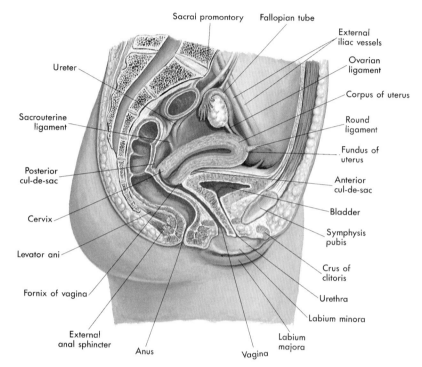

FIGURE 1-23
Midsagittal view of the female pelvic organs. (From Seidel.[23])

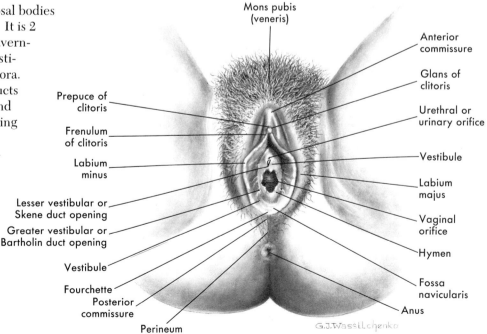

FIGURE 1-24
External female genitalia. (From Bobak et al: *Maternity and gynecologic care: the nurse and the family,* ed 4, St Louis, 1989, Mosby–Year Book.)

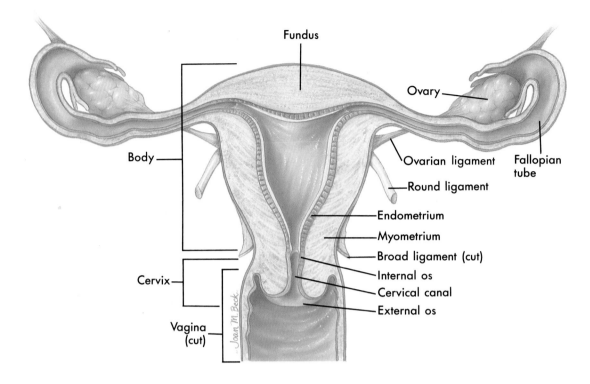

FIGURE 1-25
Uterus, vagina, uterine tubes, ovaries, and supporting ligaments. The uterus and one uterine tube are cut in section, and the vagina is cut to show the internal anatomy. (From Thibodeau GA: *Anatomy and physiology*, St Louis, 1989, Mosby–Year Book.)

VAGINA

The vagina is a fibromuscular canal that extends from the vestibule to the lower segment of the uterus (cervix). It is approximately 9 to 10 cm long. Its anterior wall is partly fused with the urethra. Mucosal secretions, menstrual fluids, and the products of conception exit the body through the vagina.

The microscopic anatomy of the vagina is characterized by four layers. The inner lining is a squamous cell epithelium with abundant mucus-producing cells. Under the influence of estrogens, the epithelium of the vagina produces rugae (wrinkles) and adequate lubrication, which allow deformation during coitus or childbirth. Beneath the epithelium is the submucosal layer, which contains vascular elements, nerves, and lymphatic channels. Smooth muscle bundles make up the third layer, and the fourth consists of connective tissue and a rich vascular network.

UTERUS AND FALLOPIAN TUBES

The uterus is a hollow, pear-shaped, muscular organ that opens into the vagina (Figure 1-25). It is approximately 9 cm deep, 6.5 cm wide, and has muscular walls 3.5 cm thick. Two principal components, the body (corpus) and neck (cervix), are visible on inspection with the unaided eye. The central cavity of the uterus is marked by three openings, the insertions of the paired fallopian tubes and the outlet (os). The top of the corpus, above the insertion of the fallopian tubes, is called the fornix. The lower portion of the uterine cavity is called the isthmus. The endocervical canal, extending from the interior to the outer aspect of the os, marks the lower outlet of the uterus.

The microscopic anatomy of the uterus consists of three layers, the endometrium, the myometrium, and the perimetrium. The endometrium, or inner lining, is made up of a functional layer of epithelial cells responsive to hormonal influences and a basal layer. The functional layer sloughs off during one phase of the menstrual cycle, and the basal layer regenerates the functional layer later in the cycle. The myometrium is a thick tunic of smooth muscle bundles. It is thickest at the layer of the fundus, possibly to facilitate efficient contractions during childbirth. The perimetrium, or outer layer, consists of the connective tissue. Unlike the cervical cavity, the endocervical canal is lined by a columnar epithelium that transforms to squamous epithelium in the vagina.

The fallopian tubes originate adjacent to the ovaries, taper, and enter the uterus just beneath the fundus. Each tube is 8 to 12 cm long and approximately 1 cm in diameter. The end nearest the ovary, called the infundibulum, flares and is marked by fimbriae that draw the ovum into the tube.

PHYSIOLOGY OF FEMALE FERTILIZATION AND IMPLANTATION

The physiology of female fertility centers on the events of the menstrual cycle. The menstrual cycle is primarily modulated by the pituitary-ovarian axis. The menstrual cycle begins at menarche (approximately 12½ years of age) and ends with menopause (often occurring within the fifth decade of life). The cycle consists of three phases, which are centered around the primary event of ovulation, or release of a mature ovum. During menstruation the functional (superficial) layer of the endometrium is sloughed and expelled through the vagina. After menstruation comes the follicular, or proliferative, phase, as a follicle of the ovary matures while the basal layer of the endometrium regenerates the functional layer. Follicular maturation occurs under the influence of follicle-stimulating hormone (FSH) released from the pituitary. The presence of FSH, in turn, stimulates the maturing follicle to release estrogens (principally estradiol), which stimulate regeneration of the functional layer of the endometrium.

The third phase of the menstrual cycle is the secretory, or luteal, phase, which begins with ovulation. During this phase the follicle, having released its ovum, converts into the corpus luteum. Under the influence of the luteinizing hormone (LH) the corpus luteum secretes progesterone. Progesterone, in turn, stimulates the invagination of blood vessels into the functional layer and the proliferation of glands that secrete a thin, glycogen-containing fluid. If fertilization occurs, the blastocyst (united ovum and spermatozoon) implants in the uterine wall and pregnancy ensues. If fertilization and implantation do not occur, the corpus luteum degenerates and stops producing progesterone and estrogen. Lacking supportive hormones, the endometrium enters an ischemic phase, marking the beginning of menstruation and another cycle.

OVARIES

The ovaries are a pair of oval organs that lie in the woman's pelvis (see Figures 1-23 and 1-25). They produce ova and female sex hormones. The ovaries are found at the lateral aspects of the uterus adjacent to the infundibula of the fallopian tubes. They are supported by the mesovarian portion of the broad ligament, the ovarian ligaments, and the suspensory ligaments. In an adult woman, the ovary is approximately 3 to 5 cm long, 2.5 cm wide, and 2 cm thick.

The microscopic anatomy of the ovary consists of a medulla and cortex. The centrally located medulla contains connective tissue, vascular elements, and lymphatic channels. The peripheral cortex comprises approximately 200,000 mature ova within immature follicles. During a woman's reproductive years, approximately 300 to 400 follicles mature and leave the ovary by means of ovulation. The remaining follicles either fail to mature completely or degenerate before maturation. Following ejection of an ovum, the follicle develops into a corpus luteum. If the extruded ovum is fertilized, the corpus luteum proliferates and generates the hormones needed to maintain pregnancy. If the ovum is not fertilized, the corpus luteum secretes relatively few hormones and soon degenerates.

CHAPTER 2

Assessment

Evaluation of the patient with disorders of the genitourinary system begins with a history, followed by systematic physical examination of the kidneys, bladder, urethra, and genitalia. These findings are combined with results of diagnostic tests, laboratory data, and a general nursing evaluation to determine relevant diagnoses and design an appropriate management plan. The historical interview and physical examination are conducted in an environment that ensures adequate privacy and a relatively relaxed, unhurried pace. Adequate supervision is crucial for the physical examination of the genitourinary system.

HISTORY

Assessment of the genitourinary system begins with the historical interview, which serves to determine the patient's complaints and to uncover potentially significant related conditions. The historical interview also provides a baseline evaluation of cognitive and psychosocial perspectives that influence the presentation, severity, and management of genitourinary dysfunction.

Begin the historical interview with an open-ended question, such as, "What has brought you to see me?" or "What kind of problem has caused you to seek help?" This question is followed by more specific inquiries about the genitourinary system and related systems.

THE ENVIRONMENT AND EQUIPMENT

Because of the sensitive nature of the evaluation of the genitourinary system, the historical interview and physical examination are completed in an environment that

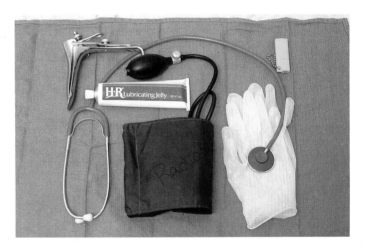

FIGURE 2-1
Equipment for genitourinary assessment.

ensures patient confidentiality and privacy. A chaperone remains a crucial element during the physical examination.

Figure 2-1 shows the equipment needed for the physical examination. The blood pressure cuff, gloves, lubricant, penlight, and specula are important components of the examination.

HEALTH HISTORY

Chief complaint: altered urinary elimination patterns (incontinence/urinary retention/dysuria)

Duration of symptoms
Bladder management program/voiding patterns
  Bladder managed by spontaneous voiding
    Diurnal frequency
    Nocturia
    Force of urinary stream
    Hesitancy to void
    Urgency to void
  Containment devices used
    Diapers (type, average number used per day)
    Pads (type, average number used per day)
    Condom catheter
  Bladder managed by intermittent catheterization
    Prescribed frequency of catheterization
    Actual schedule of catheterization
  Bladder managed by indwelling catheter
    Suprapubic or urethral type
    Time since catheter was first inserted
    Type of catheter (Teflon coated, silicone, lubricant coated)
  Incontinence
    Stress (provoked by physical exertion in absence of urgency)
    Urge (provoked by intense urgency to void)
    Continuous (dribbling leakage superimposed on normal voiding pattern versus constant leakage with failure to store urine)
    Reflex incontinence (bladder evacuation in the absence of urgency, not related to physical stress)
  Urinary retention (feelings of incomplete bladder emptying, acute inability to void requiring catheterization, documented residuals, overflow, dribbling, leakage despite inability to completely empty bladder)
Urologic history
  Dysuria (painful urination, burning or stinging with urination)
  Documented urinary tract infection (recurrence, frequency, association with fever, hematuria, precipitating and alleviating factors)
  Congenital urologic disorders, vesicoureteral reflux
  Urinary calculi (single or recurrent episodes, type of stone, passed spontaneously or treated by lithotripsy, surgery, endoscopic retrieval, follow-up treatment)
  Urinary system tumor (type, treatment)
  Hematuria (not associated with infection, cause, treatment)
Related system disorders
  Neurologic disorders
    Disorders of the brain (tumor, cerebrovascular accident, increased intracranial pressure, multiple sclerosis, parkinsonism, Alzheimer's disease)
    Disorders of the spinal cord (traumatic injury, spinovascular disease, stenosis, spina bifida, transverse myelitis, multiple sclerosis)
    Disorders of the peripheral nervous system/metabolically induced neuropathies (peripheral neuropathy related to diabetes mellitus, heavy metal toxicity, ethanol abuse–related neuropathies, zosteriform neuropathies)
  Bowel elimination patterns (fecal incontinence, frequency of bowel movements, chronic constipation, history of impaction)
  Sexual dysfunction (erectile or ejaculatory dysfunction in males)
Medications affecting continence
  Medications reducing detrusor contractility (antispasmodics, anticholinergics, antipsychotropics, antidepressants, antiparkinsonian agents, beta adrenergics, calcium channel blocking agents, narcotics, recreational drugs, cannabis)
  Medications increasing detrusor contractility (cholinergic agents)
  Medications reducing sphincter resistance (alpha blocking agents, skeletal muscle relaxants)
  Medications increasing sphincter resistance (alpha sympathomimetics)
Surgical history (genitourinary procedures, abdominopelvic surgery, neurosurgical procedures, orthopedic procedures involving the spine)

Chief complaint: pain

Onset and duration of symptoms (time since onset, gradual versus sudden occurrence of symptoms)

Location of pain

Flank pain (related to kidney, renal pelvis, upper ureter, overlying muscles, gallbladder, surgical incision)

Abdominal pain (related to midureter, small or large bowel, surgical incision, abdominal muscles)

Suprapubic pain (related to bladder, trigone, lower ureter, female reproductive organs, surgical incision)

Scrotal pain (related to testis, spermatic cord, epididymis, radiating pain from upper ureteral or midureteral obstruction, incisional pain)

Penile pain (urethra, bladder, incisional pain)

Mons pubis (urethra, bladder, vagina, symphysis pubis, reproductive organs, radiating pain from upper ureteral or midureteral obstruction)

Rectal (prostatic, rectal, perirectal)

Character of pain

Cramping, stabbing (bladder spasm, bladder inflammation, gastrointestinal cramping)

Dull, boring (incisional pain; obstruction; prostatic, testicular, or epididymal pain; interstitial cystitis)

Duration

Sudden onset, short duration (bladder spasm, gastrointestinal cramping)

Gradual or sudden onset, long duration (incisional pain, obstruction, epididymal, prostate, testicular inflammation, interstitial cystitis)

Alleviating, aggravating factors (bladder fullness, position, urination, pressure, ejaculation, bowel movement)

Urologic history

Documented urinary tract infection (recurrence, associated with fever, hematuria, precipitating and alleviating factors)

Inflammatory bladder lesions (interstitial cystitis, bladder tumors, cystitis cystica, radiation cystitis, chemotherapy-induced cystitis)

Dysuria in the absence of inflammatory lesions (urethral syndrome)

Urinary calculi (previous occurrence, number of episodes passed spontaneously, treated by lithotripsy, surgery, endoscopic retrieval, follow-up treatment)

Congenital urinary anomalies (ureteropelvic junction obstruction, retrocaval ureter, urethral valves)

Voiding dysfunction (urinary retention, incontinence, neuropathic bladder dysfunction)

Related system disorders

Metabolic disorders

Hypercalcemia disorders (hyperthyroidism, immobility, excessive dietary intake, excessive vitamin D intake, hypercalciuria)

Uric acid disorders (gouty arthritis, hyperuricacidemia)

Enzyme disorders (hyperoxaluria, xanthinuria, enteric hyperoxaluria)

Renal tubular disorders (renal tubular acidosis, cystinuria)

Endocrine disorders (hyperparathyroidism, Cushing's syndrome, hyperthyroidism)

Medications (antibiotics, vitamin and calcium supplements, drugs that influence urinary pH, reduce urinary oxalates, and uric acid)

Surgical history (surgery for urinary calculi, surgery to correct obstruction, other genitourinary procedures, abdominopelvic surgery)

Chief complaint: altered sexual function, erectile/ejaculatory dysfunction

Duration of symptoms

Erectile dysfunction (failure to initiate erection, failure to sustain erection, altered sensations, altered libido)

Ejaculatory dysfunction (failure to experience orgasm, failure to ejaculate in antegrade fashion, altered sensation, altered libido)

Related system disorders

Vascular disorders (peripheral vascular disease, tobacco abuse, trauma to pelvis, arteriosclerosis)

Neurologic disorders (disorders of the brain, spinal cord, peripheral nervous system)

Endocrine disorders (hypogonadotropic eunuchoidism, panhypopituitarism, hyperprolactinemia, hypothyroidism, testosterone deficiency)

Psychogenic disorders

Medications affecting erectile dysfunction (antihypertensives, antipsychotics, antidepressants, anticholinergics, recreational drugs, antiarrhythmic agents, diuretics)

Medications affecting ejaculatory dysfunction (alpha sympathomimetics, alpha blocking agents)

Surgical procedures (abdominopelvic procedures, genitourinary procedures, neurosurgical procedures, orthopedic procedures of the spine)

Chief complaint: altered sexual function, infertility

Duration of attempts to achieve pregnancy

Reproductive system history

    Male (erectile dysfunction, ejaculatory dysfunction, frequency of intercourse, timing of intercourse, volume and general quality of semen, history of vasectomy, history of previous pregnancy or previous partners, prior treatment for infertility)

    Female (menstrual history, frequency of menstrual periods, history of prior pregnancy, previous partners, frequency of intercourse, timing of intercourse, prior use of birth control devices, medications or surgery)

Developmental history

    Male (undescended or congenitally absent testis, orchiopexy, torsion, herniorrhaphy, bladder neck surgery, genetic or endocrine disorders)

    Female (ovarian agenesis or dysgenesis, obstructive lesions, bicornuate or septate uterus, atresia)

Prior infections (sexually transmitted diseases, mumps orchitis, pelvic inflammatory disease, infections related to intrauterine device)

Related systems

    Endocrine (hypopituitarism, hypothyroidism, gonadotropic insufficiency, hyperprolactinemia, estrogen or testosterone deficiencies, congenital adrenal hyperplasia, galactorrhea)

    Respiratory (Young's syndrome, cystic fibrosis)

    Neurologic (disorders affecting erectile, ejaculatory dysfunction; disorders affecting lubrication of vaginal vault; disorders affecting sphincter mechanism; lower spinal cord injury; spina bifida disorders)

Surgical history

    Male (bladder neck surgery, prostatectomy, transurethral surgery, retroperitoneal surgery, extensive abdominopelvic surgery, repair of varicocele, inguinal or scrotal surgery, pituitary surgery)

    Female (abdominopelvic procedures, oophorectomy, salpingectomy, tubal ligation, pituitary surgery, polypectomy, dilation and curettage, tuboplasty)

Exposure to toxins (heavy metal toxins, aniline dyes, radiation)

Drugs that affect fertility

    Chemotherapy agents

    Recreational drugs (alcohol, nicotine, marijuana)

    Antiinfectives (nitrofurantoin, sulfasalazine, metronidazole)

    Drugs that affect erectile or ejaculatory function (see page 265)

    Hormonal agents that affect menstrual cycle or spermatogenesis

GENERAL ASSESSMENT

Physical examination of the genitourinary system comprises evaluation of the abdomen and external genitalia. Before beginning the examination, ensure proper privacy for the patient. Collect materials needed for the evaluation beforehand, to avoid entering and leaving the room during the examination. Arrange for a chaperone as indicated. In general, a clinician is chaperoned at all times when examining the genitourinary system. Clearly, supervision is mandatory when examining a person of the opposite gender or an individual with mental health or cognitive disorders that may alter his ability to recall reliably the events of the evaluation.

General assessment begins with evaluation of the individual's mobility, dexterity, and cognition. Assess how the patient ambulates and the use of assistive devices, including a walker, cane, or wheelchair. Note his ability to transfer onto a chair or examining table. Evaluate dexterity by observing the patient's ability to remove clothing; specifically note his ability to manipulate zippers or buttons. Generally evaluate the patient's cognition throughout the historical interview and physical examination. Determine whether he is oriented and alert, and assess his ability to recall, store, and synthesize skills needed to perform self-care functions. This information is particularly necessary when determining a management plan requiring self-care skills.

General evaluation also includes assessment for compromised renal function. Blood pressure readings

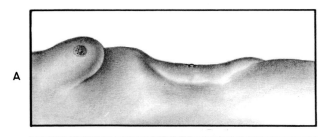

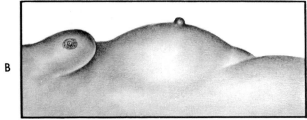

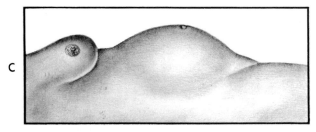

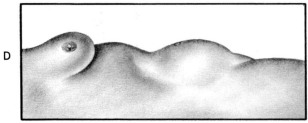

FIGURE 2-2
Abdominal profiles. **A,** Scaphoid. **B,** Fully rounded or distended, umbilicus everted. **C,** Fully rounded or distended, umbilicus inverted. **D,** Distended lower half. (From Seidel.[23])

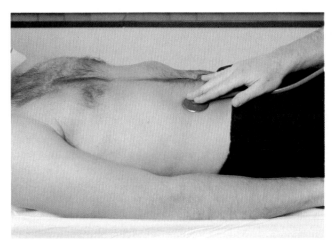

FIGURE 2-3
Auscultation of abdomen.

are obtained in the supine, sitting, and/or standing positions. Elevated blood pressure may be renovascular in origin, indicating a defect in a single kidney or primary vascular abnormalities. Skin integrity may be altered, with a proneness to bruises and slowed wound healing. Chronic anemia may be noted as pallor accompanied by general weakness and low tolerance of physical exertion. Electrolyte imbalance also may cause fatigue, nausea, and vomiting and may alter cognition in severe cases. Peripheral edema may be noted, and certain individuals may experience shortness of breath or other signs of congestive heart failure. The hair may appear thin and brittle as a result of protein wasting; weight loss and muscle wasting may be detectable.

ABDOMEN

General approach: Allow the patient to empty the bladder before the examination. Ask the patient to lie in the supine position, and help him transfer to the table and remove clothing as indicated. Approach the individual slowly and deliberately, explaining the components of the evaluation as they occur. Place the person in a relatively comfortable position, using pillows as indicated, and ask him to breathe slowly through the mouth when performing maneuvers that provoke anxiety.

Inspection: Inspect the abdomen from a seated position at the patient's right side. Observe the contour of the abdomen and the skin. The skin may be pale or tanned and may contain a fine venous network noticeable to the naked eye. Jaundice, discrete lesions, or generalized redness may indicate several specific disorders, including infection. Note the presence, size, and location of scars. They indicate trauma or surgical procedures that may affect the urinary system and adjacent structures. Abdominal scars also alert the nurse to the potential for adhesions, which may cause abdominal discomfort and may be perceived by the patient as pelvic, bladder, or renal pain.

Inspect the abdomen for contour and symmetry. The normal abdomen may appear flat, rounded with ample adipose tissue in obese individuals, or concave in thin adults. A visible mass of the upper abdominal quadrants may indicate the presence of a renal tumor or obstruction causing severe hydronephrosis. A centrally located protrusion in the suprapubic area may indicate a distended bladder (Figure 2-2).

Auscultation: After the inspection, the abdomen is auscultated *before* light and deep palpation, because these maneuvers alter normal peristalsis. Lay the warm stethoscope against the skin of the abdomen, and listen for bowel sounds, noting their presence, frequency, and character (Figure 2-3). Normal peristalsis is noted as clicks and gurgles that occur without any distinguishable pattern. As few as five and as many as 35 sounds may be heard per minute. Evaluating the presence of bowel sounds is particularly significant after urologic surgery requiring manipulation or reconstruction of the bowel.

Percussion: Percussion is included in examination of the genitourinary system when a distended bladder is suspected (Figure 2-4). Percussion of the suprapubic area follows general percussion of all abdominal quadrants to evaluate tympany versus dullness for that individual. Tympany is noted over lower quadrants, where hollow bowel predominates, and dullness is noted over the liver. Normally the bladder holding 150 ml of fluid or less remains below the symphysis pubis so that percussion reveals tympany in the suprapubic area. In contrast, dullness in the suprapubic area predominates when a large volume of urine is present in the bladder.

Palpation: Stand at the patient's side, and begin light palpation with warm hands while giving a thorough explanation (Figure 2-5). Make certain that the patient is relatively comfortable before beginning palpation. Help him overcome ticklishness by allowing him to palpate his own abdomen before your palpation.

Light palpation is used to detect areas of tenderness and muscular resistance. A significant mass or urinary system infection that causes tenderness may produce resistance on light palpation. A pelvic mass or distended bladder also may be noted as resistance on light palpation over the lower quadrants of the abdomen and suprapubic area.

Deep palpation is used to delineate the abdominal organs and to detect subtle masses. Use the palmar surface of your hand to press deeply and gently into the abdominal wall (Figure 2-6). The liver, spleen, loops of bowel, and borders of abdominal muscles may be palpable. Slight tenderness over the cecum, sigmoid colon, and aorta may be noted in normal individuals. Any mass that causes muscle guarding is evaluated for size, shape, consistency, and magnitude of tenderness provoked by palpation.

The kidneys are assessed for tenderness and masses, as are adjacent organs, including the liver, spleen, and gallbladder. To evaluate the kidneys, ask the patient to assume a sitting position. Place the palm of your right hand over the left costovertebral angle (Figure 2-7). Strike your hand lightly with the fist of the left hand. The patient should perceive this light blow as a dull thud rather than as sharp tenderness or pain. The maneuver is repeated over the right costovertebral angle.

Palpation of the kidneys is realistic only in the relatively thin adult patient. Ask the patient to assume a supine position. From the patient's right side, reach across with the left hand to his left flank to palpate the left kidney. Ask the patient to inhale deeply, elevating

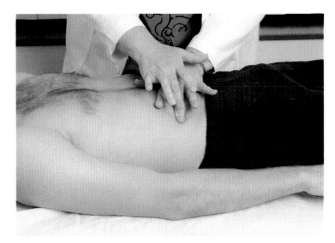

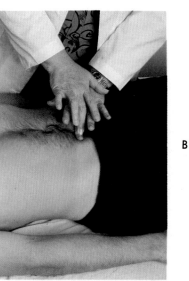

FIGURE 2-4
A, Percussion of abdomen. **B,** Percussion of bladder.

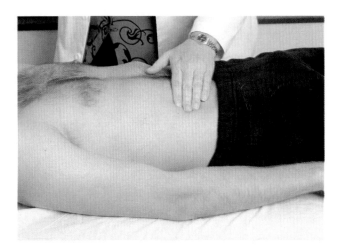

FIGURE 2-5
Light palpation of the abdomen.

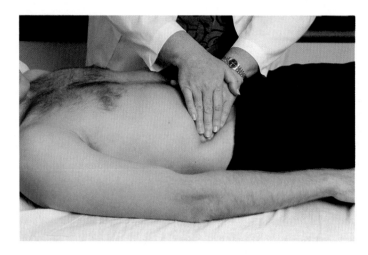

FIGURE 2-6
Deep palpation of the abdomen.

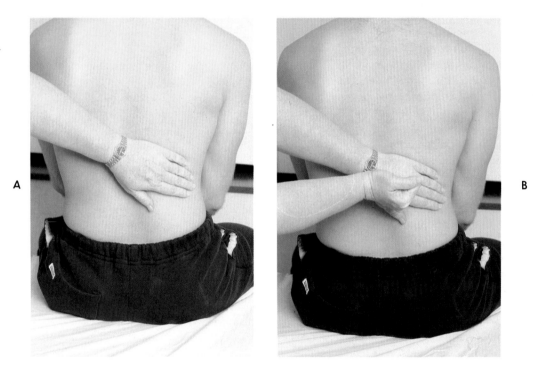

A   B

FIGURE 2-7
Test for costovertebral angle tenderness. **A,** Placement of hand. **B,** Hand is gently hit wth opposite fist.

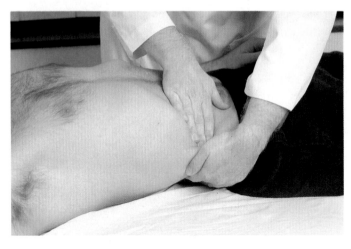

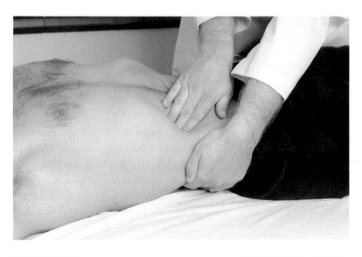

FIGURE 2-8
Palpation of the left kidney.

FIGURE 2-9
Palpation of the right kidney.

the left flank. Palpate deeply to locate the kidney. An alternate approach is to capture the kidney by asking the patient to inhale and then exhale deeply during deep palpation. Stand on the patient's left side, and place the left hand over the flank with the right hand over the costal margin. Ask the patient to take a deep breath and exhale slowly; the descending kidney will be felt between the fingers (Figure 2-8).

The right kidney often is more easily palpated than the left. Stand on the patient's right side, and place

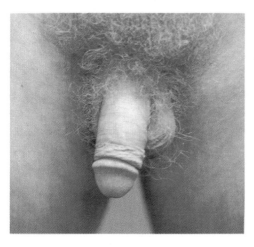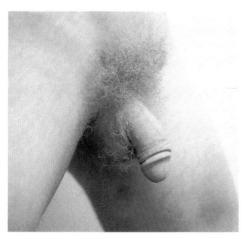

FIGURE 2-10
Inspection of male genitalia. (From Seidel.[23])

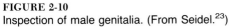

your left hand under the right flank. The left hand is placed under the right costal margin. Again, the patient is asked to inhale deeply and exhale slowly. You may feel the kidney as it slips between your fingers (Figure 2-9).

A normal kidney is firm, not tender, and smooth. Only the lower pole is palpable; hydronephrosis or masses are likely to distort size and tenderness. You may be unable to palpate the kidneys because of the patient's size, body habitus, and tenderness. Imaging studies are used to supplement information on renal size and position obtained during the physical examination.

MALE GENITALIA

General approach: Ask the patient to lie down. Men typically are quite anxious when the genitalia are examined. Approach the patient using straightforward language; avoid changing facial expressions if unexpected findings are discovered on evaluation.

Inspection: Inspect the distribution of the hair on the genitalia. Scrotal hair typically is coarser than scalp hair and assumes a triangular distribution, with the apex pointing toward the scrotum. The scrotum is lightly covered with hair and the penis relatively hair free. Examine the perineal skin for integrity; men with significant urinary leakage may have altered skin integrity and rashes related to urinary leakage (Figure 2-10).

The penis and scrotum are inspected next. The skin of the penis may be more pigmented than adjacent abdominal integument. If the man has been circumcised, examine the glans penis and corona for rashes or lesions. The glans penis is expected to be slightly dryer

than surrounding skin in the circumcised man. Gently retract the foreskin of the uncircumcised man to inspect the glans and corona for rashes or lesions. In the uncircumcised man, the glans is relatively moist and pink. The urethral meatus is examined next. It should be ovoid and located on the ventral surface of the glans several millimeters from the tip. Press the glans penis between the thumb and forefinger to inspect the mucosa of the fossa navicularis (terminal portion of the urethra). The mucosa should readily separate, exposing pink, moist tissue. Discharge, indicating urethritis, should be absent. Scarring or inability to expose distal mucosa may indicate stenosis and coexisting voiding dysfunction (Figure 2-11).

The scrotum is inspected next. It often is lightly covered with hair and may be red in fair-skinned individuals. The skin of the scrotum is characterized by wrinkles (rugae), allowing retraction of the testes toward the body. A central raphe dividing the hemiscrotums is noted. A penlight is held behind the scrotum in a darkened room. Transillumination shows the testes only. Other dark areas indicate inflammation or a tumor; a hydrocele will transilluminate (Figure 2-12).

Finally, the anal area is inspected. The perianal skin often is reddened, but it should have no lesions or rashes.

Palpation: Palpate the penile shaft for evidence of masses or tenderness. In addition to discrete masses, discrete hard nodules, indicating Peyronie's disease, may be noted.

Before you palpate the scrotum, carefully explain the procedure; then gently palpate the scrotum, using the thumb and forefinger (Figure 2-13). Warm hands and a slow, deliberate approach are necessary when do-

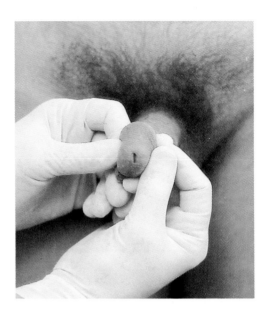

FIGURE 2-11
Examination of urethral orifice. (From Seidel.[23])

ing scrotal palpation. Determine the presence of a testis in each hemiscrotum. The testis should feel oval with a C-shaped tube, the epididymis, at its dorsal aspect. The testis should not be tender on light palpation but should be sensitive to pressure. Orchitis or epididymoorchitis produces exquisite tenderness on palpation because of the swelling and redness of the affected hemiscrotum. Testicular tenderness also is noted with torsion. The inflammation associated with orchitis or epididymoorchitis may be relieved by gentle elevation of the testis (Prehn's sign), whereas the torsive testicle remains unaffected. Testicular tumors produce a distinct nodule with sensations of scrotal fullness or pressure. Testicular examination provides an excellent opportunity to instruct the patient to perform monthly self-examination (page 312.)

Check the patient for a hernia (Figure 2-14). With the patient in a standing position, ask him to bear down, and observe the area of the inguinal canal for evidence of a bulging hernia. Next, gently insert the

A
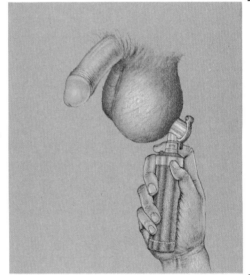
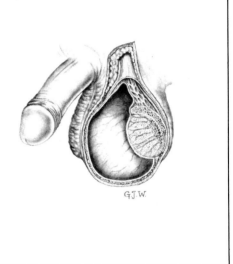

B
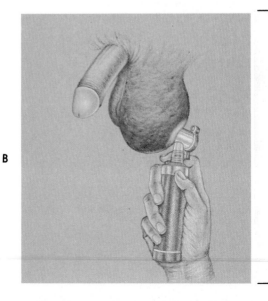
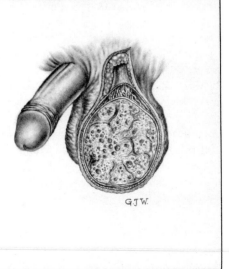

FIGURE 2-12
Transillumination of the scrotum. **A,** Hydrocele shows good transillumination. **B,** Testicular solid tumor shows no penetration of light.

gloved examining finger into the inguinal canal, using the loose skin of the scrotum dorsal to the testis. Again, ask the patient to bear down or cough, and feel for the sudden appearance of the hernia against the examining finger.

Assessing the prostate is part of the digital rectal examination (Figure 2-15). Ask the patient to lie on his side with the legs flexed at the knees or to stand up and lean over the examining table. Explain the procedure, and warn the patient that insertion of the finger causes a feeling of pressure and vague discomfort. Ask him to bear down slightly to relax the anal sphincter as the gloved examining finger is gently inserted, using adequate water-soluble lubricant. Rotate the examining finger toward the individual's bladder to palpate the prostate for size, consistency, symmetry, and contour. The posterior lobes of the prostate are amenable to palpation. The prostate is approximately 4 cm in diameter and protrudes about 1 cm into the rectal vault. The posterior lobes should be symmetric and have a firm, smooth consistency.

Benign prostatic hyperplasia (hypertrophy) causes symmetric enlargement of the gland and gives it a soft, boggy consistency. Prostatic adenocarcinoma may be detected as a discrete nodule that causes asymmetric enlargement or induration of the affected lobe. Inflammation of the gland (prostatitis) produces symmetric enlargement and moderate to exquisite tenderness on palpation.

Palpation of the prostate may cause emission of fluid into the urethra. Any secretions obtained during digital examination are cultured to test for bacterial infection of the gland.

After palpating the prostate, ask the patient to tighten the anus around your finger. Inability to tighten the anal sphincter voluntarily may indicate a neurologic abnormality, particularly when noted in combination with diminished or absent perineal sensations. The examination is completed by eliciting the bulbocavernosus reflex. Gently compress the glans penis while the examining finger remains in the rectum. In the normal individual, the anal sphincter contracts, or "winks." Absence of the bulbocavernosus reflex may indicate neurologic abnormality.

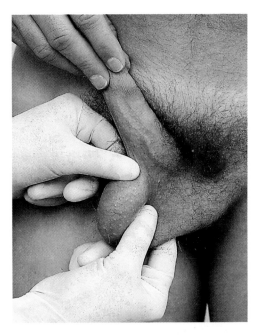

FIGURE 2-13
Palpation of scrotal sac. (From Seidel.[23])

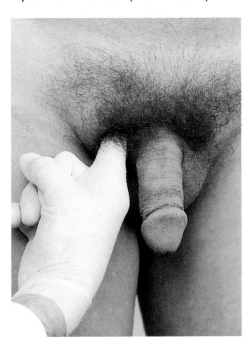

FIGURE 2-14
Assessment for inguinal hernia. (From Seidel.[23])

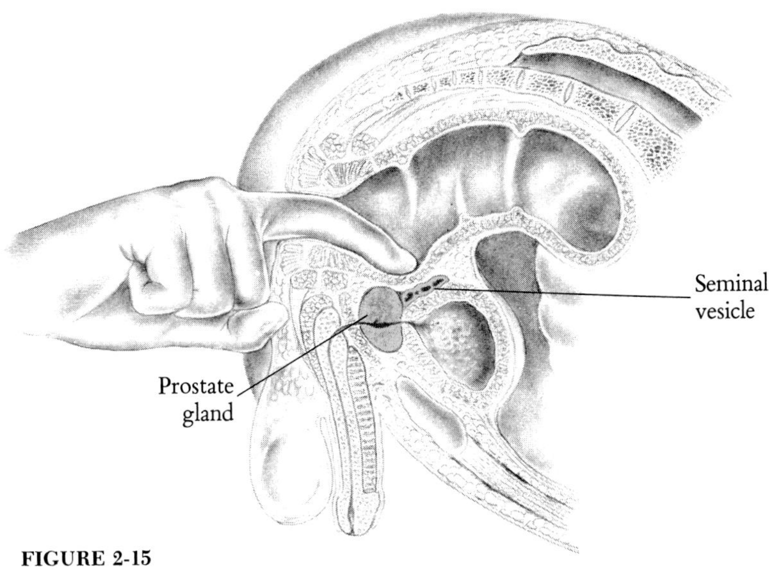

Seminal vesicle

Prostate gland

FIGURE 2-15
Digital palpation of prostate gland with gloved finger. (From Seidel.[23])

FEMALE GENITALIA

General approach: Ask the patient to lie in a dorsal lithotomy position; support the legs with stirrups. The female patient usually is anxious when the genitourinary system is examined and may recall specific, uncomfortable experiences caused by pelvic examination. Reduce the patient's anxiety by ensuring privacy through adequate draping and preventing people from entering or leaving the room during the examination. Help the patient find a comfortable position, using pillows and stirrup supports. Explain the procedure, and maintain eye contact with the patient before and during the procedure as possible. Approach the patient slowly and deliberately, and help her breathe slowly and deeply during anxiety-provoking maneuvers.

Inspection and palpation: Sitting at the end of the table, inspect the external genitalia. Observe the distribution of hair. Typically the pubic hair is coarser than scalp hair. Inspect the skin for rashes or lesions. Women with significant urinary incontinence may have altered skin integrity as a result of chronic exposure of the skin to urine. Examination of the labia majora may reveal plump- or shriveled-appearing tissue. Signs of inflammation, including edema and redness, may indicate an abscess of Bartholin's gland. Separate the labia majora gently, using the gloved fingers to inspect the labia minora, which should be soft and without tenderness. Irritation and excoriation may indicate vaginitis (Figure 2-16).

Inspect the urethral meatus (Figure 2-17). It should appear as a rosette or ovoid slit. It should lie within the midline and may be slightly within the vagina. Next, inspect the vaginal mucosa for color, presence of mucous secretions, and rugae. The well-estrogenized vaginal vault is pink and moist and has rugae. It should not be tender to the touch and should not produce an itching sensation. Evaluate the strength of the circumvaginal (pelvic floor) muscles by asking the woman to squeeze your examining finger. The circumvaginal muscles should squeeze against your finger in an anteroposterior manner, pulling the finger up towards the cervix. Pelvic floor descent or urethral sphincter incompetence may coexist with stress urinary incontinence caused by pelvic descent.

Inspect and palpate the perineum. The skin should be smooth, although an episiotomy scar may be noted on women who have delivered children. This tissue is thick and smooth in nulliparous females and thinner and more rigid in multiparous women.

Speculum examination: Lubricate the speculum, and gently insert it into the vaginal vault (Figure 2-18). Water-soluble lubricant is used unless cytologic specimens need to be obtained during the examination. Locate the cervix, and inspect it for color, position, size,

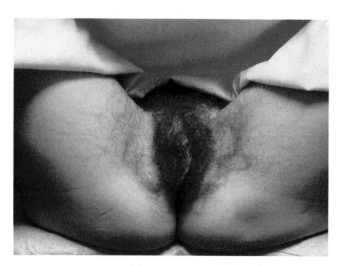

FIGURE 2-16
Inspection of female genitalia. (From Seidel.[23])

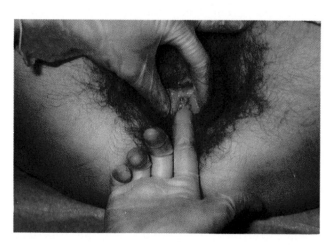

FIGURE 2-17
Examination of female urethra. (From Seidel.[23])

and shape of the os. A normal cervix is pink and moist; pregnancy may cause a more bluish appearance and anemia a paler color. The cervix should be located in the midline; remember that the position of the cervix correlates with the position of the uterus. Anterior orientation of the cervix indicates retroverted uterus, whereas posterior orientation indicates anteverted uterus. Deviation to the left or right may indicate a mass, adhesions, or pregnancy.

Note any cervical discharge. Normally cervical discharge is odorless, murky or clear, and varies in consistency from viscous to clear and thin. Discharge from bacterial or fungal infection is malodorous and yellow, gray, or green. Gently remove the speculum, specifically noting the state of the vaginal mucosa.

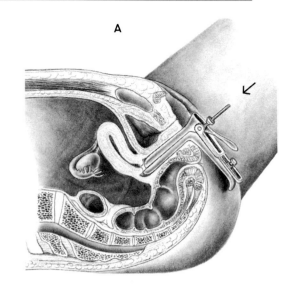

Next, insert a single blade of the speculum to inspect for signs of pelvic descent. First, orient the speculum toward the woman's rectum. Ask her to cough or bear down, and observe for herniation of the bladder into the vaginal vault. Next, orient the blade toward the bladder, and ask the woman to cough or bear down, again observing for herniation of the rectum into the vaginal space. Herniation of the anterior vaginal wall is called cystocele, and posterior wall herniation is called a rectocele. Observe the urethra for leakage (stress urinary incontinence) associated with the physical stress of coughing or bearing down. As you withdraw the speculum, inspect the cervix for evidence of forward migration, indicating uterine prolapse.

Explain to the woman that a bimanual examination will follow inspection with the speculum (Figure 2-19). Remove the glove from one hand, and lubricate the index and middle finger of your gloved examining hand. Gently and gradually insert the full length of these fingers into the vaginal vault, allowing adequate time for the patient to relax her circumvaginal muscles to the fullest extent feasible. Palpate the vaginal wall for nodules, cysts, or masses. Locate the cervix with the palmar aspect of your gloved fingers, and gently palpate it circumferentially. Inspect the cervix for size, length, and shape, which should correspond to the impression obtained on specular examination.

Grasp the cervix between your gloved examining fingers and gently move it from side to side. A normal cervix moves 1 to 2 cm without causing discomfort. A tender, fixed cervix may indicate pelvic inflammatory disease or an ectopic pregnancy. Insert the tip of the finger into the os of the cervix to assess its patency. The os should admit approximately 0.5 cm of the fingertip.

Palpate the uterus for position, size, shape, and masses. The normal nongravid uterus is pear shaped and 5 to 8 cm long. Enlargement may indicate pregnancy in a young adult woman or a mass in postmenopausal women or those who are not pregnant.

Palpate the ovaries whenever possible. They should feel firm, smooth, and ovoid and measure 3 × 2 × 1 cm. A normal ovary is tender on examination, although exquisite pain is not expected. Nodules and enlargement are abnormal.

A digital rectal examination completes the female genital evaluation. Test for anal sphincter tone and for the bulbocavernosus reflex. In the woman, gently tap the clitoris to elicit the reflex. Poor anal sphincter tone, absence of the bulbocavernosus reflex, and diminished sensations may indicate neurologic disease that is causing voiding dysfunction.

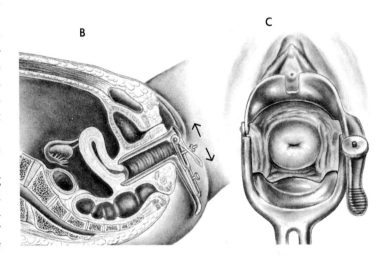

FIGURE 2-18
A, Insertion of speculum. **B,** Gentle separation of blades. **C,** Visualization of cervix. (From Seidel.[23])

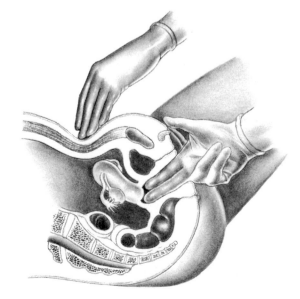

FIGURE 2-19
Bimanual palpation of uterus and ovaries. (From Seidel.[23])

CHAPTER 3

Diagnostic Procedures

KIDNEY-URETER-BLADDER X-RAY (KUB, PLAIN ABDOMINAL X-RAY)

A kidney-ureter-bladder (KUB) x-ray is an anteroposterior (oriented from front to back) film of the kidneys, ureters, and bony pelvis done without contrast material. A single film is obtained in the supine position (Figure 3-1). The KUB is used as a single study to detect the presence of radiopaque urinary calculi (Figure 3-2). The KUB also is used to detect bowel gas patterns that may be abnormal in the presence of a large abdominal, pelvic, or renal mass. The renal shadows may be noted on KUB, allowing rough determination of renal size and location and proximity to suspected calculi. An anteroposterior view of the spine is provided. Evaluation of anatomic defects of the bony spinal column may indicate neuropathic bladder dysfunction caused by dysraphism of the lower spine.

INDICATIONS

Urinary calculi
Preliminary x-ray for intravenous urogram/pyelogram
Preliminary x-ray for voiding cystourethrogram/cystogram/videourodynamic testing

CONTRAINDICATIONS

None

NURSING CARE

Preparation for a KUB varies according to the purpose of the study. Bowel preparation ("bowel prep") is required when a KUB is obtained before an intravenous pyelogram; no preparation is used when a KUB is done

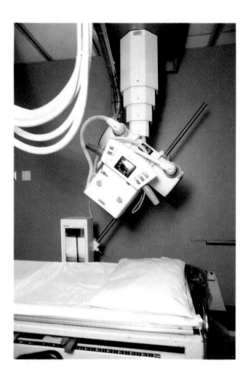

FIGURE 3-1
Equipment for KUB. (From Brundage D: *Renal disorders*, St Louis, 1992, Mosby–Year Book.)

as a single study or before a cystogram, voiding cystourethrogram, or videourodynamic testing.

PATIENT TEACHING

Explain the procedure and its purpose as a single exam or as a preliminary x-ray for an intravenous pyelogram or voiding cystogram. Assure the patient that the procedure is painless. Advise the patient that the KUB may not detect every urinary stone, particularly if the calculi are small, obscured by bowel gas, or radiolucent.

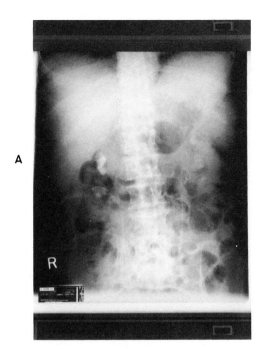
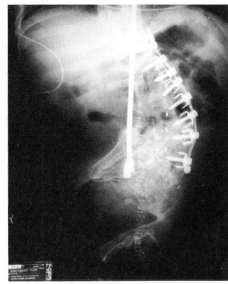

FIGURE 3-2
A, KUB image of urinary stone. **B,** KUB image of spina bifida.

INTRAVENOUS PYELOGRAM/UROGRAM (IVP/IVU) WITH NEPHROTOMOGRAMS

An intravenous pyelogram/urogram (IVP/IVU) is a series of contrast-enhanced x-rays that provide detailed information about the entire urinary tract, including the kidneys, ureters, and bladder, as well as clues to renal function through evaluation of their ability to concentrate and excrete contrast material. Information about the transport of urine from the renal pelvis to the bladder is evaluated by means of sequential x-rays of the abdomen and pelvis after contrast material has been injected intravenously (mechanical compression of the abdomen may be used to enhance the quality of the x-rays). X-rays of the partly filled bladder provide a limited cystogram; the patient's ability to empty the bladder is assessed through a postvoiding x-ray. The IVP/IVU is performed after adequate preparation of the bowel to minimize visual obscurity caused by fecal material and bowel gas in the abdomen (see Figure 3-1).

Views obtained during an intravenous pyelogram are enhanced by the use of nephrotomography that produces a series of x-rays focusing on a single plane of the kidney rather than the multiplane views obtained by the standard technique (Figure 3-3). Nephrotomograms

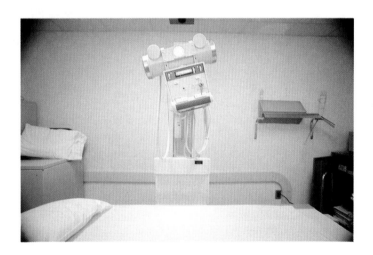

FIGURE 3-3
Equipment for IVP with tomograms.

are particularly useful for evaluating urinary calculi or renal tumors (Figure 3-4).

Radiation doses delivered during an intravenous pyelogram vary significantly, ranging from 1047 to 1465 mR (milliroentgens).

INDICATIONS

Urinary calculi

Recurrent urinary tract infection (UTI)

Febrile urinary tract infection

Hematuria

Abdominal or pelvic mass or tumor

Urinary system tumor

Obstruction

Congenital urinary system anomaly

Baseline evaluation for neuropathic bladder

CONTRAINDICATIONS

Allergy to intravenous, iodine-bound contrast material

Allergy to cutaneous iodine-based cleansing solution

Allergy to shellfish

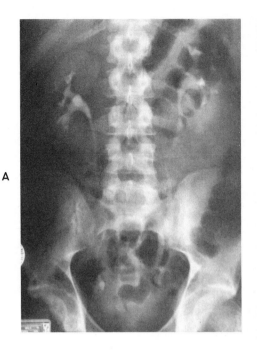 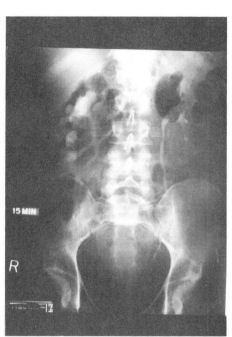

FIGURE 3-4
A, Normal IVP image. **B,** Hydronephrosis of right side.

NURSING CARE

Patients must be carefully screened for potential allergy to intravenous contrast materials. Consult the radiology department and physician about the patient with a history of allergy to shellfish. Additional contraindications for IVP/IVU include individuals at increased risk for dehydration secondary to bowel preparation or diseases that predispose the individual to rapid dehydration, such as diabetes mellitus, renal insufficiency, or multiple myeloma.

Proper preparation for IVP/IVU is affected by the patient's age, health, and patterns of bowel elimination. Preparation typically includes catharsis and dehydration. *Catharsis* usually is accomplished with the aid of an over-the-counter preparation such as Dulcolax or castor oil. In older or sedentary persons, the oral cathartic agent is combined with a suppository to stimulate more efficient evacuation of the bowel. *Dehydration* is influenced by the patient's age and general health. Young children or infants often remain NPO for only a brief period of 4 hours or less and prior overhydration is carefully avoided. Overnight dehydration may be used in adults while prior overhydration is avoided.

Individuals with chronic neuropathic constipation may require a more vigorous preparation. Traditional enemas rely on a bolus of fluid to stimulate bowel evacuation. This technique is not ideal for IVP preparation because it increases bowel gas that further obscures desired views. As an alternative, a mechanical system, such as the Avitar, may be used. The Avitar uses a pulsing motion with small volumes of saline warmed to approximate body temperature to produce effective bowel elimination.

Carefully monitor the patient for postprocedural complications, including hypersensitivity reactions and acute renal failure. *Hypersensitivity reactions* vary in severity from transient nausea, urticaria, and itching to respiratory failure and death. Allergic reactions are immediately apparent after injection of contrast material. A small amount of material is injected, and the patient is monitored carefully for urticaria, rhonchi, or shortness of breath. An antihistamine such as diphenhydramine, corticosteroids, and an emergency cart are kept readily available.

Acute renal failure is a rare but serious complication; provide adequate fluid intake, and observe for urinary output of at least 30 ml per hour after an intravenous pyelogram. Inability to retain fluids because of nausea and vomiting after an intravenous pyelogram is promptly reported; dehydration enhances the risk of renal failure in susceptible individuals.

PATIENT TEACHING

Explain the procedure and its purpose. Inform the patient that he will be taken to a radiologic suite and placed in a supine position. An intravenous needle is placed, and contrast material is injected into the vein in a single bolus after a small initial dose to determine immediate allergic response. Serial x-rays are obtained over a period of minutes to hours, depending on the patient's clinical condition and hospital protocols. Warn the patient that he may experience sensations of flushing, an unpleasant taste in the mouth, or nausea as the contrast is given. Reassure him that these responses are transient. Advise the patient that an abdominal binder, producing mild pressure against the abdomen, may be used to enhance the quality of certain images.

Advise the patient who asks specific questions about radiation exposure to discuss his concerns with the radiologist or attending physician.

RETROGRADE PYELOGRAM (RPG)

A retrograde pyelogram (RPG) is a series of x-rays that provide detailed anatomic views of the ureter, ureteropelvic junction, renal pelvis, and calyces. The procedure is performed under endoscopic visualization of the ureterovesical junction; a ureteral catheter is placed in the lower ureteral segment, and contrast material is *gently* injected or infused by means of gravity into the upper urinary tract (Figure 3-5).

INDICATIONS

Same as for intravenous pyelogram/urogram; RPG is used with patients who are allergic to iodine-bound contrast material or who have a nonfunctioning kidney incapable of concentrating and excreting contrast.

CONTRAINDICATIONS

Allergy to cutaneous iodine-based cleansing agents

NURSING CARE

Pyelonephritis, related to instrumentation and injection of material into a sterile body compartment, is a potentially serious complication. Observe the patient closely for flank pain, dysuria, chills, and fever for 24 to 48 hours after the procedure. Consult the physician promptly and obtain urine for culture and analysis should symptoms occur. Administer antiinfective agents as directed. Provide an adequate fluid intake after the procedure.

Overdistention of the renal collecting system may cause extravasation of contrast material, producing flank pain and fever. This response typically is transient and disappears within 48 hours, although a urinalysis and culture are done to rule out infection.

PATIENT TEACHING

Explain the procedure and its purpose. Advise the patient that injection of the contrast material may cause transient flank pain.

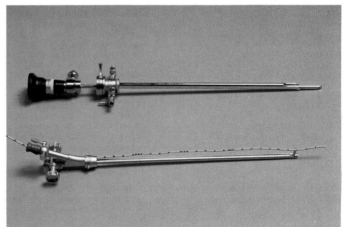

A

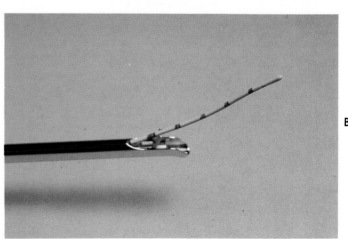

B

FIGURE 3-5
Cystoscope with McCarthy bridge for RPG. **A,** Bridge.
B, Placement of ureteral catheter.

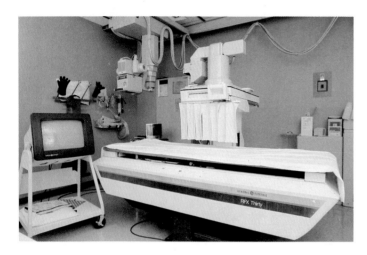

FIGURE 3-6
Fluoroscopy equipment for VCUG.

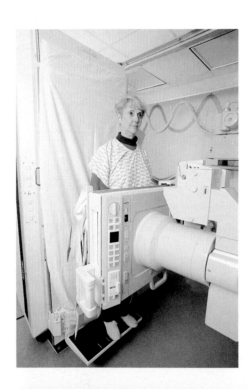

FIGURE 3-7
Position for voiding cystourethrogram.

CYSTOGRAM, VOIDING CYSTOURETHROGRAM (VCUG)

A cystogram or voiding cystourethrogram requires catheterization and instillation of contrast material into the bladder (Figures 3-6 and 3-7). A cystogram is a series of x-rays of the bladder during filling. The VCUG combines images of the cystogram with x-rays of the bladder and urethra during micturition (Figure 3-8).

INDICATIONS

Recurrent urinary tract infection (UTI)
Febrile urinary tract infection
Congenital anomaly of the urinary system
Trauma of the lower urinary tract or pelvis
Evaluating and grading vesicoureteral reflux
Unexplained gross or microscopic hematuria

CONTRAINDICATIONS

Allergy to intravesical iodine-bound contrast materials
Allergy to cutaneous iodine-based cleansing solutions
Current urinary tract infection

NURSING CARE

Urinary tract infection is a contraindication for a cystogram or VCUG. Obtain a urine culture before the test and administer antiinfective agents as directed. The principal complications of the test are urinary tract infection and urethral or bladder discomfort. Help the patient relieve discomfort by encouraging plenty of fluids and by having him sit in a tub filled with warm water to above the waist. Teach the patient the signs of urinary tract infection (dysuria, frequency, and odorous, discolored urine), and advise him to contact his referring physician should symptoms occur. Reassure the patient that discomfort after the test should disappear within 24 hours.

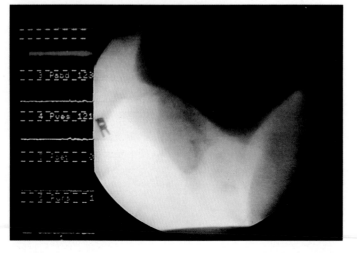

FIGURE 3-8
Normal VCUG.

RETROGRADE URETHROGRAM (RUG)

A retrograde urethrogram (RUG) requires instillation of a relatively small volume of iodine-bound contrast material into the male urethra from a retrograde direction. The fluid is instilled in one of three ways: through a catheter-tipped syringe, through a Foley catheter snuggled into the fossa navicularis with the balloon inflated with approximately 1 ml of fluid, or through a holder specially designed to prevent exposure of the clinician's hand to radiation during the procedure. Oblique x-rays of the urethra are obtained after instillation of approximately 15 to 30 ml of contrast material (Figure 3-9).

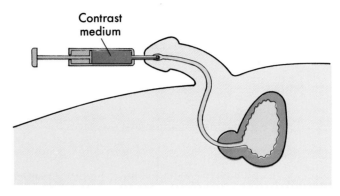

FIGURE 3-9
Technique for retrograde urethrogram.

INDICATIONS

Urethral stricture
Urethral fistula
Urethral trauma
Urethral diverticulum
Urethral tumor

CONTRAINDICATIONS

Allergy to intravesical iodine-bound contrast material
Allergy to cutaneous iodine-based cleansing solutions

NURSING CARE

Urinary tract infection is treated before a retrograde urethrogram whenever possible. Care after the test centers on preventing complications. Mild dysuria and urethral burning typically are transient; help the patient reduce the discomfort by encouraging plenty of fluids and by having him sit in a tub filled with warm water to his waist.

PATIENT TEACHING

Explain the procedure and its purpose. Reassure the patient that the discomfort he may feel during and after the test is transient. Inform him of the signs and symptoms of lower urinary tract infection, and advise him to contact his referring physician promptly should symptoms occur.

COMPUTED TOMOGRAPHY (CT SCAN) OF THE ABDOMEN AND PELVIS

A computed tomography (CT) scan provides computer-generated, axial images of the abdominal contents, including the kidneys, ureters, bladder, and major renal vessels. The CT scan also provides axial images of the male genitalia, including the pelvic lymph nodes. CT images of the pelvis are useful for detecting and evaluating urinary system tumors and enlarged lymph nodes caused by metastatic invasion or pelvic abscess, or distortion caused by a primary pelvic mass. The CT scan provides an estimate of tissue densities expressed as Hounsfield units; normal parenchyma measures 80 to 100 Hounsfield units. Fluid-filled cysts have a lower density, whereas solid tumors have a density similar to normal parenchyma. Evaluation may be enhanced by injection of contrast material.

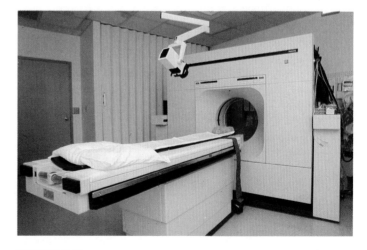

FIGURE 3-10
CT equipment.

The procedure is performed by having the patient lie in a supine position while a belt mechanism moves the body precise distances to obtain needed images (Figure 3-10). A single longitudinal view outlines the location of subsequent cuts (Figure 3-11).

INDICATIONS

Abdominal mass
Detecting and staging genitourinary tumors

CONTRAINDICATIONS

Allergy to intravenous iodine-bound contrast material (when an injection is needed to enhance imaging)

NURSING CARE

Hypersensitivity reactions may occur when contrast materials are injected (see nursing care of the patient undergoing IVP/IVU). Because the patient must remain still during the procedure, sedation sometimes is used for those who cannot cooperate or understand directions.

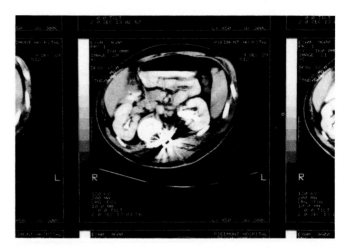

FIGURE 3-11
Normal abdominal CT demonstrating kidneys.

PATIENT TEACHING

Explain the procedure and its purpose. Advise the patient that contrast material may be injected to obtain the needed images. Discuss the need to remain still during the procedure so that serial images are adequately obtained.

MAGNETIC RESONANCE IMAGING (MRI)

MRI uses radio waves that alter the magnetic field produced by human tissue rather than roentgen rays (x-rays) for imaging. Because of the uneven proton counts of living tissues, each creates a small magnetic field. When exposed to a stronger electromagnetic field, the protons align along the field produced by the stronger magnet at the lowest possible energy state. Disturbing the body's normal equilibrium with radiofrequency pulses causes a brief rise in the energy state of these protons. When the radiofrequency is discontinued, the protons rapidly return to a lower energy state, producing a signal that a computer can detect and convert into an image (Figure 3-12).

The MRI study is useful for visualizing kidneys and structures of the pelvis, including the prostate, scrotal contents, and penis in males. Views can be generated from coronal, sagittal, and transaxial planes (Figure 3-13). MRI has not proved useful for detecting urinary calculi or calcified tumors.

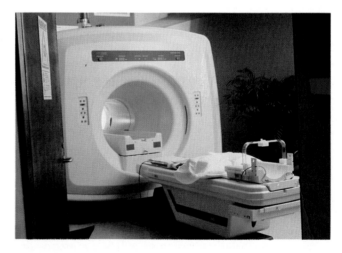

FIGURE 3-12
MRI equipment.

INDICATIONS

Abdominal or pelvic mass
Genitourinary system tumor

CONTRAINDICATIONS

Pacemaker (MRI may interfere with mechanism)
History of aneurysm surgery requiring surgical clips

NURSING CARE

Preparing a patient for an MRI scan includes carefully explaining that MRI scanning requires the patient to lie still in an enclosed tube that contains the electromagnet needed for realignment of the body's magnetic field. Consult the radiologist about sedating patients with a history of claustrophobia. Patients who cannot cooperate or understand directions may require deeper sedation.

PATIENT TEACHING

Explain the procedure and its purpose. Reassure an anxious patient that MRI scanning is not painful and that a technologist will be in verbal communication with him throughout the procedure, although the tech-

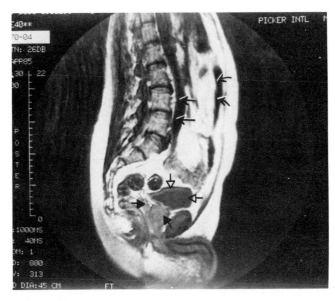

FIGURE 3-13
MRI of pelvic contents of male. (From Gillenwater JY et al: *Adult and pediatric urology*, ed 2, St Louis, 1991, Mosby−Year Book.)

nologist will not be in the room with him. Advise the patient to remove all metal objects that may be drawn to the magnet.

ENDOSCOPY

Endoscopy is the visualization of hollow viscera within the body by means of light-enhanced telescopic or fiberoptic imaging. Endoscopy of the urinary system allows direct visualization of the renal pelvis and calyces (nephroscopy); ureters (ureteroscopy); and bladder, urethra, and ureterovesical junctions (cystoscopy or cystourethroscopy) (Figure 3-14). Rigid endoscopy requires insertion of a metal sheath followed by introduction of telescopes attached to a powerful light source for visual inspection. Flexible endoscopy uses fiberoptic technology for visualization through a relatively small, one-piece system. Both flexible and rigid endoscopic instruments provide working ports for obtaining biopsy specimens, for catheterization of ureters, and for other procedures requiring direct visualization of the urinary system.

Nephroscopy is a procedure that allows visualization of the renal pelvis and calyces from an antegrade perspective. A percutaneous tract is obtained before the

nephroscope is inserted. Nephroscopy often is combined with percutaneous nephrolithotomy or ureterolithotomy.

Ureteroscopy allows direct visualization of ureters and ureterovesical junctions. The procedure typically is performed from the retrograde perspective, and the ureteroscope is designed to dilate and visualize each ureter. Flexible instruments have significantly improved the quality and clinical utility of ureteroscopy.

Cystourethroscopy is the most commonly used endoscopic procedure in urology. The urethra, bladder urothelium, trigone, and ureterovesical junctions are visualized from the retrograde perspective. Rigid cystourethroscopy requires introduction of a metal sheath into the bladder via the urethra followed by insertion of a telescope attached to a powerful light source for direct visualization. Urethroscopic images are obtained during insertion or withdrawal of the sheath. Flexible cystoscopy uses a softer, flexible sheath that contains a fiberoptic system attached to a powerful light source. Flexible instruments also allow visualization of the bladder outlet from an antegrade perspective by reorienting the scope on itself. Fiberoptic images may be slightly less clear than those produced by rigid instruments.

INDICATIONS

Urinary calculi
Recurrent urinary tract infection (UTI)
Febrile urinary tract infection
Vesicoureteral reflux (selected cases)
Obstruction of bladder outlet
Urethral stricture
Urethral or bladder fistula
Urinary incontinence (selected cases)
Neuropathic bladder (selected cases)
Congenital anomalies of the urinary system

CONTRAINDICATIONS

Current urinary tract infection

NURSING CARE

Careful preparation may include a preanesthesia checklist as well as assurance of sterile urine. Before the test, obtain a urine culture, and treat bacteriuria with sensitivity-guided antiinfective agents under a physician's direction. Advise the patient that nephroscopy demands percutaneous access to the renal pelvis, requiring spinal or general anesthesia during dilation. Ureteroscopy requires dilation of the ureters, requiring significant sedation or anesthesia. Cystourethroscopy may or may not require sedation or anesthesia, depending on the type of instrument used (rigid systems cause more discomfort than do flexible ones) and the procedures performed as part of endoscopy. For example, flexible cystoscopy typically is done with intraurethral instillation of a water-soluble lubricant that may or may not contain lidocaine. In contrast, rigid cystoscopy combined with transurethral resection of a bladder tumor or prostate requires spinal or general anesthesia.

Complications after endoscopy include bleeding and infection. Assess the patient's urinary output after endoscopy for signs of *hematuria*. After routine cystourethroscopy, the urine may be pink tinged; reassure the patient that even small amounts of blood can discolor a significant volume of urine. Promptly report evidence of frank bleeding or clots to the physician.

Infection may affect only the lower urinary tract or may enter the systemic circulation through minute tears in the urinary mucosa. Assess the patient for signs of systemic infection and potential septic shock, including fever, chills, rapid pulse, and tachypnea, followed

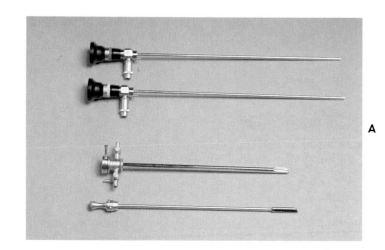

A

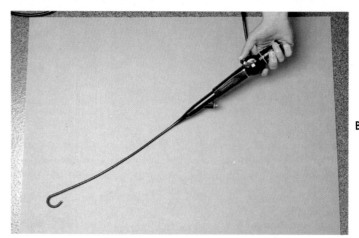

B

FIGURE 3-14
Endoscopy equipment. **A,** Rigid. **B,** Flexible.

by hypothermia and decreasing blood pressure during later stages of shock. Immediately report fever and signs of systemic infection, before potentially irreversible septic shock occurs. Administer intravenous or oral prophylactic antibiotics after endoscopy as directed. Lower urinary tract infection is noted as persistent dysuria and lower abdominal or back discomfort without fever or chills after the first 24 hours following evaluation.

PATIENT TEACHING

A careful explanation of the procedure and its purpose is essential before endoscopy. Consult the physician and anesthesiologist about forms of anesthesia and/or sedation expected during the procedure. Anesthesia may range from local insertion of lidocaine impregnated with lubricating jelly to spinal or general anesthesia, depending on the patient's clinical condition and anticipated procedures. Explain to the patient that he will be placed in a lithotomy position for rigid endoscopy and in a lithotomy or supine position for flexible endoscopy. Advise the patient that he will be placed in a lithotomy position for ureteroscopy, or in a prone position for nephroscopy, which will be performed after a tract has been established through the flank. Patients who do not require systemic, spinal, or general anesthesia typically are prepared by local anesthesia of the urethral wall. Advise the patient that a water-soluble lubricant of 2% lidocaine is placed in the urethra. Explain to men that the medication will be held in place for a brief period using a penile clamp.

After the procedure, teach the patient to watch for signs of urinary tract infection (dysuria, frequency, and urgency) and systemic infection (signs of urinary tract infection accompanied by malaise and fever). Advise him to contact his physician promptly should symptoms occur.

URODYNAMIC TESTING (CYSTOMETRICS)

Urodynamics is a set of tests that measure urinary system transport, storage, and elimination functions. Screening urodynamics implies uroflowmetry or uroflowmetry combined with a single-channel cystometrogram. Multichannel urodynamic studies combine several parameters for evaluating lower urinary tract function. Videourodynamic testing combines multichannel urodynamic variables with fluoroscopy of the lower urinary tract, similar to techniques used during voiding cystourethrography, to assess lower urinary tract physiology and morphology (Figure 3-15).

Uroflowmetry (urinary flow study, uroflow study, flow study) is a dynamic study of urinary flow rate. The patient urinates into a funnel connected to a flow rate apparatus. Uroflowmeters rely on one of several systems to produce analog or computer-generated graphic results. The von Garrelts flowmeter uses a weight transducer to produce results, whereas other systems use spinning disks, capacitance, or air displacement meters. Uroflowmetry is useful as a screening measure to detect abnormal flow patterns indicating possible outlet obstruction or deficient detrusor contractility. It also is used before a pressure-flow study as a quality control measure, which provides a "normal" flow pattern before the invasive instrumentation required for detailed testing.

A cystometrogram (CMG) is a dynamic test of bladder filling that compares volume and intravesical pressure by means of an analog or computer-generated graph (Figure 3-16). The patient is placed in a supine position, and one or more catheters are introduced into the bladder through the urethra or via suprapubic access. The bladder is filled with a liquid such as water, saline, or contrast material or with carbon dioxide (not recommended by the International Continence Society). A filling CMG is obtained in supine and upright positions. The filling CMG typically is followed by a voiding pressure study that combines CMG with flow data.

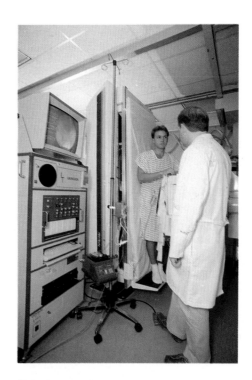

FIGURE 3-15
Videourodynamics.

Testing is accomplished by means of a one-catheter, multichannel, or two-catheter technique. A one-catheter technique is technically simple but prone to artifact produced by infusion and pressure measurement through a single-lumen tube. Multichannel or two-catheter techniques avoid this artifact, although the two-catheter technique is technically more demanding. A two-catheter technique offers the potential advantage of allowing removal of the filling tube, enhancing the quality of the pressure-flow study.

Insertion of an abdominal pressure catheter enhances testing by detecting artifact produced by changes in abdominal pressure caused by position changes or movement. A small tube with a fluid-filled balloon is placed in the lower portion of the rectum using clean technique. The tube is connected to a pressure transducer, and values are recorded on a polygraph or computer. Subtracting the abdominal pressure from the intravesical pressure produces a variable called detrusor pressure, which provides an approximate representation of the contribution of the smooth muscle of the bladder wall to filling and micturition bladder pressures. In women, placement of an intravaginal balloon device may be substituted for the rectal balloon.

When intravesical, abdominal, and detrusor pressures are simultaneously measured, the clinician remembers that only the intravesical pressure variable is considered "absolute" or without inherent error. The abdominal pressure is prone to artifact, which may come from the walls of the balloon needed to obtain the variable from an air-filled chamber (rectal or vaginal vault) or from potential contraction of the smooth muscle of the rectal vault or striated circumvaginal muscles. The artifact in the abdominal pressure tracing also renders the detrusor pressure prone to error. Therefore when a three-channel CMG is performed, the intravesical pressure is measured with an empty bladder, and the abdominal pressure is set to equal the intravesical pressure. Since the bladder is empty, the detrusor pressure is set at 0 cm H_2O and filling is begun.

The CMG is useful in determining bladder capacity, the compliance of the bladder wall, the stability of the detrusor muscle, and sensations of filling. Bladder and rectal pressures measured during micturition contribute to the voiding pressure study.

Cystometric techniques also may be adapted to evaluate dynamic characteristics of continent diversions, including capacity, compliance, the presence of bolus contractions, and the competence of continence mechanisms. Because the bowel has the potential to reabsorb water and electrolytes, continent diversions routinely are filled with an isotonic solution such as saline or a slightly hypertonic solution (iodine-bound contrast material). A filling CMG often is combined with continuous pressure measurement of the continent nipple (see the section on the urethral pressure study). A sphincter electromyogram and abdominal pressure measurement are useful in some cases. Cystometric measurements commonly are combined with fluoroscopy for videourodynamic testing of the continent diversion; this allows assessment of the shape of the pouch, its anatomic relationships, and the presence of abnormal findings such as extravasation of contrast or reflux of urine to the kidneys.

A **sphincter electromyogram** (EMG) measures the electrical activity of the pelvic floor musculature. Graphic, oscilloscopic, and/or audible data provide information about the response of the pelvic floor muscles

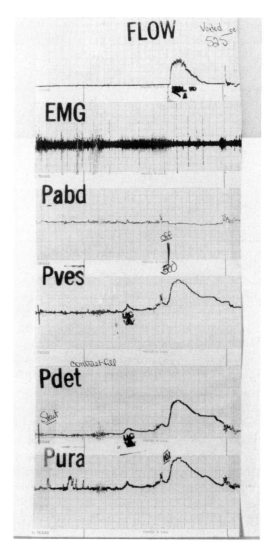

FIGURE 3-16
Analog urodynamic tracing.

to bladder filling and micturition. Additional information is provided by eliciting the bulbocavernosus response. Three EMG techniques are commonly used. Patch electrodes allow evaluation by means of an analog or computer-generated graph. After adequate skin preparation, electrocardiogram (ECG) patches are placed over the perineal area. This technique offers the advantage of allowing the patient to be mobile during testing and avoids discomfort through use of noninvasive patch electrodes. It provides assessment of gross muscle action during bladder filling and micturition (kinesiologic assessment) but is limited by significant artifact, which is caused by impedance from the skin and underlying fatty tissue.

Percutaneous wire electrodes provide a more artifact-free analysis of gross muscle action during bladder filling and micturition. Monitoring of audible signals produced by action potentials (AP) at muscle level is useful for distinguishing true contraction from artifact. Wire electrodes also allow the patient to be mobile during testing and have the potential for analysis of individual AP waveforms.

Bipolar needle EMG with oscilloscopic monitor offers the most detailed EMG information, including summation of gross muscle action and analysis of individual AP waveforms. Its disadvantages are the discomfort caused by needle placement and the limited patient mobility.

The sphincter EMG typically is performed during the filling cystometrogram and voiding flow study.

A **voiding pressure study** (pressure flow study, micturition study) combines uroflowmetry, cystometrogram, and sphincter electromyogram data to provide a detailed assessment of micturition. The voiding pressure study is obtained immediately after the filling cystometrogram. The filling catheter is removed, and the patient voids into a urinary flowmeter while the intravesical, intraabdominal, and detrusor pressures, sphincter EMG, and uroflowmetry are measured simultaneously. Fluoroscopic monitoring is added in the case of videourodynamic testing (Figure 3-17). A graphic comparison is used to evaluate detrusor contractility, urinary flow rate, and pelvic floor muscle response to voiding. Analysis is enhanced by computer-generated pressure-flow plotting or calculation of detrusor energy factors.

A **urethral pressure study** produces a graphic representation of sphincter closure pressure, functional length, continuous response to bladder filling and micturition, or response to a specific provocative maneuver such as a cough. The urethral pressure profile (UPP) is obtained by slowly withdrawing a catheter through the urethra while side ports simultaneously perfuse the urethral wall and measure urethral closure pressure. Maximum urethral closure pressure (MUCP) provides a static measurement of the dynamic sphincter mechanism. Functional length provides an estimate of the length of the urethra affected by the sphincter mechanism. A microtip catheter also may be pulled through the urethra to obtain a urethral pressure profile.

Continuous urethral pressure monitoring uses a multichannel catheter to measure urethral pressure during bladder filling and micturition or in response to a specific provocative maneuver such as a cough.

The **Whitaker test** (upper tract urodynamics) provides graphic tracings of the pressure gradient between the renal pelvis and ureterovesical junction. A percutaneous cannula that is attached to a constant-rate infusion pump and a pressure transducer is inserted into the kidney by a surgeon or interventional radiologist. A second tube is inserted into the bladder via the urethra

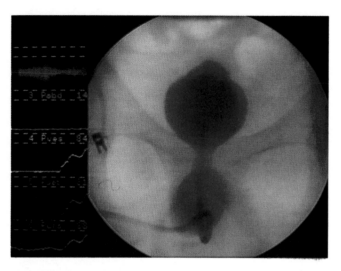

FIGURE 3-17
Videourodynamic image.

and attached to a second pressure transducer. Fluid is infused at a rate of 10 ml per minute until the renal pelvis, ureter, and bladder are relatively full or until flank pain and obvious obstruction are noted. After the test has been completed, the cannula (perfusion) pressure and bladder pressure are subtracted to determine the presence or absence of upper urinary tract obstruction. The Whitaker test is useful in markedly dilated systems and when DTPA testing fails to evaluate potential obstruction adequately. Its principal disadvantage is the invasive nature of a test that requires percutaneous placement of a cannula. The results depend on use of a continuous infusion rate; 10 ml per minute typically is recommended.

INDICATIONS

Urinary incontinence
Voiding dysfunction in the absence of incontinence
Neuropathic bladder dysfunction
Bladder outlet obstruction
Urinary retention of unknown cause
Suspected ureteral obstruction

CONTRAINDICATIONS

Current urinary tract infection (UTI)
Acute, debilitating illness limiting mobility

NURSING CARE

A urinary tract infection is a relative contraindication to urodynamic testing. A urine culture and sensitivities are obtained, and the urinary system is rendered sterile *before* testing. Consult the urologist or referring physician for rare exceptions. Encourage fluid intake, and ask the patient to abstain from voiding for 1 to 4 hours before testing for an optimum urinary flow study. Pre-procedure anxiety rarely requires light sedation.

After the test, monitor the patient for discomfort related to urethral instrumentation and for infection. Administer prophylactic antibiotics to reduce the risk of infection as directed. Help the patient relieve discomfort through forcing fluids, frequent voiding as required, and a warm bath filled to waist level.

PATIENT TEACHING

Careful instruction before the test is necessary to alleviate anxiety. Advise the patient that urodynamic testing involves very little pain. Catheterization is required, but the catheters are smaller than a rigid cystoscope and soft. Teach the patient the importance of relaxation during urethral catheterization, and help him practice breathing techniques before the procedure. Advise the patient that catheterization is followed by placement of a rectal tube, and reassure him that the tube will not cause the bowels to move. Rather, counsel the patient that he is likely to perceive slight pressure and a transient desire to defecate.

Consult with the urodynamics laboratory about the methodology for sphincter EMG. When appropriate, advise the patient that patch electrodes are painless and that needle or wire electrodes are painful only at the moment of insertion. If patch electrodes are used, advise the patient that ECG-type patches are placed near the anus after skin preparation. Reassure him that the procedure is not painful when patches are used.

Inform the patient that several fills with sterile water or other liquid will be accomplished. Explain that the voiding study requires micturition into a uroflowmeter after the filling tube has been removed if a two-catheter technique is used.

After the procedure, teach the patient the signs and symptoms of urinary tract infection, including frequency and dysuria persisting beyond the first 24 hours after the test. Instruct the patient to contact the physician promptly should symptoms occur.

IMAGING URINARY DIVERSIONS

Imaging urinary diversion requires infusion of contrast material into some type of urinary diversion such as a continent pouch or Bricker ileal conduit. These images provide detailed information about the anatomy of the pouch, anatomic relationships to adjacent structures, and any abnormal findings such as extravasation or reflux. The pouchogram may be combined with urodynamic evaluation to assess the capacity, compliance, and continence mechanisms of the diversion. A KUB may be performed before the procedure to detect radiopaque calculi.

INDICATIONS

Baseline evaluation for subsequent comparison
Recurrent pouchitis (infection of urine in the pouch)
Febrile urinary tract infection (UTI)
Incontinence of continent diversion
Obstruction of the pouch
Urinary calculi

CONTRAINDICATIONS

Allergy to cutaneous iodine-based cleansing solution
Allergy to intravesical iodine-bound contrast material

NURSING CARE

Before the procedure, screen the patient for allergy to contrast material. Consult the radiology department, and allow the patient to self-catheterize a continent diversion whenever possible. This reduces the patient's anxiety and the risk of trauma to continent stoma if radiologic personnel do not have extensive experience with continent diversions.

Care after the procedure centers on preventing complications. Potential complications include infection and extravasation, particularly for the patient with a continent diversion. Monitor the patient for signs of infection, including leakage, discomfort, or cramping with malodorous, cloudy urine. Promptly contact the physician if symptoms occur.

PATIENT TEACHING

Preparation for the procedure includes a brief explanation of the test and reassurance that the diversion will not be overfilled to the point of causing pain. Instruct the patient with a Bricker ileal conduit to bring an extra pouch, since testing requires exposure of the stoma for catheterization. Instruct the patient with a continent diversion to bring an ostomy catheter, since the radiology department may not have the appropriate type of catheter readily available.

After the test, instruct the patient in the signs and symptoms of pouchitis (bacteriuria in the incontinent or continent diversion). Advise the patient to contact the physician promptly should symptoms occur.

DYNAMIC INFUSION CAVERNOSOMETRY AND CAVERNOSOGRAPHY (DICC)

Dynamic infusion cavernosometry and cavernosography (DICC) is a set of diagnostic tests that measure the neurovascular elements of penile erection (Figure 3-18). The study is divided into four phases. In phase 1, the patient is given an intracavernous injection of a vasodilator (e.g., papaverine or prostaglandin E_1), and cavernous response is measured by means of a single pressure transducer placed in the corporal body. In phase 2, penile venous competence is measured. Heparinized saline is infused rapidly into the penis until a predetermined suprasystolic pressure is attained. The infusion then is abruptly halted, and the rate of venous runoff is assessed. Phase 3 evaluates arterial competence. Heparinized saline is rapidly infused into the corporal body several times, and right and left cavernosal artery occlusion pressures are determined using Doppler ultrasound. In phase 4, contrast material is infused slowly into the corpora cavernosa, and serial x-ray images are obtained.

DICC is used to determine the cause of erectile dysfunction. The test can evaluate dysfunction caused by venous leakage or incompetence, arterial insufficiency, and neuropathic dysfunction and has the potential to assist in diagnosis of psychogenic erectile dysfunction, although those results are best combined with other diagnostic methodologies. DICC is particularly useful in determining the cause of erectile dysfunction among males who do not respond to a pharmacologic erection program.

INDICATIONS

Erectile dysfunction

CONTRAINDICATIONS

Allergy to intravenous iodine-bound contrast material

NURSING CARE

DICC is an invasive and valuable evaluation of neurovascular influences governing penile tumescence. Nursing care centers on ensuring safety during testing and avoiding complications. Any history of allergy is obtained before the test. The patient is attached to cardiac (three-lead ECG) and automatic blood pressure monitors. Baseline vital signs, pulse, respirations, and blood pressure are obtained. Lidocaine is injected subcutaneously before the test to ablate the pain of having needles inserted into the cavernosal bodies. Two butterfly needles are placed in each corpus cavernosus; one is for measuring intracavernosal pressure, and the other is for infusion of heparinized saline or contrast material after

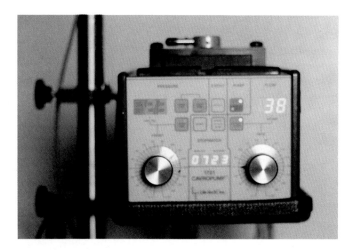

FIGURE 3-18
Pump for DICC.

the local anesthetic has been given. During the first phase a vasodilator is given, and the cavernosal response is monitored. The drug requires 12 minutes or longer to act; cavernosal pressure, ECG, and blood pressure are monitored continuously. Ideally the intracavernosal pressure will approximate mean arterial pressure, indicating competent vascular control of erectile function. Failure to approximate mean arterial pressure indicates venous incompetence, arterial insufficiency, or a combination of these problems.

During the second phase, heparinized saline is infused by means of a continuous pressure pump to a suprasystolic level. Once the pressure has been established, the infusion is stopped and the rate of pressure fall is monitored over a 30-second period. The patient probably will perceive sensations of intense pressure, and the pump should be designed to automatically stop infusion when the desired pressure has been obtained. Overshooting this suprasystolic pressure is potentially harmful and must be meticulously avoided. Blood pressure and ECG are monitored throughout phase 2.

During the third phase the cavernosal pressure is raised to just above mean arterial pressure, and then the infusion is stopped. The nurse ensures silence in the testing suite while both the nurse and physician listen for the return of Doppler sounds, indicating arterial occlusion pressure. The occlusion pressure should approximate mean arterial pressure.

Nursing care during the final phase centers on preventing or rapidly reversing any allergic reaction to infusion of the contrast material. During the first minute of phase 4, contrast material is infused very slowly and the patient's response is monitored. The patient is closely monitored for evidence of allergic response throughout the final phase, and intracavernosal pressures are closely monitored to prevent overfilling and ischemia of local tissues.

After the examination, the needles are removed and an occlusive dressing is placed on the penis. Nursing care centers on preventing complications. Reassure the patient that analgesic or narcotic pain relief is rarely needed. Injection of a vasoconstricting agent occasionally is indicated, when persistent or painful tumescence is noted.

PATIENT TEACHING

Carefully explain the purpose of the procedure and the need for several clinicians in the room throughout the test. Review each of the four phases before the procedure, and inform the patient as each is finished. Warn the patient that the initial injection of lidocaine causes discomfort but that it prevents subsequent pain.

Teach the patient to monitor himself for priapism (prolonged painful erection) after the test. Tell the patient to contact the physician promptly if his erection does not subside within several hours after the procedure has been completed. Advise the patient to leave the occlusive dressing in place for 2 hours after the test and to monitor himself for bleeding for another 2 hours after that. Counsel the patient that he should avoid strenuous activities for the evening after the test and that a hematoma (bruise) of the penis may be noted for several days.

Advise the patient that priapism (painful erection) is a significant but rare complication. Teach him that an erection that persists for 6 hours after DICC constitutes a medical emergency; advise him to contact his physician immediately and arrange transport to an emergency treatment facility for pharmacologic reversal of the erection. Explain that pharmacologic reversal of priapism typically involves local injection of a vasoconstrictive agent such as an alpha sympathomimetic.

RADIONUCLIDE IMAGING (NUCLEAR IMAGING)

Nuclear imaging produces computer images of urinary tract structures obtained by means of intravenous or intravesical infusion of a radionuclide tracer substance (Figure 3-19). Renal scans use radionuclide substances injected intravenously that are either bound to renal tubular cells or excreted by glomerular filtration. Renal scans are used to evaluate functional aspects of the urinary system, including the mass of functioning parenchyma, differential function between kidneys, and semiquantitative function of excretory and transport functions.

Technetium 99m diethylenetriamine pentaacetic acid (DTPA) is principally excreted through glomerular filtration. It is injected in an intravenous bolus, and sequential, computer-generated images are obtained. An initial 30-second image may be taken to determine cortical blood flow. Subsequent images are obtained at 1 minute, and two images are obtained at 5, 10, 15, and 20 minutes. DTPA will image the kidneys, ureters, and bladder. The scan is used primarily to assess upper urinary tract obstruction, although the glomerular filtration rate (GFR) and effective renal plasma, renal flow, and differential renal function may be estimated using the DTPA radionuclide. Radionuclide scans provide

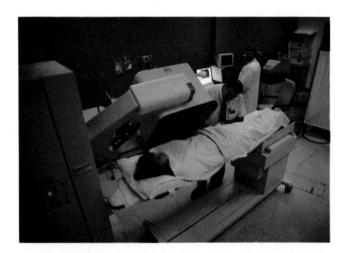

FIGURE 3-19
Radionuclide equipment.

more functional information than does an intravenous pyelogram, but they show less anatomic detail (Figure 3-20). Evaluation of obstruction is enhanced by injecting a diuretic agent, such as furosemide, followed by serial images, allowing qualitative analysis of radionuclide washout from each kidney. The computer provides a semiquantitative estimate of washout by producing a graph comparing radionuclide concentration in each kidney over time.

Technetium 99m dimercaptosuccinic acid (DMSA) is bound to the basement membrane of the proximal renal tubule. It allows evaluation of the renal cortex. An intravenous bolus of radionuclide is injected, and computer-generated, serial images of the renal parenchyma are obtained (Figure 3-21).

Iodine 131 orth-iodohippurate (OIH) (Hippuran) is excreted in the urine by glomerular filtration (20%) and by tubular excretion (80%). Its use is limited because of the higher doses of radiation (particularly gamma energy) involved compared to other radionuclides.

Technetium 99m antimony colloid is an investigational pharmaceutical agent that may prove useful in evaluating ileopelvic lymph nodes.

Technetium 99m mercaptoacetyltriglycine (MAG₃) is an experimental radionuclide that purports to combine the properties of DTPA and DMSA tracers, specifically the ability to detect differential renal function accurately and to evaluate a possible obstruction of the upper urinary tract.

The nuclear cystogram is useful for patients who are allergic to intravesical iodine-bound contrast materials. It can adequately assess vesicoureteral reflux, but lacks the anatomic detail of the voiding cystogram.

INDICATIONS

DTPA renal scan:
    Obstruction
    Differential renal function
    Calculating the glomerular filtration rate (GFR)
DMSA renal scan:
    Differential renal function
    Detecting renal scars
Hippuran scan:
    Renal insufficiency
Nuclear cystogram:
    Vesicoureteral reflux

CONTRAINDICATIONS

None

NURSING CARE

Radionuclide tracer substances are injected intravenously for renal scans. Observe the site for signs of irritation from the nuclear tracer substance. Bowel prepa-

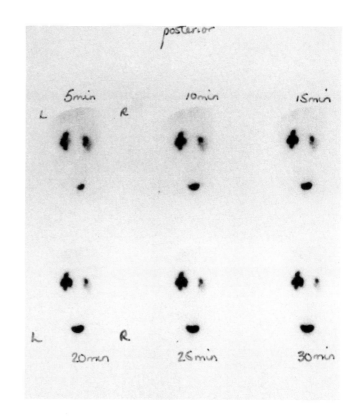

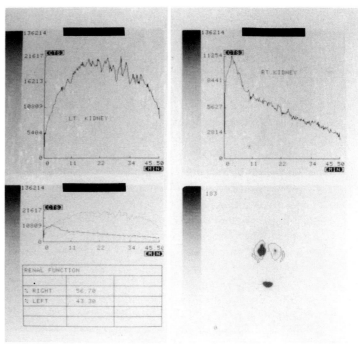

FIGURE 3-20
DTPA scan showing left ureteropelvic junction obstruction and hydronephrosis. The right kidney is normal.

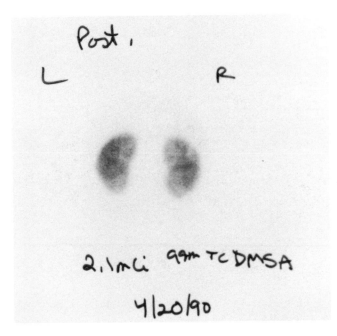

FIGURE 3-21
Normal DMSA scan.

ration is not required. Patients are exposed to significantly less radiation compared with intravenous pyelogram. Nonetheless, since a radionuclide is injected intravenously and excreted via the urine, pregnant women are advised to refrain from caring for these patients for the first 24 hours after a radionuclide scan. Consult the radiology department for hospital policies on disposal of incontinent containment or collecting bag devices immediately after radionuclide testing.

PATIENT TEACHING

Explain the procedure and its purpose, and advise the patient that the radionuclide scan will provide more detailed information about renal functioning than does the intravenous pyelogram/urogram. Inform the patient of the hospital's policy on disposal of incontinent pads or diapers after the radionuclide scan or nuclear cystogram.

ULTRASONOGRAPHY OF THE URINARY AND MALE REPRODUCTIVE SYSTEMS

Ultrasonography uses high-frequency sound waves (varying from 5,000 to 20,000 Hertz [Hz]) rather than radionuclide counts or x-ray beams to image the organs of the urinary and reproductive systems. These organs include the kidneys, ureters, bladder, prostate, and testes (Figure 3-22). Ultrasonography offers distinct advantages over radiographic techniques. Since radiation exposure is avoided, several images can be obtained, and repeat studies over a brief period of time carry negligible risk. Lack of radiation exposure also expands the possible setting for testing to an outpatient office or clinic, which may not have the lead-shielded rooms needed for x-ray and radionuclide techniques.

Renal scan: Images of the kidneys, renal pelvis, and proximal ureters are obtained from the prone and supine positions (Figure 3-23). A conducting jelly is spread on the patient's abdomen or back, and axial (transverse) and longitudinal (sagittal) images are obtained. A renal scan will image renal parenchyma, including the pyramids, calyces, and renal pelvis. Longitudinal and sagittal measurements of the kidneys may be obtained. Hydronephrosis can be detected, as can dilated renal pelves and ureters, which produce more

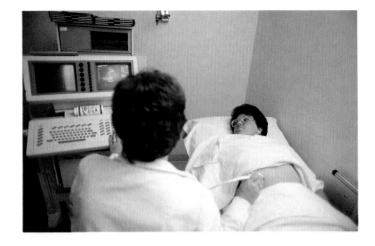

FIGURE 3-22
Ultrasonography of the genitourinary tract.

sonolucent images than do adjacent structures. Calculi are noted when they block transmission of ultrasonic waves, producing a shadow below the area of the stone. Solid tumors are detected when they produce distortion of the renal collecting system and when they contain calcified walls; cysts are noted because of their sonolucent, fluid-filled centers and loculated architecture.

Bladder scan: Sonolucent bladder images are obtained when urine is present in the lower urinary tract. The patient is placed in a supine position, and the suprapubic area is scanned. The relative thickness of the bladder and some of its architectural features also are noted. Dilated ureters are visible, although a normal ureter cannot be distinguished. Comparison of full and postvoid bladder volumes allows evaluation of efficiency of micturition. A quantitative estimation of bladder volume may be obtained.

Prostate scan: The prostate scan is obtained by gently inserting a probe into the rectum. Because the prostate is not a fluid-filled organ (unlike the kidneys and bladder), a fluid-filled balloon is used to enhance images of the organ. Axial and longitudinal views are obtained by using one or two probes (Figure 3-24).

Testicular scan: Imaging of the testicular parenchyma is used to detect masses.

INDICATIONS

Abdominal mass
Urinary calculi
Recurrent urinary tract infection (UTI)
Febrile urinary tract infection
Asymmetric enlargement of the prostate
Testicular mass

CONTRAINDICATIONS

None

NURSING CARE

Bowel preparation is not required for renal or bladder sonogram. Preparation for a prostatic sonogram usually consists of a low enema and evacuation of the bowel immediately before the scan.

PATIENT TEACHING

Explain the procedure and its purpose, and reassure the patient that renal, bladder, or testicular scans are

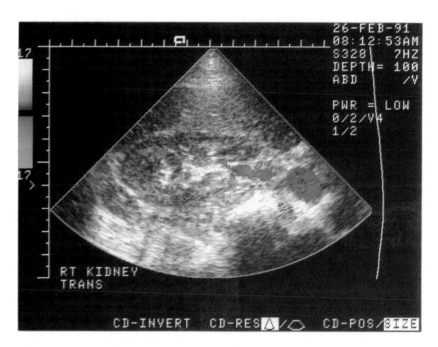

FIGURE 3-23
Ultrasound image of kidney. (From Brundage D: *Renal disorders*, St Louis, 1992, Mosby–Year Book.)

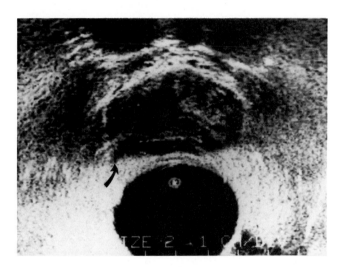

FIGURE 3-24
Prostate ultrasound image showing invasive adenocarcinoma. (From Gillenwater JY et al: *Adult and pediatric urology*, ed 2, St Louis, 1991, Mosby–Year Book.)

painless and noninvasive. Reduce the patient's anxiety about a prostatic sonogram by explaining that the probe is inserted gently into the rectum with adequate lubrication. Explain that this procedure is not painful; rather, the patient is likely to feel gentle pressure against the prostate and a desire to defecate.

RENAL ARTERIOGRAM

A renal arteriogram is a series of radiographic films that provide a detailed evaluation of the arterial supply of the kidneys. The patient is taken to a radiologic suite, and the skin over the femoral artery is prepared and anesthetized. A radiopaque catheter is threaded through the femoral artery into the abdominal aorta and then into the renal artery, where contrast material is injected. (If passage to the renal artery via the femoral artery proves technically impossible, the axillary artery is used as an alternative.) Serial radiographic images are obtained over the first 2 to 4 seconds after the injection, allowing visualization of the renal arterial system. A nephric phase follows that lasts 15 to 20 seconds; it is marked by opacification of contrast in the renal parenchyma. The final, venous phase has limited diagnostic value because of extensive renal extraction and concentration of the contrast material.

Digital subtracted angiography enhances the quality of the study by allowing smaller doses of radiation than are used with conventional techniques.

INDICATIONS

Renal mass or tumor
Renal trauma
Renal vascular hypertension

CONTRAINDICATIONS

Allergy to intravenous iodine-bound contrast material

NURSING CARE

Preparation for the procedure often includes injection of a narcotic or antianxiety medication to reduce fear. Care after the procedure focuses on preventing complications, including bleeding at the arterial puncture site and allergic reactions to the contrast material. Assess the pedal pulses and capillary filling of nail beds regularly (at least every 1 to 2 hours). The puncture site is covered with a pressure dressing and is assessed for signs of frank bleeding until the dressing is removed, 24 to 48 hours after the procedure. The patient is placed on strict bed rest for 4 to 8 hours or more, depending on the physician's judgment and the hospital protocol. Advise the patient to expect a hematoma (bruise) at the puncture site that will resolve over the next several weeks. Monitor the patient for hypersensitivity reactions, including shortness of breath, wheezing, and rhonchi during and immediately after injection of the contrast material (see the section on intravenous pyelogram/urogram, page 33).

PATIENT TEACHING

Explain the procedure and its purpose, and address the patient's anxiety about the prospect of intraarterial access. Advise the patient that the discomfort caused by the intraarterial contrast material is transient. Discuss postprocedural care with the patient, including the need for bed rest and limited movement of the affected limb during the first 4 to 8 hours after the procedure.

RENAL VENOGRAM

A renal venogram is a set of x-rays of the kidneys' venous drainage system. A radiopaque catheter is placed in the right femoral vein and carefully advanced to the opening of the left renal vein. Contrast material is injected, and the catheter is directed upward into the contralateral (right) renal vein, where the process is repeated. Imaging may be enhanced by injecting epinephrine into the renal artery, followed by venography approximately 10 seconds later.

INDICATIONS

Renal vascular hypertension
Renal vein thrombosis
Renal mass or tumor
Congenital anomalies of the urinary system

CONTRAINDICATIONS

Allergy to intravenous iodine-bound contrast material

The patient may be given an injection of a narcotic or antianxiety medication before the procedure. Care after the procedure focuses on preventing or managing complications, including bleeding at the puncture site and allergic responses (see the preceding section on Renal arteriogram).

Explain the procedure and its purpose, and reassure the patient that the discomfort caused by injection of the contrast material is transient (see Renal arteriogram).

BIOPSY PROCEDURES

Biopsy of the urinary system involves obtaining a small amount of tissue for microscopic examination.

Renal calyx, pelvis, ureter: A brush biopsy technique typically is used. A ureteral catheter is inserted into the ureter under endoscopic visualization, and a steel or nylon brush is gently rubbed against the area of interest. The tissue trapped within the brush is retrieved and then analyzed by the pathologist.

Bladder, urethra: A bladder or urethral biopsy is obtained during an endoscopic examination. A small grasping forceps is inserted into the working port of a rigid or flexible cystoscope, and a small cut of tissue is obtained for pathologic examination. Biopsy typically includes several specimens from the area of interest and at least one from a normal-appearing, distant bladder or urethral wall.

Prostate: Prostate tissue is obtained by a hollow needle guided by ultrasound. A transrectal route is used, and a biopsy "gun" is inserted into a holder attached to the ultrasonic probe. As with the bladder biopsy, several specimens from the area of interest are supplemented by biopsy of distant, apparently normal tissue.

INDICATIONS

Renal calyx, pelvis, ureter:
    Obstructing tumor or mass
Bladder, urethra:
    Tumor
Inflammatory lesion
Prostate
    Asymmetric enlargement
    Nodule
    Induration

CONTRAINDICATIONS: None

Careful handling of the tissue after a biopsy is crucial to the success of the examination. Consult the pathology department, hospital policy manual, or the physician about proper handling of specimens. Label all specimens with the patient's name, the date the specimen was obtained, the source of the specimen, and any other information required by the pathology department. Clearly label any tissue specimen obtained from a mass from apparently normal tissue. Provide the pathologist with a brief clinical history in consultation with the physician. Renal biopsy may cause temporary discomfort, and sedation may be used before or during the procedure. A brief explanation of the procedure will help allay the patient's anxiety.

Complications after a biopsy include infection of the puncture site or kidney. Monitor the patient for signs of a urinary tract infection, including urinary frequency and dysuria, with fever and chills caused by upper urinary tract involvement. Routinely assess the puncture site for signs of inflammation, including redness and purulent discharge.

See the section on retrograde pyelogram, page 35, for nursing care following brush biopsy of the renal pelvis or calyx.

See the section on endoscopy, page 39, for nursing care following a bladder or urethral biopsy.

Preparation for a prostatic biopsy includes a cleansing enema, which reduces the risk of tracking fecal material while obtaining a transrectal specimen. Prophylactic antibiotics may be given before the procedure. Consult the physician about short-term therapy with a fluoroquinolone, such as norfloxacin or ciprofloxacin, before a prostatic biopsy.

Care after the biopsy may include prophylactic antibiotic therapy for 24 to 72 hours or more. Teach the patient the signs of systemic infection (fever, malaise) or acute prostatic inflammation (exquisite perineal pain and dysuria). Advise the patient to consult the physician promptly should symptoms occur.

CHAPTER 4

Inflammations of the Genitourinary System

The incidence of genitourinary system infections is second only to that of respiratory infections. Bacteriuria may affect the bladder, renal pelvis and ureters, and renal parenchyma. Discrete inflammatory lesions are found in the urethra, bladder wall, and trigone. Infections of the male reproductive system may involve the testis, epididymis, and prostate. Infectious agents, including bacteria, viruses, and parasites, as well as exposure to radiation and irritating pharmacotherapeutic agents, may cause inflammation of the urinary system.

Cystitis/Urinary Tract Infection

Cystitis is an inflammation of the bladder wall. The term has been used synonymously with urinary tract infection, although the two conditions are not identical. **Urinary tract infection** (UTI) is a nonspecific term referring to infection anywhere in the system, including the urethra and upper urinary tract.

PATHOPHYSIOLOGY

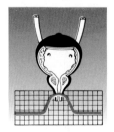

The pathogenesis of cystitis depends on the causative agent. In this discussion cystitis is divided into three categories:

1. Infectious cystitis
   Bacterial
   Viral
   Fungal
   Tubercular
   Parasitic
2. Chemotherapy- and radiation-induced cystitis
3. Inflammatory lesions of the bladder
   Cystitis cystica
   Cystitis glandularis
   Eosinophilic cystitis
   Cystitis emphysematosa

BACTERIAL CYSTITIS

Bacterial cystitis is the most common form of infectious cystitis. The most common causative pathogen in both women and men is *Escherichia coli*. Other common pathogens include strains of *Klebsiella, Enterobacter, Proteus, Pseudomonas,* and *Serratia;* gram-positive organisms such as staphylococci and streptococci occasionally are seen.[56]

The three routes of bacterial invasion into the bladder are ascension through the urethra, the hematogenous route, and via lymphatic channels; the most common is the ascending urethral pathway. Bacteria are commonly forced into the bladder without necessarily causing infection. The determinants of bacterial cystitis depend on the virulence and inoculum size of invasive bacteria and the adequacy of the host's defense mechanisms. Data concerning the number of bacteria needed to produce a bladder infection are based solely on animal studies, which show that an extremely large inoculum (over 1 million) is needed to produce cystitis if host defense mechanisms are not compromised. Fortunately, the normal number of bacteria that enter the bladder through the urethra is considerably smaller (fewer than 100).

The human body has two primary defense mechanisms that oppose the establishment of infection when bacteria enter the bladder. The first is the urine itself, which is bacteriostatic or bactericidal to the most common pathogens associated with cystitis, such as *E. coli* and a number of other anaerobic bacteria commonly found in urethral flora. The efficiency of this antibacterial activity depends on the size of the bacterial inoculum, the osmolality of the urine, and the concentration of urea nitrogen and ammonium in the urine. A urinary pH of 6 or greater adversely affects antibacterial activity, but the presence of specific antibodies in the urine such as IgA and IgG has not been shown to cause significant effects.

The bladder wall is the second line of defense for bacterial invasion from the urethra, bloodstream, or lymphatic route. Inflammatory changes within the bladder wall are apparent within 30 minutes of invasion when polymorphonucleocytes (PMNs) begin to migrate to the bladder mucosa. Within 2 hours the entire mucosal lining is injected by PMNs, and significant antibacterial activity is measurable by the fourth hour. Inspection at 24 hours reveals clumps of PMNs throughout the mucosal lining, and urine culture is negative.

The most important defense against bacterial cystitis is the unobstructed flow of urine throughout the urinary tract and regular, complete evacuation of the bladder. This important concept is the basis of the rationale for clean intermittent catheterization. Regular emptying of the bladder flushes bacteria that would ultimately colonize the urine if allowed to remain within the bladder.

Abnormalities that interfere with natural host defenses against urinary tract infection include the presence of residual urine, which provides an opportunity for bacteria to reproduce and overwhelm other inherent antibacterial mechanisms. Vesicoureteral reflux also compromises the body's defense mechanisms by allowing the spread of bacteria from the urine into the upper tracts and possibly into the renal parenchyma. Urinary calculi are often obstructive to urinary outflow and serve as a nidus for infection during antibiotic therapy. In addition, any disease or circumstance that interferes with the body's immune system decreases the efficiency of the bladder wall's reaction to bacteriuria.[42]

Women and Bacterial Cystitis

Women are particularly susceptible to bacterial cystitis for a number of reasons. Stamey[55] studied the problem of bacterial cystitis in women and concluded that much of the nomenclature used to describe the condition does not adequately define this condition. He described four bacteriurial states in women: (1) first infection, (2) unresolved bacteriuria during therapy, (3) bacterial persistence, and (4) reinfection (recurrence).

1. The etiology of first infection is unclear but is presumed to be similar to reinfections. Unlike recurrent episodes of cystitis, bacteria from the first infection are typically sensitive to any antibiotic and are unlikely to recur within a 2- to 3-year period unless other predisposing factors are present.

2. Unresolved bacteriuria during therapy may arise from several causes. The bacteria may be resistant to the antibiotic chosen for therapy, or selection of a secondary strain may become predominant as the primary form of bacteria is eliminated. In approximately 6% of patients treated, resistant, mutant bacteria develop and proliferate. Renal insufficiency may cause inadequate concentrations of antibiotic in the urinary tract, although the correct agent has been chosen. A staghorn calculus may be large enough to support a critical mass of bacteria too great for antibiotics to resolve.

3. True bacterial persistence may arise after 5 to 10 days of therapy, resulting in culture-proven nonsterile urine from one of two causes. Men with chronic bacterial prostatitis have a persistent focus for ascending urethral infection from the prostatic ductal system. Women or men with struvite stones in the urinary tract have a site of persistent bacteria even after antibiotic therapy.[56]

4. Reinfection of the bladder accounts for most occurrences of bacterial cystitis among women.

The most common route for bacteria to gain access to the bladder is from the urethra. The colonization of the urethra arises from the vaginal introitus and vestibule rather than from the rectum, as is commonly assumed. Longitudinal studies show that cultures of the vaginal vestibule and distal urethral mucosa are more predictive of recurrent bacterial cystitis than analysis of rectal flora. Ascending infection in the female is particularly problematic because of the relatively short, straight course of the urethra and plentiful flora in the genital area. The relationship between vaginal flora and urethral bacteria is further supported by examining the close anatomic relationship of these two structures, which are confined by the distal labia minora.[56]

The role of sexual intercourse in recurrent urinary infections has been studied repeatedly. Sexual intercourse is associated with an increased incidence of recurrent urinary tract infections, and some women specifically correlate intercourse and recurrence. It is interesting to note that nuns have a 0.4% to 1.6% incidence of urinary tract infection, which is lower than the general population, and that married women have a higher incidence than single women. Although sexual intercourse does not cause bacterial cystitis, it does promote the milking of bacteria into the bladder and can cause minor urethral injury that may result in infection among women predisposed to the condition.[55]

Changes in the urinary tract unique to pregnancy increase a woman's likelihood for having recurring urinary tract infections or experiencing a first infection of the bladder. The primary urologic change noted with pregnancy is the "physiologic hydroureter of pregnancy," which is the reversible dilation of the ureters and renal pelvis. This dilation often begins as early as the seventh week of gestation and progresses until delivery. The right ureter is more extensively affected than the left, and ureteral peristalsis is significantly slowed after the second month of gestation, so that intraureteral volume may be as great as 25 times normal.[30]

Bacteriuria is more common among pregnant women than in nonpregnant women in the same age group. Ureteral dilation may play a role in this increased incidence. It is known that pregnant women with bacteriuria are at a significantly increased risk (20% to 40%) for developing pyelonephritis and that this risk is dramatically reduced by treating the bladder infection. In addition, catheterization during pregnancy is associated with increased risk of subsequent bacterial cystitis. Although the association between premature delivery and pyelonephritis is well documented, no correlation exists between bacteriuria and premature delivery.[30]

Bacterial cystitis is likely to result in urinary frequency, urgency, and dysuria. Women in particular may complain of suprapubic discomfort and a feeling of pressure in the perineal area. Nocturia and low back pain are also caused by bladder infection. Urge incontinence may take the form of detrusor instability with subsequent painful bladder "spasms" and associated leakage, or it may occur as urethral instability, allowing urine passage into the posterior urethra and causing a perception of intense urgency and urinary leakage. Gross hematuria, chills, fever, and flank pain occur only occasionally with cystitis unless it is also associated with pyelonephritis. Approximately half of patients with significant bacteriuria are asymptomatic. Women with dysuria and frequency who have no bacteriuria or a colony count of fewer than 10,000 per milliliter are typically diagnosed as having an "acute urethral syndrome."[55,56]

VIRAL CYSTITIS

Viral cystitis causes symptoms similar to those of bacterial infections; hematuria is particularly common. Papovaviruses and adenoviruses are the most common causative agents. Immunosuppressed or immunocompromised individuals are at particular risk of developing viral cystitis, as are children. Because viral cultures generally are not available, diagnosis is based on clinical exclusion: urine cultures for bacteria are negative, and inflammation causes bladder wall thickening, detectable on ultrasound.

FUNGAL CYSTITIS

Cystitis caused by fungal infection is much less prevalent than bacterial cystitis, but its incidence and recognition have greatly increased within the past 25 years. The most common fungal infection of the bladder is candidiasis. The *Candida* organism is endemic to the human body and can often be found in the pharynx, stomach, intestinal tract, and vaginal vault (particularly in pregnant women). The increasing incidence of candidal overgrowth is related to the use of antibiotics. Administration of antibiotics is thought to stimulate the production of *C. albicans* by altering the pH of gastrointestinal mucosa, suppressing normal bacterial flora that competes with the fungus for food, and inhibiting polymorphonuclear phagocytosis, which helps the body guard against overgrowth.

The body's defenses against candidal infection of the urinary tract include normal bacterial flora that inhibits fungal growth and polymorphonuclear leukocytes in the mucosa of the urethra and bladder that have marked anticandidal effects. In addition, prostatic fluid in men is fungicidal, which helps explain the relatively low incidence of candidal cystitis in men compared to women. Cell-mediated immunity and other white blood cells also help the body prevent candidiasis.

Candidal cystitis often occurs because of predisposing factors such as diabetes mellitus, obstructive prostatic enlargement, and pregnancy and is often noted after the patient has undergone antibiotic therapy for bacterial infection. The symptoms are similar to those of bacterial cystitis and include urgency, marked frequency, dysuria, suprapubic pain, and nocturia. Pneumaturia (the expression of gas or air through the urethra during or after micturition) may be seen. The mucosal lining of the bladder is marked by grayish white spots that result in mucosal bleeding if removed. The ureteral orifices may be affected so that cystoscopic findings may resemble tubercular infection of the bladder. In certain cases asymptomatic candidal colonization of the urine without inflammation of the bladder may be seen.[46]

TUBERCULAR CYSTITIS

Tuberculosis of the bladder results from the implantation of the tubercle bacilli into the wall, causing an uneven mix of inflamed areas interspersed with normal mucosal segments. The cystoscopic picture of the bladder may resemble interstitial cystitis or candidal infection with patches of inflamed tissue and reddened ureteral orifices. The anterior urethra is not affected by the infection, but the posterior urethra and prostate are heavily involved in men, representing progression from prostate to bladder. The trigone is relatively spared from inflammatory changes, but the dome of the bladder is extensively affected, resulting in a marked loss in capacity.

The primary symptom of tubercular cystitis is marked frequency and urgency. Bladder volume rapidly decreases and may result in irreversible changes in advanced stages of the infection.[56] Urodynamic assessment in advanced cases may reveal poor compliance of the bladder wall and a functional capacity of 60 milliliters of urine or less.

PARASITIC CYSTITIS

Although schistosomiasis is relatively rare in the United States, it is relatively common elsewhere in the world. The ova of this parasite enter the bloodstream by penetrating the skin. The veins of the bladder are a popular breeding site for the parasites. The eggs are then extruded into the vesicle for further spread of the parasitic organisms. The healing of the affected areas of the bladder causes thickening and contraction of the bladder wall. Damage of the ureterovesical junction often occurs, resulting in vesicoureteral reflux. Contracted bands mar the bladder and may extend into the lower ureter. Urinary calculi may be present because of urinary stasis and ova in the urine.[55]

CHEMOTHERAPY- AND RADIATION-INDUCED CYSTITIS

Chemotherapy- or radiation-induced cystitis is characterized by inflammatory changes in the bladder wall in the absence of infection. The symptoms are similar to those of infectious cystitis and include urgency, frequency, and suprapubic pain. Detrusor instability and urge incontinence may occur.

Although the bladder is relatively resistant to radiation, therapeutic doses greater than 6,000 to 7,000 rad over a 6- to 7-week period may result in cystitis. The bladder's tolerance to radiation is significantly compromised if schistosomiasis is present. Chemotherapy-induced cystitis may arise from systemic cyclophosphamide or intravesical antineoplastic drugs such as mitomycin. The diagnosis is made when symptoms of cystitis are reported with a normal culture and positive history of exposure to radiation or a chemotherapeutic agent.[38,57]

INFLAMMATORY CYSTITIS

Cystitis emphysematosa is a rare form of bladder inflammation resulting from infection by gas-forming urinary bacteria or (more commonly) vesicoenteric fistula. The condition may also be observed after urologic instrumentation or urodynamic testing using carbon dioxide. Pneumaturia is associated with this form of cystitis.[32]

Inflammatory lesions of the bladder cause intense, irritative symptoms, including dysuria, frequency, and urgency. Lesions may represent a complication of chronic bacterial infection or outlet obstruction. Inflammatory lesions often resemble malignant tumors, and certain lesions are considered premalignant. Table 4-1 summarizes three of the most common types of lesions.

COMPLICATIONS

Infectious cystitis:
- Upper urinary tract infection (pyelonephritis)
- Systemic infection
- Septicemia, septic shock
- Men: epididymitis, prostatitis
- Women: vaginitis

Inflammatory bladder lesions:
- Bladder malignancy
- Infectious cystitis

Table 4-1

INFLAMMATORY LESIONS OF THE BLADDER

Lesion	Gross appearance	Malignant potential
Cystitis cystica	1 cm cysts in bladder base, may extend into upper urinary tracts	May resemble tumor
Cystitis glandularis	Generalized inflammation of bladder wall	May represent premalignant lesion or coexist with cancer
Eosinophilic cystitis	Polypoid lesions with generalized bladder wall inflammation	Not considered premalignant

Table 4-2

BACTERIAL PATHOGENS COMMONLY ENCOUNTERED IN THE URINARY TRACT AND TREATMENT OPTIONS

Pathogen	Commonly effective antibiotic agents*
Escherichia coli	Trimethoprim-sulfamethoxazole, ampillicin, norfloxacin, amoxicillin clavulanate, nitrofurantoin, ciprofloxacin
Pseudomonas	Carbenicillin, gentamicin,† norfloxacin, ciprofloxacin
Klebsiella	Cephalexin, tetracycline, trimethoprim-sulfamethoxazole, norfloxacin
Proteus mirabilis	Ampicillin, tetracycline, trimethoprim-sulfamethoxazole, norfloxacin, amoxicillin clavulanate, nitrofurantoin
Morganella morganii	Trimethoprim-sulfamethoxazole, norfloxacin
Serratia	Trimethoprim-sulfamethoxazole, norfloxacin, carbenicillin
Group D *Streptococcus*	Ampicillin, nitrofurantoin, amoxicillin clavulanate
Staphylococcus	Cephalexin, tetracycline, trimethoprim-sulfamethoxazole
Staphylococcus saprophyticus	Cephalexin, trimethoprim-sulfamethoxazole, tetracycline

From Gray ML. and Dobkin KA. In Thompson J: *Mosby's manual of clinical nursing*, ed 2, St. Louis, 1989, Mosby–Year Book.
*Antibiotic therapy is guided by individual culture and sensitivity reports.
†Requires parenteral administration.

Table 4-3

ANTIBIOTIC THERAPY FOR BACTERIAL CYSTITIS

Type of therapy	Antibiotic agents*
Single-dose therapy	Amoxicillin (Amoxil), 3 g
	Trimethoprim-sulfamethoxazole (Bactrim DS, Septra DS), 1 or 2 double-strength tablets
	Sulfisoxazole (Gantrisin), 1-2 g
Short-term therapy (5-14 days)	Ampicillin (Amcil), 2 g in 4 divided doses
	Amoxicillin (Amoxil), 2 g in 4 divided doses
	Trimethoprim-sulfamethoxazole (Bactrim DS, Septra DS), 1 double-strength tablet bid
	Nitrofurantoin (Macrodantin), 50-100 mg qid
Suppressive therapy for recurrences (6-24 mo)	Trimethoprim-sulfamethoxazole (Bactrim DS, Septra DS), 1 regular-strength tablet daily
	Nitrofurantoin (Macrodantin), 50-100 mg/day

Modified from Farrar.[36]
*Antibiotic therapy is guided by individual culture and sensitivity reports.

DIAGNOSTIC STUDIES AND FINDINGS

Diagnostic Test	Findings
Urinalysis	Color: dark yellow, pink or red, sediment commonly present
	Nitrate/nitrite: positive when bacteriuria present
	Glucose oxidase: positive when bacteriuria present
	Hemoccult: positive in complicated cases
	Microscopic examination: positive for bacteria, fungi, and parasites (eosinophils noted in eosinophilic cystitis); and pyuria (more than seven WBCs per high-power field) in infectious cystitis; RBCs may be present; RBCs, WBCs, and no bacteria with viral cystitis
Urine culture	>100,000 (10^5) colony-forming units (CFU) per milliliter of agar indicates clinically significant infection; lesser colony counts are significant when associated with symptomatic cystitis; sensitivity disks indicate appropriate antiinfective drug therapy
	Urine culture negative for parasitic, fungal, or chemotherapy- or radiation-induced therapy
Cystoscopy	Infectious cystitis: reddened, inflamed bladder wall and trigone
	Tubercular cystitis: alternating areas of normal and inflamed bladder mucosa
	Cystitis cystica, cystitis glandularis: multiple inflammatory cysts of bladder neck and trigone
	Eosinophilic cystitis: multiple, nonmalignant, polypoid bladder wall lesions
Bladder wall biopsy	Infectious cystitis: consistent with acute inflammation
	Cystitis cystica: negative
	Cystitis glandularis: may demonstrate cancer
	Eosinophilic cystitis: extensive eosinophilic infiltration
	Chemotherapy- or radiation-induced cystitis: chronic inflammation of bladder mucosa
Voiding diary	Reduced functional capacity, urinary frequency, nocturia
Urodynamics	Infectious cystitis, cystitis cystica, cystitis glandularis, eosinophilic cystitis: urodynamics contraindicated except in special cases
	Tubercular cystitis: small capacity with poor bladder wall compliance
	Chemotherapy- or radiation-induced cystitis: sensory urgency with low capacity; bladder wall compliance may be compromised; unstable detrusor may be noted
Voiding cystourethrogram	Cystitis emphysematosa: lucent filling defect produced by gas-producing bacteria

MEDICAL MANAGEMENT

GENERAL MANAGEMENT

Provide copious fluid intake

Ensure regular, complete bladder evacuation

DRUG THERAPY

Administer urinary analgesic, phenazopyridine hydrochloride (Pyridium) or Urised

Administer antiinfective medications, guided by culture and sensitivity report (Table 4-2)

Treatment of choice is short-term oral antibiotic therapy (Table 4-3)

COMMON SIDE EFFECTS OF URINARY ANTIINFECTIVE DRUGS

Trimethoprim/sulfamethoxazole (Bactrim, Septra)

Side effect: Renal toxicity

Nursing management: Administer with water, maintain adequate fluid intake

Nitrofurantoin (Macrodantin)

Side effect: Nausea/gastrointestinal upset

Nursing management: Administer with meals or snack

Carbenicillin (Geocillin, Geopen)

Side effect: Diarrhea

Nursing management: Administer with Lactinex, 2 tablets, given with antibiotic

Side effect: Nausea related to medication odor, foul taste

Nursing management: Administer with iced water; advise patient to swallow rapidly and avoid smelling drug; drug may need to be discontinued if intolerance is marked

Cephalexin (Keflex)

Side effect: Nausea, mild diarrhea

Nursing management: Administer with meals or snack

HYPERSENSITIVITY REACTIONS

Signs/symptoms

Rash
Urticaria
Anaphylaxis
Diaphoresis
Wheezing/bronchoconstriction
Nausea/vomiting
Pounding headache
Stevens-Johnson syndrome (rare, potentially lethal sloughing of skin)

Nursing management

Prevention
    Obtain careful history of drug allergies.
    Teach patient signs and symptoms of hypersensitivity response and their management.
Management of ongoing reaction
    Stop medication immediately.
    Seek emergency medical care if symptoms of wheezing/bronchoconstriction and anaphylaxis occur.
    Promptly contact health care professional for management of symptoms and alternate drug therapy.
    Administer steroidal antiinflammatory drugs, antihistamines, and cardiorespiratory drugs as directed for severe response with anaphylaxis.
    Single-dose therapy is an alternative to short-term antibiotic therapy (Table 4-3).
    Administer parenteral medications when oral drugs are not tolerated or when pathogens are resistant to oral agents.
    Administer parenteral fluids when oral fluids are not tolerated because of fever, nausea, and vomiting.
    Administer suppressive antibiotic drugs for 6-24 mo for recurrent infections.

1 ASSESS

ASSESSMENT	OBSERVATIONS
Urinary elimination patterns	Increased frequency, nocturia; recurrence of incontinence in patients with unstable bladder
Location and character of pain	Suprapubic discomfort; lower back pain relieved temporarily by urination; burning pain on urination (dysuria)
Possible renal infection	Fever, chills, flank pain when upper urinary tract is involved
Possible sepsis	Fever followed by chills, hypothermia; signs of impending shock, including hypotension and tachycardia

2 DIAGNOSE

NURSING DIAGNOSIS	SUBJECTIVE FINDINGS	OBJECTIVE FINDINGS
Altered patterns of urinary elimination related to bladder inflammation	Complains of urinary urgency, frequency of urination, nocturia	Frequency of urination with reduced functional capacity, nocturia; urge incontinence may recur in individuals with history of unstable bladder
Pain related to bladder inflammation	Complains of dysuria (burning pain on urination), lower back pain, suprapubic pain	Tenderness in suprapubic area and costovertebral angle; tenderness and flank pain with upper urinary tract infection (pyelonephritis)
Potential noncompliance related to drug therapy	Reports discontinuing antibiotics after symptoms subsided or because of side effects	Repeat urine culture demonstrates recurrent or persistent bacteriuria

3 PLAN

Patient goals

1. The symptoms of urgency to urinate will dissipate.
2. Diurnal urinary frequency will return to preinfection patterns.
3. Episodes of nocturia will return to premorbid patterns.
4. Lower back pain and suprapubic pain will be resolved.
5. Febrile urinary tract infection (pyelonephritis) will be avoided.
6. Persistent urinary tract infection will be avoided.
7. Recurrence of urinary tract infection will be minimized or rapidly managed.

4　IMPLEMENT

NURSING DIAGNOSIS	NURSING INTERVENTIONS	RATIONALE
Altered patterns of urinary elimination related to bladder inflammation	Encourage copious fluid intake (at least 1,500 ml/day for the average adult).	Fluids flush the urinary system, enhancing the body's most important mechanical defense mechanism against urinary tract infection (UTI).
	Discourage patient from limiting fluids despite fears that copious intake will aggravate urinary frequency.	Limiting fluids concentrates urine, aggravating rather than alleviating frequency and urgency.
	Reassure patient that urinary frequency is temporary, and urge her not to postpone urination during acute infection.	Although urinary frequency interferes with other ADL, regular, complete bladder evacuation rids the urinary system of pathogens.
	Administer oral, intramuscular, or intravenous antiinfective medications, or teach patient to administer these agents herself.	Antiinfective agents reverse symptoms of bladder inflammation by helping the body rid itself of pathogens.
	Reassure patient with a history of an unstable bladder that recurrence of urge incontinence is temporary.	Even when adequately managed through medication and timed voiding, bladder instability (and its symptoms of urgency, frequency, urge-induced incontinence, and nocturia) may recur when inflammation is present.
	Administer intravenous fluids as directed when patient cannot tolerate oral beverages because of fever and nausea.	Urinary system needs adequate fluid intake to rid itself of pathogens; patients with symptoms of nausea and vomiting related to febrile UTI require parenteral fluids until these symptoms subside and oral beverages can be tolerated.
Pain related to bladder inflammation	Encourage patient to take a sitz bath in water above waist level.	Warm water relieves lower back and suprapubic discomfort associated with bladder inflammation.
	Provide external applications of heat to lower back as needed.	Applying moist, warm heat (in addition to sitz bath) temporarily relieves lower back pain associated with bladder inflammation.
	Administer prescribed urinary analgesics, or teach patient to administer these agents herself.	Urinary analgesics reduce irritative bladder symptoms through their direct effect on the bladder mucosa and their antispasmodic actions.
	Encourage patient to void regularly and not to attempt to postpone micturition during episodes of acute inflammation.	Bladder filling increases irritative symptoms caused by infection; micturition reduces this discomfort.
	Encourage intake of clear, caffeine-free beverages; discourage excessive intake of citrus beverages.	Caffeine and citrus juices may irritate the bladder mucosa, aggravating frequency and discomfort.

NURSING DIAGNOSIS	NURSING INTERVENTIONS	RATIONALE
	Administer nonsteroidal antiinflammatory analgesic medications as indicated, or teach patient to administer them herself.	Irritative symptoms caused by inflammatory bladder lesions may respond to nonsteroidal antiinflammatory drugs.
	Administer antispasmodic agents, or teach patient to administer these drugs herself according to medical direction.	Antispasmodic agents reduce irritative bladder symptoms and enhance functional capacity through their anticholinergic effects; these agents may be useful for patients with chronic symptoms of cystitis caused by inflammatory bladder lesions, in contrast to persons with acute infection.
	Prepare patient for cystoscopy with resection or fulguration of specific lesions, if indicated, and biopsy.	Inflammatory bladder lesions may respond to endoscopic treatments such as fulguration (similar to cauterization), typically administered in combination with antiinflammatory and antiinfective medications.
	Advise women patients of potential for vaginitis caused by antiinfective drug therapy.	Antiinfective drug therapy may affect normal vaginal bacterial flora, producing overgrowth of fungus ("yeast infection"); whenever possible, antiinfective medications that exert minimum effect on vaginal bacterial flora are chosen; antifungal creams obtained by prescription or over the counter are used to manage symptoms of discomfort and to eradicate vaginal inflammation and infection.
Potential noncompliance related to drug therapy	Administer one-time IM dose or ongoing IV/IM medications for UTI.	Recurrence of UTI or persistent infections may be due to incomplete eradication of urinary system pathogens.
	Teach patient who is self-administering oral medications the schedule and length of time antiinfective medications are to be taken.	Relief from symptoms of acute cystitis often precedes complete eradication of urinary pathogens; stopping medications before the prescribed 7-10 days has elapsed increases the risk of recurrent or persistent infections. (See Patient Teaching.)
	Teach patient potential side effects of oral antiinfective medications and strategies to counteract these effects.	Patients may stop taking antiinfective agents because of potential side effects; teaching the patient strategies to reduce or avoid side effects increases the probability of compliance with medication regimen. (See Patient Teaching.)
	Counsel patient about symptoms and signs of hypersensitivity response to antiinfective or analgesic medications; advise her to discontinue the drug immediately should these symptoms occur and to contact her health care provider promptly.	Hypersensitivity to antiinfective or analgesic drugs requires prompt discontinuation to avoid serious complications; eradication of infection and inflammation requires treatment with an alternate drug.

➔ ❯ ❯ ❯

NURSING DIAGNOSIS	NURSING INTERVENTIONS	RATIONALE
	Advise patient about potential for recurrence, including specific risk factors identified.	Potential for recurrent infection and inflammation is enhanced by coexisting conditions; prompt treatment of recurrence minimizes course of distressing symptoms and potential for complications, including pyelonephritis.
	Teach patient to self-administer suppressive antibiotics for 6-24 mo prescribed by physician.	Daily dose of suppressive antibiotics may reduce incidence of urinary system infections.
	Advise patient to have regular checkups (including repeat cystoscopic examination when advisable) for inflammatory bladder lesions.	Inflammatory lesions may represent uncertain risk for malignant degeneration and may coexist with cancerous tumors; routine evaluation may be indicated to ensure early intervention should cancer be detected.
Knowledge deficit	See Patient Teaching.	

5 EVALUATE

PATIENT OUTCOME	DATA INDICATING THAT OUTCOME IS REACHED
The symptoms of urgency to urinate have dissipated.	Voiding patterns have returned to preinfection norms; symptoms of urgency have disappeared.
Diurnal urinary frequency has returned to preinfection patterns.	Diurnal frequency is no greater than q 2 h.
Episodes of nocturia have returned to premorbid patterns.	Nocturia is once or less for individuals under 65 years of age or twice or less for older persons.
Lower back pain and suprapubic pain have resolved.	The patient reports that symptoms of suprapubic and lower back pain have been relieved.
Febrile urinary tract infection (pyelonephritis) has been avoided.	The patient's body temperature remained below 38.3° C (101° F) as bacteriuria was eradicated.
Persistent urinary tract infection has been avoided.	Urine culture shows no bacterial colonies after completion of antiinfective therapy.
Recurrence of UTI is minimized or rapidly managed.	The patient understands specific strategies to avoid recurrence of infection and a plan to manage recurrent infection if it develops.

PATIENT TEACHING ▪▪▪▪▪▪▪▪▪▪▪▪▪▪▪▪▪▪▪▪▪▪▪▪▪▪▪▪▪▪▪▪▪▪

1. Teach the patient the causes of cystitis, including the most common pathogens (bacteria, fungi).
2. Explain the body's defense mechanisms against infection and inflammation of the bladder, including regular urinary elimination, adequate hygiene, and the role of the immune system.
3. Advise the patient of controllable and genetic factors that affect her predisposition to cystitis.
4. Teach the patient to recognize the signs and symptoms of recurrent cystitis and strategies to manage recurrent infection.
5. Advise the patient who experiences recurrent infectious cystitis to obtain a urine specimen at a nearby medical facility and to contact her health care professional when a specimen has been obtained.
6. Teach the patient to self-administer medications whenever possible, and emphasize the importance of adherence to a 7- to 10-day course.
7. Teach the patient to administer suppressive medications immediately before bedtime to ensure an anti-infective drug effect during the longest period of urinary retention they are likely to experience.
8. Discuss potential side effects of medications and strategies to avoid these untoward effects (see box on side effects, page 58).
9. Explain signs and symptoms of hypersensitivity response to medications and strategies for managing these signs (see box on hypersensitivity reactions, page 58).

Interstitial Cystitis

Interstitial cystitis is a pancystitis of the bladder wall that results in small capacity, frequency, nocturia, and a chronic, burning pain that may significantly alter the individual's life-style. Unlike acute inflammations, interstitial cystitis is a chronic, unabating condition that may persist for years or a lifetime.

The incidence of interstitial cystitis is unknown. Approximately 20,000 to 90,000 individuals in the United States have been diagnosed with interstitial cystitis; some investigators believe that as many as 450,000 Americans may have the condition but remain undiagnosed or incorrectly diagnosed. Among hospitalized patients, it has been reported in 0.02% to 4.8% and in 1 in 300 to 400 individuals seeking medical treatment for urinary system pain. The rate of occurrence among women compared to men is approximately 10 to 1. Its occurrence in children remains controversial, although suspicious cases have been described.[41,44]

PATHOPHYSIOLOGY

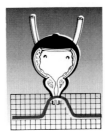

The principal symptom of interstitial cystitis is pain accompanied by marked urinary frequency and nocturia. The onset of symptoms is rather abrupt, although they persist for months or years. The pain of interstitial cystitis is typically characterized as burning with sharp, stabbing sensations. The marked discomfort of bladder filling is temporarily relieved by micturition, only to return with minimum bladder distention. Analgesics and narcotics offer only modest, temporary relief.

The voiding dysfunction caused by interstitial cystitis is characterized by marked diurnal urinary frequency, nocturia, and intolerance of postponement of micturition. Individuals with interstitial cystitis frequently void every hour or more often and may void as regularly as every 10 to 15 minutes during certain periods. These individuals may have more than four episodes of nocturia a night, resulting in fatigue. They have a marked intolerance of postponing micturition because of the severe pain caused by bladder filling. These sensations are magnified during diagnostic procedures, including cystoscopy and urodynamics, that require relatively rapid bladder filling.

CHARACTERISTIC SIGNS AND SYMPTOMS OF INTERSTITIAL CYSTITIS*

Symptoms

- Urinary frequency more than five times during 12 waking hours
- Nocturia more than twice
- Symptoms present longer than 1 year
- Urgency
- Pain with bladder distention and fullness, temporarily relieved by urination
- Suprapubic, pelvic, vaginal, and/or perineal pain
- Laboratory studies
  No bacteriuria
  No fungal or parasitic infection
- Cystoscopy/biopsy
  Hunner's ulcer
  Petechiae of bladder mucosa noted on cystoscopic examination under general anesthesia
  No inflammatory bladder lesions
  No malignant tumors of the bladder wall
  No urethral diverticula
- Urodynamic findings
  No detrusor instability
  Small capacity (less than 400 ml)
  Poor bladder wall compliance (advanced cases)

*Adapted from Holm-Bentzen M: Workshop on interstitial cystitis, Bethesda, Md 1987.

INTERSTITIAL CYSTITIS ASSOCIATION (ICA)*

Goals

1. To share common experiences among those affected by the disease.
2. To provide information for interstitial cystitis patients and their families.
3. To foster research related to interstitial cystitis, its causes, care, and cure.

East Coast: PO Box 1553, Madison Square Station
New York, NY 10159
West Coast: PO Box 151323
San Diego, CA 92115

*Modified from Slade.[52]

Chronic pain, voiding dysfunction, and fatigue probably produce the anxious disposition characteristic of people with interstitial cystitis. In their desperation to obtain relief from bladder pain, they often seek help from several caregivers, bolstering their image as anxious and irritable. Unfortunately, the disorder's complex of symptoms and uncertain origin have made misdiagnosis a significant problem.[52]

The cause of interstitial cystitis is still the subject of debate. Interstitial infection, extravesical infection, hormonal abnormalities, psychogenic factors, autoimmune disorders, lymphatic obstruction, and ischemia-induced pain have been implicated in the pathogenesis.

Autoimmune disorders have certain characteristics that resemble the symptom complex of interstitial cystitis. Antiinflammatory agents have been used to treat interstitial cystitis with modest success. Bladder antibodies and antinuclear antibodies have been identified in tissue biopsies and the bloodstream. Other investigators have focused on dysfunction of the glycosaminoglycan (GAG) layer that is postulated to protect the bladder mucosa and contribute to its impermeability to re-

absorption of urinary constituents or water. Still others perceive interstitial cystitis as a disorder caused by ischemia, comparable to reflex sympathetic dystrophy. Psychogenic disturbances also have been postulated to produce the symptoms of interstitial cystitis, although it seems much more likely that the symptoms of anxiety, the fatigue, and the perceptions of desperation are the result of the significant pain and voiding dysfunction caused by bladder inflammation, rather than the source of the condition.[31,41,49]

The long-term clinical course of interstitial cystitis is one of protracted voiding dysfunction and pain, often lasting for many years. As the condition progresses, the bladder wall becomes fibrotic and poorly compliant. At this point the frequency and diffuse pain persist, although the pain related to bladder filling may subside. Unfortunately, even urinary diversion may fail to relieve the pain caused by interstitial cystitis, although these procedures undeniably relieve severe urinary frequency and nocturia.

COMPLICATIONS

Bacteriuria
Bladder instability with urge incontinence
Poor compliance of bladder wall with upper urinary tract infection (pyelonephritis)

DIAGNOSTIC STUDIES AND FINDINGS

See box above.

MEDICAL MANAGEMENT

GENERAL MANAGEMENT AND DRUG THERAPY

Urinary analgesics and antispasmodics: To maximize bladder capacity.

Steroids and nonsteroidal antiinflammatory agents (e.g., indomethacin [Indocin]) or antihistamines: To reduce pain and inflammation.

Intravesical instillation of medications, commonly dimethyl sulfoxide (DMSO), silver nitrate (AgNO$_3$), heparin, oxychlorosene (Chlorpactin), natrium chromoglucate, or steroids (prednisolone).

Sodium pentosan-polysulfate (Elmiron): An oral agent designed to reduce GAG layer dysfunction.

Tricyclic antidepressant (e.g., amitriptyline [Elavil]): To relieve ischemic pain.

Analgesics, narcotics, or tranquilizers: To relieve pain.

Transcutaneous, transvaginal, or transrectal electrostimulation: To relieve pain.

CYSTOSCOPIC MANAGEMENT

Hydraulic bladder distention under general anesthesia: Up to six treatments.

Cystoscopic resection or fulguration of ulcers; laser resection of bladder mucosa.

SURGICAL MANAGEMENT

Surgical reconstruction of urinary tract, including augmentation enterocystoplasty with extensive resection of bladder wall; continent or incontinent diversion.

Surgical denervation of the bladder, including sacral rhizotomy, resection of hypogastric plexus, and perivesical denervation or transvaginal denervation.

---

1 ASSESS

ASSESSMENT	OBSERVATIONS
Location, character, and duration of pain	Localized to bladder, mons pubis, vagina, or suprapubic area; chronic burning or dull, boring pain (may resemble pain caused by peripheral neuropathy) intensified by bladder filling and postponement of micturition, temporarily relieved by micturition
Patterns of urinary elimination	Marked diurnal frequency; nocturia; urgency; urge incontinence rare

→ > >

2 DIAGNOSE

NURSING DIAGNOSIS	SUBJECTIVE FINDINGS	OBJECTIVE FINDINGS
Pain related to bladder inflammation of uncertain etiology	Complains of bladder, suprapubic, or vaginal pain	Intolerance of bladder filling despite absence of inflammatory lesions of bladder, infectious cystitis, tumor, stones, or other identifiable condition
Altered patterns of urinary elimination related to bladder pain and inflammation	Complains of urinary frequency, nocturia, and inability to postpone micturition	Bladder diary, urodynamic testing demonstrate compromised capacity despite absence of detrusor instability or urge incontinence
Ineffective individual coping related to chronic pain, fatigue	Reports sense of hopelessness in search for relief from symptoms; distrustful of caregivers, family, or friends who fail to "understand" the condition	Fails to identify sources of help from health care professionals or through patient advocacy and support groups
Sexual dysfunction related to pain or fear of pain produced by intercourse	Expresses fear of engaging in intercourse and of pain related to intercourse	Documented reduction in satisfaction and frequency of intercourse

3 PLAN

Patient goals

1. The patient will obtain relief of pain related to interstitial cystitis.
2. The patient will have reduced diurnal frequency (q 2 h or less often).
3. The patient will have two or fewer episodes of nocturia.
4. The patient will be able to identify sources of support for individuals with interstitial cystitis, including the Interstitial Cystitis Association's patient advocacy and support group. (See box on page 64.)
5. The patient will maintain sexual relationship.

4 IMPLEMENT

NURSING DIAGNOSIS	NURSING INTERVENTIONS	RATIONALE
Pain related to bladder inflammation of uncertain etiology	Administer or teach patient to self-administer prescribed systemic medications to alleviate pain caused by bladder filling.	Analgesics or narcotics may offer temporary relief, reducing anxiety and providing rest; tricyclic antidepressants may reduce pain from ischemia similar to indication for use in peripheral neuropathy–induced discomfort; antiinflammatory drugs, steroids, and antihistamines may offer relief from discomfort by reversing inflammatory process affecting bladder wall; antispasmodics and urinary analgesics may offer relief from pain by enhancing bladder capacity and reducing sensory discomfort at level of bladder wall.

NURSING DIAGNOSIS	NURSING INTERVENTIONS	RATIONALE
	Administer intravesical medications as directed; instill a 2% lidocaine water-soluble lubricant 2-3 min *before* catheter insertion; gently insert a small catheter, using aseptic technique; drain the bladder, and instill the medication; instruct the patient to remain relatively still on the table in the supine position while the solution is retained for 15-30 min; the medication is then drained either by micturition or from a catheter.	Instillation of dimethyl sulfoxide (DMSO) produces temporary relief of bladder pain, possibly by dilation of local blood vessels or through its antiinflammatory properties; steroids may provide pain relief by reversing inflammation; heparin may provide relief through vasodilatory effects or by stabilizing mast cells and inhibiting fibrin production; silver nitrate may produce relief by its astringent-caustic effects, reversing inflammation, or by its bactericidal effects.
	Administer or teach patient to self-administer sodium pentosan-polysulfate (Elmiron) as prescribed.	Elmiron may relieve pain by reducing inflammation caused by altered permeability of the GAG layer coating the bladder's inner epithelium.[41,49]
	Prepare patient for hydraulic distention performed under anesthesia; explain that the bladder will be filled until intravesical pressure reaches a constant value, either 80 mm Hg or the patient's systolic blood pressure; this pressure is maintained for 5-15 min, and then the water is drained; reassure patient that the procedure is completed using general anesthesia.	Hydraulic distension may relieve bladder pain by destroying local sensory nerves and enhancing capacity.
	Perform electrostimulation, and teach patient to repeat this therapy with a home unit; set pulse width, frequency, stimulation duration and rest period, and total session length in consultation with physician; teach patient to increase intensity to point of discomfort, then reduce intensity to just below this level.	Electrostimulation applied via transcutaneous, transvaginal, or transrectal routes may relieve bladder pain by activating a gating mechanism that reduces pain and/or by enhancing bladder capacity.[41,44]
	Advise patient that caffeinic beverages, citrus juices, carbonated drinks, alcoholic beverages, and cigarette smoking may exaggerate bladder pain; inform her that certain patients tolerate these fluids well, whereas others do not; instruct her to eliminate one particular beverage at a time and judge the results; only beverages that prove irritable for her need to be reduced or eliminated.	Beverages containing caffeine, carbonated beverages, or citrus juices may cause mild sensory urgency (even among normal individuals); this urgency may be particularly intolerable for the chronically irritated, painful bladder of interstitial cystitis.[52]
	Advise patient that she may have to avoid certain types of exercise because they intensify bladder pain; running, jumping, high-impact aerobics, and weight-lifting may be particular problems.	Certain forms of physical exertion may intensify pain caused by interstitial cystitis, possibly because they jar the bladder, magnifying sensations of filling.

→ › ›

NURSING DIAGNOSIS	NURSING INTERVENTIONS	RATIONALE
	Advise patient that some individuals can reduce pain by changing their diet; instruct her to refer to the book by L. Gillespie, *You Don't Have to Live with Cystitis!* (New York, 1986, Rawson Associates) for dietary advice on reducing acidic foods and specific amino acids; remind patient that dietary measures, like all treatments, help only a certain number of individuals with interstitial cystitis.	Certain acidic or spicy foods and particular amino acids may cause mild bladder irritation; cutting back on these foods without compromising a well-balanced diet may reduce pain.
	Advise patient to avoid clothing that fits tightly at the waist.	Tightly fitting garments may exaggerate bladder and genital pain.
	Advise patient that a warm bath with water above waist level, heat to bladder area (heating pad), or assuming a knees-to-chest position may relieve pain temporarily.	Applying warmth to affected area and positional changes provide temporary relief from dull, aching pain.
	Advise patient that biofeedback techniques, hypnotherapy, relaxation therapy, and other nontraditional coping techniques may reduce bladder pain.	Nontraditional pain-relief techniques work in several ways, including selective imaging, relaxation of strained muscles used to guard against pain, and diversional methods.
	Prepare patient for reconstructive urologic surgery, either augmentation enterocystoplasty procedure or continent or incontinent diversion procedure, as directed.	Reconstructive urologic procedures may relieve bladder pain in a limited group of patients with severe symptoms.
Altered patterns of urinary elimination related to bladder pain and inflammation	Advise patient that prolonged, severe restriction of fluid is not helpful when attempting to reduce frequency caused by interstitial cystitis.	Some patients may reason that reducing fluid intake will alleviate bladder pain by slowing the process of bladder filling; however, limiting fluids exposes urinary system to greater risk of bacteriuria by interfering with mechanical antegrade of urine flushing bacteria from the system; bacteriuria produces an additional source of inflammation, intensifying urinary frequency and bladder pain; in addition, limiting fluids concentrates solutes in the urine, which may further irritate the mucosa.
	Advise patient that *temporary* limitation of fluids is advisable when access to toileting facilities is limited.	Although prolonged, severe limitation of fluids is potentially harmful to the urinary system and bladder, temporary limitation helps prevent pain caused by inability to urinate when a toilet is not available.

NURSING DIAGNOSIS	NURSING INTERVENTIONS	RATIONALE
	Help patient ensure that she has access to a toilet whenever possible; specific strategies include prior knowledge of location of toilets, placing a collection device in the car while on long trips or in locations without easy access to a toilet, or keeping the device at the bedside.	Marked urinary frequency accompanies pain and intolerance of postponement of micturition in interstitial cystitis; attempts to behaviorally expand bladder capacity have not met with particular success or patient acceptance.
Ineffective individual coping related to chronic pain, fatigue	Give patient the name and address of interstitial cystitis patient advocacy and support groups (see box on page 64).	A support or advocacy group can help patient identify others who share her experiences with pain and urinary frequency; it also provides a resource for coping strategies and peers who can evaluate effectiveness of these strategies; the support group also functions to encourage research and education of health care providers who interact with individuals who have interstitial cystitis.
	Encourage patient to identify and maintain diversional or recreational activities, exercise, and social events.	Social isolation and aversion to pleasant activities intensify isolation and reduce ability to cope with chronic pain.
	Reassure patient that frequent voiding is necessary and acceptable; advise her that others have "used the bushes" or other nontraditional toilet facilities when necessary.	Coping with bladder pain necessitates frequent voiding; enabling the individual to be assertive about this aspect of her life reduces guilt and subsequent social isolation.[52]
	Reassure patient that it is acceptable and necessary to turn down certain activities that markedly aggravate pain or make toilets unreasonably inaccessible.	Marked pain may render some activities intolerable.
	Counsel patient's family on the symptoms and chronic nature of interstitial cystitis.	Family relationships may become strained if symptoms of interstitial cystitis are interpreted as "craziness" or "refusing to tolerate a little desire to urinate."
	Teach family to help patient cope with lifestyle adjustments necessitated by interstitial cystitis; specific strategies include helping with household duties, tolerating frequent toileting, helping her identify toileting facilities, helping her identify support groups, and helping her obtain medical treatment.	Family support helps patient identify and use individual coping mechanisms needed to combat pain and frequency.
	Encourage patient to use humor to deal with chronic bladder pain.	Humor helps patient express feelings related to bladder pain and altered voiding patterns; it also alerts others to patient's experience in a positive, readily acceptable manner.[52]

→ > >

NURSING DIAGNOSIS	NURSING INTERVENTIONS	RATIONALE
	Reassure patient that expression of negative feelings is entirely acceptable and necessary when coping with chronic pain.	Feelings are neutral, neither good nor evil; suppressing negative feelings to avoid guilt or unpleasant reactions from others leads to greater emotional and spiritual distress, whereas expressing these feelings helps the individual cope with the issue at hand and move on to other concerns.
	Reassure patient that assertiveness in seeking health care is entirely appropriate and necessary; encourage patient to seek care from a urologic specialist with experience in interstitial cystitis when suspicious symptoms are present; advise patient that care from other health care providers such as nurses, pain management specialists, and hypnotherapists is entirely appropriate for specific interventions to help her cope with pain and altered urinary elimination patterns.	Misdiagnosis of interstitial cystitis is not uncommon (a survey of persons with interstitial cystitis showed that victims seek care for 2-4½ yr before a correct diagnosis is established; these individuals sought care from two to five health care providers before diagnosis); many individuals report being told their symptoms were of psychogenic origin.[52]
Sexual dysfunction related to pain or fear of pain produced by intercourse	Reassure patient that frequency of intercourse is not the sole expression of sexual intimacy.	Intercourse is one behavior in a spectrum of human responses that define sexuality and intimacy.
	Discuss alternate expressions of sexual intimacy, including hugging, sensual massage, shared bathing, or other activities that provide mutual stimulation and satisfaction.	Alternate expressions of sexual intimacy provide satisfaction without aggravating bladder pain.
	Reassure patient that it is entirely acceptable to refuse sexual intercourse when symptoms of pain render him or her unable to achieve any satisfaction from the experience.	Sexual intercourse is appropriate only when *both* partners seek the experience.
	Advise patient's partner that diminished tolerance of frequency of intercourse and certain positions or maneuvers is a result of chronic pain rather than a rejection of intimacy.	Educating the partner is likely to increase empathy and open communication needed to maintain an intimate relationship.
	Consult a therapist or sexuality specialist when appropriate.	Counseling and therapy concerning specific techniques for intercourse or alternate behavior may require specific interventions for severe cases; certain patients also associate sexual arousal with bladder pain; therapy from an expert is needed to help the patient reverse this association.

5 EVALUATE

PATIENT OUTCOME	DATA INDICATING THAT OUTCOME IS REACHED
Bladder pain has been reduced.	The patient reports subjective relief from bladder pain; the patient can be distracted from bladder pain for certain periods of time.
Diurnal frequency has been reduced.	The patient's voiding diary demonstrates greater diurnal frequency (q 2 h or less often is considered ideal).
Nocturia has been reduced.	The patient's voiding diary demonstrates reduction of episodes of nocturia (no more than one episode per night is considered ideal).
The patient can identify coping strategies for pain and frequency.	The patient can describe coping strategies and can identify diversional activities used to cope with bladder pain.
Intimate sexual relationships have been maintained.	The patient can identify alternatives to sexual intercourse and mechanisms for avoiding or reducing pain during intercourse; the patient evaluates intimate relationships and sexual acts as satisfying.

PATIENT TEACHING ■

1. Discuss the various suspected causes of interstitial cystitis. Explain that although a cure is not a realistic goal, treatment and pain relief are obtainable.
2. Teach the patient the side effects of the systemic or intravesical medications used to treat interstitial cystitis. Specifically, inform the patient that DMSO produces an odor of garlic that can easily be detected by anyone close to the patient. Heparin may cause blood in the urine.
3. Instruct the patient in the side effects of hydraulic distention therapy, including blood in the urine, bladder rupture, and the potential adverse effects of general anesthesia.
4. Inform the patient with severe interstitial cystitis that surgical reconstruction is an alternative therapy; *however*, consult the urologist *first*, because surgery is an acceptable alternative for only a limited group of patients with severe, chronic symptoms. Inform the patient that surgery can increase bladder capacity but may not completely relieve bladder pain.

Prostatitis

Inflammation of the glandular portion of the prostate is called prostatitis. The inflammation affects the gland and the prostatic urethra, causing discomfort in the rectal and suprapubic areas and altering patterns of urinary elimination.

Inflammation of the prostate is commonly divided into four types: acute bacterial, chronic bacterial, nonbacterial, and prostatodynia. Each form of prostatitis has a distinctive clinical presentation and is managed differently.[55]

Prostatitis is most commonly observed in males after the onset of pubescence, but rare cases of the disease have been reported among children and infants. Nonbacterial prostatitis (also named prostatosis) is the most common form of the disease. Acute and chronic bacterial prostatitis is less commonly seen. Rarer forms include viral, fungal, parasitic, and allergic prostatitis.

PATHOPHYSIOLOGY

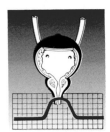

Acute bacterial prostatitis is caused by the ascent of bacteria via the urethra or the hematogenous route. Acute infection may be precipitated by urethral instrumentation or prostatic massage in the presence of chronic bacterial prostatitis. Common causative pathogens include *Escherichia coli*, *Proteus*, *Klebsiella*, *Pseudomonas*, and *Enterobacter* organisms. An acute episode of prostatitic infection is characterized by sudden onset of fever, chills, myalgia, arthralgia, and general malaise. These symptoms rapidly progress to localized discomfort in the perineal area or low back associated with irritative voiding symptoms, including urgency, frequency, nocturia, dysuria, and a persistent burning sensation in the urethra after micturition. Pain in the prostate results in varying degrees of functional bladder outlet obstruction that may cause significant urinary hesitancy or even acute urinary obstruction.

Histologic examination of prostatic tissue reveals diffuse glandular inflammation with edema and hyperemia of the stroma. Abscesses are common and may hemorrhage in severe cases. Polymorphonuclear leukocytes, bacteria, and cellular debris are present within the acini of the gland. Rectal palpation of the prostate reveals an exquisitely tender organ. Vigorous massage is contraindicated because of the associated pain and the danger of bacteremia. Because acute bacterial cystitis is typically associated, urine culture provides an excellent clue to the causative prostatic pathogen. An objective diagnosis of acute bacterial prostatitis is made with evidence of inflammation on expressed prostatic secretions (more than 10 leukocytes per high-power field), positive bacterial culture of this expressed prostatic secretion, positive bacterial cystitis, and an abnormal rectal examination.[56,57]

Chronic bacterial prostatitis commonly occurs as a result of ascending infection from the urethra. The condition may arise after an inadequately treated episode of acute bacterial prostatitis, or it may occur through hematogenous bacterial invasion. However, the precise cause of chronic bacterial prostatitis remains unclear.

The clinical symptoms of chronic bacterial prostatitis vary widely. Some men have no symptoms of prostatitis other than recurrent urinary tract infections or asymptomatic bacteriuria. More commonly, men with prostatitis note recurring irritative voiding symptoms such as urgency, frequency, dysuria, nocturia, and urethral irritation. Perineal pain, postejaculatory pain, hematospermia, and a mucoid urethral discharge may also be noted.

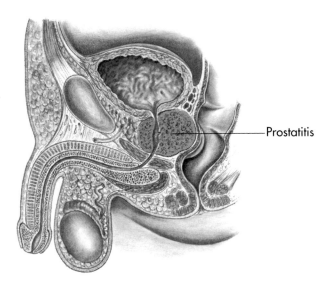

Prostatitis

Rectal palpation of the prostate may reveal prostatic calculi or may be unremarkable. Histologic examination of the prostate shows moderate inflammatory changes that are less localized than in acute infections. Objective diagnosis of chronic bacterial prostatitis requires the finding of inflammatory cells on microscopic examination of expressed secretions, a positive culture of these secretions, and a nontender gland on rectal examination.

Unlike with acute bacterial prostatitis, the chronically infected prostate is relatively resistant to antibiotic treatment because of the poor absorption of non-lipid-soluble substances into the prostatic fluid. The chronically infected prostate has deficient levels of prostatic antibacterial substance. Prostatic calculi may also lower antibiotic susceptibility by serving as a nidus for persistent infection. Thus even extended periods of oral antibiotics may not cure chronic bacterial prostatitis.[55]

Nonbacterial prostatitis is the most common form of symptomatic prostatic inflammation. Although the causative agent of nonbacterial prostatitis has not been identified, *Chlamydia* organisms have been implicated as a possible pathogen. Unfortunately, cultures are difficult to obtain, so verification of this suspicion requires further investigation.

The symptoms of nonbacterial prostatitis are similar to those of chronic bacterial prostatitis and include pelvic area pain and irritative voiding symptoms. Objective diagnosis is made by demonstrating inflammatory cells in expressed prostatic secretions with negative prostatic secretion and bladder urine cultures. Rectal examination is normal.[35,55]

Prostatodynia is the presence of symptoms of prostatitis without the physical findings. The cause of this form of prostatitis is unknown. Objective diagnosis is made by demonstrating negative inflammatory cells in expressed prostatic secretions, negative bacterial culture of these secretions, negative urine cultures despite recurrent perineal pain, and irritative voiding symptoms.

Other forms of prostatitis occur rarely and include viral prostatic inflammation after an upper respiratory infection, tubercular prostatitis, or mycotic prostatitis from blastomycosis, coccidioidomycosis, histoplasmosis, and candidiasis. Symptoms are similar to bacterial prostatitis with perineal area pain and inflammation of the prostate associated with irritative voiding symptoms.[55]

COMPLICATIONS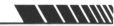

Acute bacterial prostatitis: Systemic infection; sepsis; bacteriuria; acute urinary retention; urethritis; constipation

Chronic bacterial prostatitis: Bacteriuria; urethritis; systemic infection (rare); urinary retention; constipation; bladder neck obstruction

Chronic nonbacterial prostatitis: Urethritis; urinary retention; constipation

Prostatodynia: Constipation; bladder neck obstruction

DIAGNOSTIC STUDIES AND FINDINGS

Diagnostic Test	Findings
Prostatic secretion culture: divided specimen	>5,000 bacteria/ml on prostatic culture with <3,000 bacteria/ml on urethral and bladder specimens (The prostatic divided specimen is obtained by asking the patient to urinate an initial 10-15 ml of urine into a sterile cup and then switching to another cup without interrupting the stream. The next 50-100 ml of urine is collected in the second cup. When urination has been completed, the patient is advised to avoid expressing the last few drops. The prostate is then milked for an expressed secretion. The first container of urine is labeled "urethral specimen" and divided into three portions. One portion is examined microscopically, one is cultured, and one is dry mounted on a slide using alcohol. The specimen in the second cup is labeled "bladder specimen" and submitted for routine urinalysis and culture. The third portion, labeled "prostatic expression," is divided into two portions for culture and microscopic examination.)
Urine culture	Acute bacterial prostatitis: >100,000 colony-forming units (CFU)/ml Chronic bacterial prostatitis: >100,000 CFU/ml Nonbacterial prostatitis: no bacterial growth Prostatodynia: no bacterial growth
Voiding diary	Small functional bladder capacity with diurnal frequency greater than q 2 h, nocturia, and urgency to urinate may be noted; urge incontinence may be noted with prostatodynia; retention may be present
Urinary flow study	Poor flow pattern with hesitancy to void.
Urodynamics or videourodynamics	Evidence of irritative voiding symptoms with small cystometric capacity and sensory urgency; unstable bladder contractions may be noted (particularly with prostatodynia) Evidence of mild bladder outlet obstruction with poorly filled prostatic urethra noted on fluoroscopy during voiding pressure study and postvoid residual; bladder neck dyssynergia may be noted in certain cases of prostatodynia
Prostatic ultrasound study	Inflamed tissue may resemble prostatic adenocarcinoma on ultrasound study; prostatic calculi may be noted as bright, white areas producing shadow; ultrasound study is *not* typically used for imaging in prostatitis
White blood cell count (WBC)	Elevated WBCs, indicating systemic bacterial infection in acute bacterial prostatitis

MEDICAL MANAGEMENT

GENERAL MANAGEMENT/DRUG THERAPY

Antiinfective agents are administered on the basis of culture and sensitivity reports for acute bacterial and chronic bacterial prostatitis. Intravenous medications are administered for acute bacterial infection until fever has resolved and the patient can tolerate oral fluids. When fluids can be tolerated orally, oral medications are begun. Chronic bacterial prostatitis is typically treated by oral agents, although parenteral (IV, IM) agents are used for severe cases. Mild cases of acute bacterial prostatitis are also managed by oral antiinfective drugs when oral fluids are tolerated and fever is relatively low grade. Nonbacterial prostatitis is empirically treated as a chlamydial infection with a long-acting tetracycline.

Oral antibiotics are administered for 30 days to achieve adequate intraductal penetration of the drug. An antiinfective agent that is lipid soluble with a reasonable ability to penetrate prostatic fluid (pKa) is chosen (Table 4-4).

Antipyretics are administered to reduce fever in acute prostatitis with fever.

Intraprostatic injection of antiinfective agents has been done experimentally. This is a promising technique, because it has the potential to increase ductal concentrations of the drug, negating the need for long-term administration of oral agents.

A suprapubic catheter may be required for acute urinary retention associated with acute bacterial prostatitis.

A stool softener may be given to reduce constipation and discomfort associated with straining to defecate.

Dietary restriction may reduce the discomfort of prostatodynia or chronic nonbacterial or bacterial prostatitis.

SURGERY

Open prostatectomy with removal of seminal vesicles is expected to be curative, but this treatment is limited because of its invasive nature and associated complications of impotence, infertility, and incontinence.

Partial resection of prostatic tissue by means of extensive transurethral resection is an alternative to open prostatectomy; the risk of associated complications is reduced with this approach.

Transurethral or open prostatectomy is indicated when prostatitis coexists with benign hyperplasia of the gland.

Transurethral resection of prostatic calculi may reduce infection by removing nidi for bacteria.

Table 4-4

ANTIINFECTIVE DRUG CHOICES FOR PROSTATIC INFECTION*

Drug	Dosage schedule
Trimethoprim (TM)	bid
TM/sulfamethoxazole	bid
Nitrofurantoin	qid
Tetracycline	qid
Doxycycline	bid
Minocycline	bid
Erythromycin	qid

*Medication choices based on lipid solulility and favorable pKa. From Fowler JE.: Prostatitis. In Gilenwater JY et al: *Adult and pediatric urology,* ed 2, St Louis, 1991, Mosby–Year Book.

1 ASSESS

ASSESSMENT	OBSERVATIONS
Acute bacterial prostatic infection	Positive divided culture and bacteriuria (digital examination is deferred because of pain and risk of spreading bacteria in acute bacterial infection)
Systemic infection	Fever, nausea and vomiting, positive blood cultures
Chronic bacterial prostatitis	Bacteria noted on divided specimen; bacteriuria may be found on urine culture; urethral pain or discharge is rare; digital examination reveals variable tenderness, evidence of symmetric enlargement with boggy character; irritative voiding symptoms (diurnal frequency, nocturia, urgency to void); pain during or immediately after ejaculation
Nonbacterial prostatitis	Symptoms similar to those of chronic prostatitis with negative bacteria on divided culture; or, urine culture urinalysis shows evidence of WBCs; digital examination demonstrates symmetric enlargement with tenderness; urethral discharge may be noted; culture demonstrates no bacterial growth; irritative voiding symptoms and ejaculatory discomfort
Prostatodynia	Symptoms similar to those of chronic or nonbacterial prostatitis; no bacteria or WBCs (pus) on urine culture and divided specimen; digital examination demonstrates no obvious enlargement, although tenderness often is noted; evidence of voiding dysfunction (detrusor instability with frequency and urgency) or possible bladder outlet obstruction caused by bladder neck (smooth muscle dyssynergia) or detrusor–striated sphincter (striated sphincter dyssynergia); ejaculatory discomfort is common
Location, character, and intensity of prostatitic pain	Acute bacterial prostatitis produces exquisite pain in rectal and suprapubic areas; pain is intensified by urination, pressure, or constriction against area (such as that produced during defecation) Pain caused by chronic nonbacterial prostatitis and prostatodynia is described as burning, constant, dull ache aggravated by urination, pressure against area, or defecation; discomfort is aggravated by ejaculation, although release of seminal fluids may produce some relief by relieving pressure caused by excess fluid
Urethral pain	Dysuria; burning pain centered in urethral area aggravated by urination and ejaculation
Altered urinary elimination patterns	Acute urinary retention may be present in acute bacterial infection; irritative symptoms (diurnal frequency and nocturia, urgency to void, dysuria) or obstructive symptoms (hesitancy to void, poor force of stream, sensations of incomplete bladder evacuation) may be noted

2 DIAGNOSE

NURSING DIAGNOSIS	SUBJECTIVE FINDINGS	OBJECTIVE FINDINGS
Pain related to prostatic inflammation	Complains of burning sensation in rectal or suprapubic area aggravated by pressure, straining to defecate, and ejaculation	Evidence of prostatic inflammation with or without bacterial infection; symptoms of prostatic inflammation without objective evidence of inflammation in prostatodynia
Hyperthermia related to systemic infection from acute bacterial prostatitis	Complains of malaise, nausea, fatigue, and sensations of warmth or chills	Increased systemic temperature, nausea and vomiting, impaired judgment or impaired cognition in severe cases

→ 〉 〉

NURSING DIAGNOSIS	SUBJECTIVE FINDINGS	OBJECTIVE FINDINGS
Altered patterns of urinary elimination related to prostatic inflammation	Complains of irritative voiding symptoms (diurnal frequency, nocturia, urgency to void, dysuria) or obstructive symptoms (hesitancy to urinate, poor force of stream, feelings of incomplete bladder evacuation)	Urinary frequency on voiding diary, nocturia, poor urinary stream with hesitancy to start stream on urinary flow test; urodynamics may demonstrate detrusor instability and/or evidence of bladder outlet obstruction with urinary residual
Noncompliance with medical therapy (potential) related to long-term antiinfective therapy for prostatitis	Patient reports he discontinued antiinfective therapy because there was no obvious improvement of symptoms, or improvement in symptoms prompted him to stop therapy prematurely	Persistence of positive culture with persistence or recurrence of symptoms of inflammation

3   PLAN

Patient goals

1. Symptoms of bacterial infection will disappear.
2. Symptoms of pain related to prostatic inflammation will resolve.
3. Urethral discharge and discomfort will resolve.
4. Discomfort associated with or immediately following ejaculation will disappear.
4. Irritative voiding symptoms will resolve.
5. Symptoms of obstructive voiding dysfunction (or dysfunction related to unstable detrusor in prostatodynia) will resolve.
6. The patient will self-administer long-term antiinfective drugs for the period prescribed by the physician.

4   IMPLEMENT

NURSING DIAGNOSIS	NURSING INTERVENTIONS	RATIONALE
Pain related to prostatic inflammation	Administer parenteral antiinfective drugs for treatment of acute bacterial prostatitis as prescribed.	Acute infection may be associated with nausea or vomiting and high fever; parenteral antiinfective drugs typically are required because of systemic infection and inability to tolerate oral medications; antiinfective medications relieve pain by helping the body rid itself of infection.
	Administer or teach patient to self-administer prescribed oral antiinfective drugs.	Oral antiinfective agents are used for chronic bacterial prostatitis, resolving acute infections, or for mild cases of acute infection when oral fluids are tolerated; oral antiinfective drugs are used empirically in cases of nonbacterial prostatitis to eliminate probable chlamydial infection; antiinfective medications relieve pain by helping the body rid itself of infection, which causes inflammation.

NURSING DIAGNOSIS	NURSING INTERVENTIONS	RATIONALE
	Implement temporary pain relief strategies (e.g., applying local warmth with a moist compress or by sitting in a bath with water above waist is helpful).	Warmth temporarily relieves burning pain associated with prostatitis.
	Perform gentle prostate massage, or prepare patient for prostate massage to be performed by physician on a weekly or less frequent schedule.	Gentle prostate massage relieves pain by evacuating excessive fluids from the prostate; this relieves pressure within the gland that contributes to suprapubic and rectal discomfort.
	Advise patient that ejaculation may relieve pressure in cases of chronic prostatitis; warn him that initial discomfort may be noted, but long-term relief is expected.	Ejaculation relieves prostatic discomfort by flushing secretions from the gland, similar to massage.
	Teach patient to maintain adequate fluid intake and adequate dietary fiber, and to consume fresh fruits and fruit juices.	Constipation requires straining and pressure to evacuate bowel, aggravating pain produced by prostatitis; softening stool through dietary measures lessens this discomfort.
	Administer or teach patient to self-administer stool-softening medications.	Pharmacologic stool softeners are used to prevent constipation and associated discomfort when dietary measures alone prove inadequate.
	Advise patient that certain elements of the diet may aggravate discomfort of prostatitis; spicy foods, including those containing chili powder, hot peppers, and curry, are particularly likely to aggravate prostatic pain; teach patient to eliminate these foods from the diet one at a time and judge results.	Spicy foods may aggravate discomfort of chronic bacterial or nonbacterial prostatitis or prostatodynia; eliminating these foods is advised to detect which (if any) affect an individual's pain.
	Advise patient to limit alcohol intake to 2-3 oz/day.	Excessive alcohol intake aggravates discomfort produced by prostatitis.
	Administer or teach patient to self-administer antiinflammatory agents as prescribed.	Antiinflammatory drugs may relieve prostatic pain by countering inflammatory process.
Hyperthermia related to systemic infection from acute bacterial prostatitis	Administer or teach patient to self-administer antipyretics.	Antipyretics reduce fever associated with acute infection.
	Administer parenteral or oral medications.	Systemic antiinfective drugs help the body eliminate bacterial infection producing fever.
	Administer IV fluids as prescribed, or help patient obtain adequate fluid intake (IV fluid therapy may be required for severe cases of acute bacterial prostatitis).	Dehydration exacerbates fever produced by infection.

NURSING DIAGNOSIS	NURSING INTERVENTIONS	RATIONALE
	Ensure adequate nutritional intake of carbohydrates and other nutrients during acute febrile episodes.	Fever and infection increase metabolic demands on the body; adequate nutrition helps the body rid itself of infection.
Altered patterns of urinary elimination related to prostatic inflammation	Advise patient to maintain adequate daily fluid intake (1,500-2,500 ml/day for the average adult).	Irritative voiding symptoms may be caused by bacteriuria; patients with bacterial prostatitis are particularly prone to bacteriuria; adequate fluid intake helps the urinary system flush out pathogens.
	Monitor fluid intake and urinary output in patient with acute bacterial prostatitis; regularly percuss bladder for signs of overdistension; promptly inform physician of acute retention so that suprapubic catheter can be placed for short-term drainage of urine.	Acute inflammation causes marked prostatic pain that may result in inability to urinate and acute urinary retention.
	Monitor fluid and urinary output in patient with suprapubic tube.	Suprapubic tube is placed to temporarily drain bladder in cases of acute bacterial infection with acute urinary retention; kinking of tube produces acute overdistension and intensifies pain.
	Teach patient to relax pelvic floor muscles using biofeedback and contraction-relaxation exercises in consultation with physician.	Prostatodynia and chronic bacterial and nonbacterial prostatitis may cause urinary retention from discomfort.
	Apply perianal patches, and teach patient to isolate and contract the periurethral (pelvic floor) muscles on command; help him isolate periurethral muscles from distant muscle groups, including abdominals and thighs; instruct patient to contract muscles for 10 sec, then relax muscles for 40 sec, for a total of two sets of 10 repetitions at home; instruct patient to do these exercises daily; following mastery of this skill, teach patient to combine this exercise with urination.	Patient normally uses local muscle groups to guard against pain (in this case increased tone of pelvic floor muscles acts as a guarding response to prostatic discomfort); unfortunately, this guarding may cause poor relaxation of the striated sphincter mechanism during voiding, resulting in urinary retention; retraining muscles to relax assists in complete bladder evacuation.
	Advise patient with urinary retention and documented residuals to avoid over-the-counter decongestants, diet pills, and significant alcohol intake; warn patient to urinate on a regular schedule.	Over-the-counter decongestants and diet pills contain alpha-sympathomimetic agents that increase tone in prostatic urethra and rhabdosphincter that may exacerbate urinary retention; excessive alcohol or prolonged postponement of micturition also predisposes individual with bladder outlet obstruction to acute retention.

NURSING DIAGNOSIS	NURSING INTERVENTIONS	RATIONALE
	Advise the patient with an unstable detrusor to void on a given schedule (typically q 1½-3 h) based on knowledge of diurnal urine elimination patterns obtained from voiding diary.	A timed voiding schedule may prevent unstable contractions by ensuring micturition before onset of these contractions.
	Advise patient with marked irritative voiding symptoms or an unstable bladder to institute a fluid management pattern; instruct him to ensure adequate fluid intake (1,500-2,500 ml/day) but to avoid bolus intake of fluid with meals; counsel patient to sip beverages throughout the day, limiting fluids to 8 oz with meals; advise patient to restrict beverages to sips starting 1-2 h before sleep.	Spreading fluid intake throughout the day may help reduce frequency of unstable contractions or feelings of pronounced urgency by preventing bolus fluid intake that provokes these symptoms; fluid management technique is combined with timed voiding pattern.
	Administer or teach patient to self-administer antispasmodic and anticholinergic medications as prescribed to reduce unstable bladder contractions.	Antispasmodic medications may prevent unstable muscle contractions, increase bladder capacity, and reduce irritative voiding symptoms; they are successful *only* when combined with fluid management and timed voiding.
	Institute electrostimulation therapy for irritative voiding symptoms and unstable bladder contractions using a transrectal or transcutaneous route in patient with prostatodynia; teach patient to perform therapy with a home unit; set pulse frequency, duration of stimulation and rest period, and total time of therapy in consultation with physician.	Electrostimulation therapy can reduce irritative bladder symptoms and alleviate symptoms related to an unstable detrusor in patients diagnosed with prostatodynia; therapy would not be expected to have significant benefit for patients with clinically demonstrable prostate inflammation and infection; therapy may best be reserved for patients with demonstrated unstable detrusor and no urinary retention.
Noncompliance with medical therapy (potential) related to long-term antiinfective therapy for prostatitis	Advise patient that antiinfective therapy requires him to take medications for 30 days or longer to effectively eradicate bacteria; offer a careful explanation of problems with penetration of antibiotics into prostate gland, using terms patient can understand; inform patient that relief of symptoms may not indicate complete eradication of infection and that compliance with the full term prescribed for therapy provides the greatest chance for complete cure and prevention of recurrence.	Antiinfective medications only partly penetrate the non-acutely infected prostate gland; the ideal antibiotic must be lipid permeable and its pH must be within an appropriate range to effectively penetrate the prostate (Table 4-4); thus prolonged therapy is required.
	Consult physician about using medications that are given fewer times per day.	Compliance with long-term, self-administered medications is enhanced by a relatively infrequent dosage schedule; thus medications given daily or twice daily are preferred to those given tid or qid.

NURSING DIAGNOSIS	NURSING INTERVENTIONS	RATIONALE
	Call patient at home to encourage compliance with medication regimen; offer to answer questions and evaluate progress toward resolution of symptoms.	Personal contact enhances compliance with therapy by reemphasizing importance of adherence to prolonged administration schedules; it also provides an opportunity to identify patients who do not tolerate a particular antiinfective drug regimen because of adverse effects or nonresponse, so that alternate agents can be instituted.
Knowledge deficit	See Patient Teaching.	

5 EVALUATE

PATIENT OUTCOME	DATA INDICATING THAT OUTCOME IS REACHED
Symptoms of bacterial infection have disappeared.	Divided specimen and urine cultures are free of bacteria.
Pain related to prostatic inflammation has resolved.	Dull, burning pain in the rectal and suprapubic areas has disappeared.
Urethral discharge and discomfort have resolved.	Urethral discharge has stopped; swab culture of urethra shows negative bacteria; dysuria and urethral burning pain have disappeared.
Discomfort associated with or immediately following ejaculation has disappeared.	There is no evidence of bloody ejaculate; the patient notes relief of discomfort associated with ejaculation.
Irritative voiding symptoms have resolved.	Diurnal frequency returns to q 2 h or less often; nocturia is reduced to once or less per night (documented by voiding diary); the patient states that symptoms of urgency are improved or have disappeared.
Symptoms of obstructive voiding dysfunction (or dysfunction related to unstable detrusor in prostatodynia) have resolved.	Voiding diary shows diurnal frequency of q 2 h or less often and nocturia once a night or less; urinary flow study shows improved peak and mean flow rate and postvoid residual volume less than 25% of total bladder capacity; urodynamic testing demonstrates absence of bladder outlet obstruction on pressure-flow study.
Patient can self-administer long-term antiinfective drugs for period prescribed by physician.	Bacterial infection has resolved; the patient reports that he is complying with regimen, as assessed through telephone conversations and follow-up visits.

PATIENT TEACHING ▪▪▪▪▪▪▪▪▪▪▪▪▪▪▪▪▪▪▪▪▪▪▪▪▪▪▪▪▪▪▪▪▪▪▪▪▪▪

1. Teach the patient the dosage, scheduling, and potential side effects of antiinfective, antipyretic, and antiinflammatory drugs used for therapy.
2. Instruct the patient that prostatitis is not associated with an increased incidence of prostatic cancer.
3. Provide anticipatory guidance for management of acute urinary retention.
4. Warn the patient with chronic bacterial prostatitis of the limited potential for systemic spread of infection, and teach him management strategies should symptoms of systemic infection occur.
5. Reassure the patient and significant other than prostatodynia is not a sexually transmissible disorder. Instruct the sexual partner to consult the physician for advice on intercourse.
6. Teach the patient the dosage, schedule, and side effects of antispasmodic medications. Explain the relationship between the timed voiding schedule, the fluid management program, and the antispasmodic medication regimen.

Scrotal Inflammation

Scrotal inflammation is a response to infection of the epididymis (epididymitis) or testis (orchitis). Similar symptoms are produced by torsion of the testis. Torsion is the twisting of the vascular pedicle of the spermatic cord, testis, or one of the testicular appendages, causing ischemia and potential infarction.

PATHOPHYSIOLOGY

Epididymitis

Epididymitis is defined as any inflammation of the epididymis; it may be caused by bacteria, viruses, parasites, chemicals, or trauma. Epididymitis is divided into three categories: nonspecific, specific, and traumatic. Epididymitis is the most common intrascrotal lesion. It is almost always unilateral and must be differentiated from testicular torsion, tumor, or trauma.[40] An estimated 600,000 cases occur in the United States each year. In men under 35 years of age, epididymitis is most often associated with a sexually transmitted disease. It accounts for 20% of all inpatient admissions in military urologic practices. In men over 35 years of age, gram-negative rods associated with some abnormality of the urinary tract or performance of some urologic procedure constitute the most common presentation of the condition. Epididymitis is rare in prepubertal boys.[39]

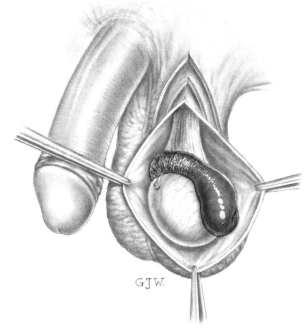

EPIDIDYMITIS (ACUTE)

Epididymitis occurs most frequently as a result of reflux of urine or some pathogenic agent through the posterior urethra, prostatic ducts, or seminal vesicles. In rare instances the causative pathogen may reach the epididymis via retrograde lymphatic pathways from the wall of the vas deferens or via hematogenous or metastatic routes. In its earlier stage, epididymitis occurs as a type of cellulitis associated with local pain and edema. In the acute stage the entire hemiscrotum becomes a single erythematous, exquisitely painful mass often associated with an inflammatory hydrocele produced by the tunica vaginalis. Later changes include peritubular fibrosis and occlusion of the epididymis, which may result in sterility.[47,53]

Nonspecific epididymitis refers to a group of common pathogens that typically gain access to the organ via urethral-vasal reflux with infected urine. Bladder outlet obstruction (requiring the individual to strain to void) is a predisposing factor to this condition. Nonspecific epididymitis is a common complication of prostatitis, urethral stricture disease, and seminal vesiculitis. Occasionally a nonspecific epididymitis arises from a septic focus such as a pharyngitis. Reflux of sterile urine into the epididymis has been reported to result in inflammation,[55,57] although others dispute this possibility.[48] Strenuous exercise has also been connected with nonpyrogenic epididymitis.[55]

Nonspecific epididymitis also occurs as a complication of certain urologic procedures, particularly transurethral resection of the prostate and urethral catheterization. Postprocedural epididymitis may occur as late as several months after instrumentation because of the persistence of subclinical amounts of bacteria in the urine. It is significant to note that the rate of epididymitis following transurethral resection of the prostate has dropped from 20% to 4% following the institution of routine prophylactic antibiotics after the procedure. Vasectomy has been advocated as a prophylactic measure for men undergoing prostatectomy, but the efficacy of this intervention remains unproven.[57]

Traumatic epididymitis (also referred to as epididymoorchitis) arises from straining, with reflux of urine into the organ. The cause of this form of epididymitis remains unclear. Some argue that the trauma only inflames an already present subclinical inflammation of the epididymis, whereas others propose that the trauma lessens resistance to some more distant foci of infection, allowing invasion of pathogens into the area.

Specific epididymitis refers to a group of known pathogens that invade the epididymis from a urinary focus or via the hematogenous route. The causative organisms most commonly associated with sexually transmitted epididymitis are *Neisseria gonorrhoeae* and *Chlamydia trachomatis* among heterosexual men and *Escherichia coli* among homosexual men. Prompt, aggressive treatment of these sexually transmitted diseases helps curtail the incidence of subsequent epididymitis, as demonstrated by the decreasing incidence of gonococcal epididymitis.

Syphilitic epididymitis may occur more often than has been suspected. This form of epididymal inflammation is typically asymptomatic and connected with the second stage of the disease. Diagnosis of syphilitic epididymitis is presumptive and established when other evidence of syphilis is present while urinary tract infection, prostatitis, and urethritis are absent.

Many forms of specific epididymitis have been reported that have spread to the organ via the hematogenous route. In cases of brucellosis, epididymitis may be the initial symptom of the condition. Meningococcal septicemia, pneumococcal pneumonia, *Haemophilus influenzae,* and other bacterial diseases have been associated with epididymal invasion. Various parasites such as amebae, schistosomes, and fungi are known to invade the epididymis.

Tubercular epididymitis arises from involvement of the prostate and is one of the few painless forms of the disease. Tuberculosis of the epididymis produces a thickened, beaded organ on palpation and leads to occlusion of the epididymal lumen.

The most common complication of epididymitis is orchitis, so the term "epididymoorchitis" is used. Infertility is a serious long-term complication of epididymitis. Sterility among men with chronic or recurrent bilateral epididymitis is 40%, and men with unilateral epididymitis have a 25% chance of infertility. Recurrences of epididymitis are particularly likely when the underlying disease process (e.g., prostatitis) remains unresolved.[39,57]

Orchitis

Orchitis typically arises from blood-borne infection; by far the most common form is pyogenic orchitis coexisting with epididymitis, as described previously. Systemic viral infections, such as mumps or coxsackievirus B infection, may also involve the testis. Granulomatous orchitis occurs as a complication of syphilis, mycobacterial infection, actinomycoses, or other fungal infections.

Testicular inflammation causes pain and enlargement; in severe cases nausea, vomiting, and fever occur. Pyogenic orchitis typically is limited to one hemiscrotum. In contrast, 50% of men affected by mumps or other forms of viral orchitis develop infection of the contralateral testis within 1 to 9 days. Inflammation may be followed by atrophy and loss of spermiogenic function unless prompt treatment is instituted. Approximately 50% of all men with nonbacterial orchitis develop atrophy detectable on palpation; a much smaller percentage experience oligospermia and infertility problems.[54]

Torsion of Testis

Torsion is the rotation or twisting of the vascular pedicle of the testis or its appendages, causing tissue ischemia and damage. Three forms of torsion threaten the testis: *extravaginal torsion* is rotation of the spermatic cord, producing ischemia of the testis, epididymis, and tunica vaginalis; *intravaginal torsion* involves the testis and epididymis but spares the surrounding tunica vaginalis; *torsion of a testicular appendage* (remnant of the wolffian or müllerian ducts) causes scrotal pain and inflammation but does not directly threaten the sperm-

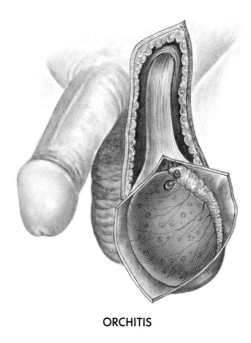

ORCHITIS

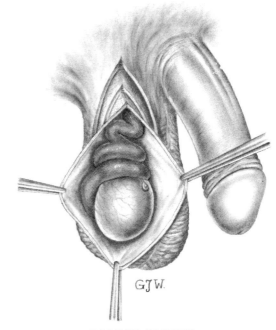

GJW.

TORSION OF TESTIS

producing tissue of the testis. Although most cases of torsion occur in males before the onset of puberty, as many as 30% of all cases affect men over 20 years of age.

The ischemia produced by testicular torsion causes scrotal inflammation and pain that may have a sudden or gradual onset. The condition may be accompanied by nausea, vomiting, and irritative voiding symptoms (urgency, diurnal frequency, dysuria, and nocturia). Left untreated, the ischemic tissue of the tunica vaginalis, testis, and/or appendage causes irreversible damage

in as little as 1 to 2 hours. Ischemic damage obliterates effective testicular function after 4 to 6 hours.[43]

COMPLICATIONS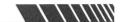

Epididymitis: Systemic infection; bacteriuria; urethritis; infertility
Orchitis: Systemic infection; bacteriuria; urethritis; infertility
Torsion: Testicular infarction; scrotal infection; infertility

DIAGNOSTIC STUDIES AND FINDINGS (DIFFERENTIAL DIAGNOSIS)

Diagnostic test	Findings		
	Epididymoorchitis	Viral orchitis	Torsion
Urine culture	>100,000 CFU*	No bacterial growth	No bacterial growth
Urinalysis	Bacteriuria Pyuria	Rare pyuria	Rare pyuria
Urethral swab culture	Negative or associated urethritis	No discharge noted	No discharge noted
Prostatic secretion culture	Negative or positive with associated prostatitis	Negative	Negative
Doppler ultrasound	Increased sound waves caused by hyperemia	Increased sound waves caused by hyperemia	Diminished sound waves caused by ischemia
Nuclear scan	Increased uptake with hyperemia	Increased uptake with hyperemia	Poor uptake with ischemia
Fever	Common	Common	Rare
Vomiting	Common	Common	Rare

*Colony-forming units.

MEDICAL MANAGEMENT

GENERAL MANAGEMENT AND DRUG THERAPY

Epididymitis

Antiinfective medication: To eradicate infection (antiinfective drug choice guided by sensitivity reports whenever feasible).

Parenteral antibiotics: May be required for severe cases.

Antiinflammatory agent: To reduce inflammation and pain.

Spermatic cord lidocaine (Xylocaine) or procaine hydrochloride (Novocain): To relieve pronounced pain caused by advanced infection.

Antipyretics: To reduce associated fever.

Antiemetics with parenteral fluids: Used when vomiting is severe or compromises fluid and electrolyte balance.

Orchitis

Medical management is identical to that for epididymitis for pyogenic (bacterial) orchitis.

Antiinflammatory agent with bed rest: Used for viral orchitis.

Penicillin or tetracycline: Used for granulomatous orchitis related to syphilis.

SURGERY

Epididymitis

Epididymectomy: Sometimes performed to eradicate chronic tubercular epididymitis.

Torsion

Corrective surgery (orchiopexy): Performed on an emergency basis.

Orchiectomy with or without removal of tunica vaginalis and implantation of prosthesis: Used when testis is found to have irreversible damage.

1 ASSESS

ASSESSMENT	OBSERVATIONS
Scrotal pain (character, onset, and duration)	**Epididymitis:** gradual onset of pain with irritative voiding symptoms and dysuria; Prehn's sign (elevating scrotum alleviates pain caused by epididymitis)
	Torsion: sudden onset of scrotal pain, no dysuria or irritative voiding symptoms; pain may be absent in rare cases

ASSESSMENT	OBSERVATIONS
Scrotal inflammation	**Epididymoorchitis:** Scrotum reddened and warm to touch; enlarged scrotum with hydrocele, dry, flaky skin with flattened rugae; hemiscrota are indistinguishable *(definitive diagnosis requires imaging studies to differentiate hyperemia of infection from ischemia of torsion)*
	Torsion: Scrotal enlargement with less prominent skin changes, no Prehn's sign *(definitive diagnosis requires imaging studies to differentiate hyperemia of infection from ischemia of torsion)*
Testicular enlargement	Testicular enlargement with torsion, epididymoorchitis, or orchitis; exquisite tenderness often contraindicates palpation or manipulation
Nausea, vomiting	Acute nausea and vomiting are common with torsion and severe cases of epididymitis and orchitis
Fever	Fever is present in severe cases of epididymitis and orchitis related to systemic infection
Altered patterns of urinary elimination	Irritative voiding symptoms are noted with epididymitis and orchitis
Urethral pain and discharge	Urethritis may be associated with pyogenic epididymoorchitis
Painful prostate	Bacterial prostatitis may be associated with pyogenic epididymoorchitis

2 DIAGNOSE

NURSING DIAGNOSIS	SUBJECTIVE FINDINGS	OBJECTIVE FINDINGS
Pain related to scrotal inflammation	Reports intense, exquisite pain in one or both testes	Inflammation of one or both hemiscrota, aggravated by manipulation or palpation; Prehn's sign may be present
Altered peripheral tissue perfusion related to ischemia of torsion	Reports scrotal pain (torsion may mimic discomfort produced by epididymitis or orchitis)	Testicular enlargement involving one or both hemiscrota
Hyperthermia related to systemic infection	Reports warmth, fatigue, malaise	Body temperature >37° C (98.6° F); may have nausea and vomiting
Potential fluid volume deficit related to nausea and vomiting	Reports nausea, vomiting, and inability to tolerate oral fluids or food	May have clinical signs of dehydration (poor skin turgor, dry mucous membranes) when nausea and vomiting are severe or persistent
Altered patterns of urinary elimination related to lower urinary tract infection	Reports frequency of urination, urgency, nocturia, and dysuria	Reduced functional capacity; diurnal frequency less than q 2 h; nocturia more than one episode per night among individuals under 65 years of age, two or fewer episodes among older adults

→ › ›

NURSING DIAGNOSIS	SUBJECTIVE FINDINGS	OBJECTIVE FINDINGS
Sexual dysfunction (potential for infertility) related to ischemia of torsion or inflammation of epididymitis or orchitis	Expresses fears or concerns about infertility or other sexual dysfunction	Oligospermia, aspermia, altered motility, and morphology noted on sperm analysis

3 PLAN

Patient Goals

1. Scrotal (testicular, or epididymal) pain will be resolved.
2. Ischemia caused by torsion will be reversed.
3. Inflammation caused by epididymal or testicular infection will be resolved.
4. Fever related to epididymitis, orchitis, or systemic infection will disappear.
5. Fluid volume deficits will be avoided or reversed.
6. Irritative voiding symptoms will resolve.
7. Infertility potential related to testicular damage will be avoided or successfully managed.

4 IMPLEMENT

NURSING DIAGNOSIS	NURSING INTERVENTIONS	RATIONALE
Pain related to scrotal inflammation	Institute temporary pain relief methods, minimize movement of scrotum, and avoid tight clothing; advise bed rest during acute phase of epididymitis or orchitis.	Movement and tight clothing aggravate pain caused by torsion, epididymitis, or orchitis.
	Minimize testicular palpation to necessary examinations performed by experienced health care providers.	Palpation of inflamed scrotum causes exquisite pain.
	Apply a Bellvue bridge or scrotal support for epididymitis or epididymoorchitis.	Scrotal support alleviates pain by altering dependent position of scrotum, promoting venous and lymphatic return and relieving edema.
	Apply ice pack to scrotum for patient with epididymitis or orchitis, ensuring adequate protection for skin.	Application of ice pack reduces hyperemia and provides temporary pain relief; application is *contraindicated* for the patient with torsion.
	Administer (or teach patient with epididymitis or orchitis to self-administer) antiinflammatory medications as prescribed.	Antiinflammatory drugs alleviate pain by reducing edema and inflammation caused by scrotal infections.
	Administer (or teach patient to self-administer) antiinfective agents for pyogenic epididymitis or orchitis.	Infection of the testis and/or epididymis produces inflammation and pain; antiinfective agents alleviate pain by helping the body rid itself of infection.

NURSING DIAGNOSIS	NURSING INTERVENTIONS	RATIONALE
	Administer analgesic or narcotic drugs during the acute postoperative period after corrective surgery for torsion.	Analgesics or narcotics alleviate pain caused by surgical incision and manipulation or removal of testicular tissue.
Altered peripheral tissue perfusion related to ischemia of torsion	Help patient experiencing scrotal pain obtain emergency medical care and proper diagnosis.	Ischemia and resulting infarction may compromise fertility in as little as 1 hour; systemic infection stemming from untreated torsion is a significant potential complication; urgent care is crucial to minimize or avoid these complications.
	Consult physician about differential diagnosis of testicular torsion versus epididymitis or orchitis.	Pain relief measures appropriate for scrotal infections (epididymitis or orchitis) are contraindicated for torsion, where discomfort is caused by ischemia rather than inflammation and hyperemia.
	Prepare patient for surgery to correct testicular torsion; review results of diagnostic tests, and consult physician about most likely surgical procedure required (orchiectomy or orchiopexy); reinforce that the procedure preserves all viable, functioning testicular tissue, and explain that a small scrotal incision will be necessary and that the entire procedure will be relatively brief (less than 2 h).	Orchiopexy (surgical manipulation of the scrotum intraoperatively with fixation to prevent recurrence) is the procedure of choice; orchiectomy (surgical removal of the testis and spermatic cord) is done only when orchiopexy is impossible because of massive tissue damage.
	Reassure patient that a prosthetic device to maintain normal appearance of the scrotum is available if orchiectomy is required.	Testicular prosthetic devices maintain the appearance of a normal scrotum.
	Advise patient that any pain experienced during immediate postoperative period will be managed aggressively.	Postoperative incisional pain is managed by a combination of bed rest, minimizing movement, and analgesic or narcotic drugs.
	Prepare patient for manual manipulation for torsion; reassure him that adequate sedation will be provided.	Occasionally torsion can be manually corrected without surgery; sedation is essential, since this manipulation causes intense pain.
	Advise patient that, in rare cases, torsion of contralateral testis may occur; teach patient to recognize cardinal signs and symptoms of torsion (acute onset of testicular or scrotal pain without irritative voiding symptoms) and importance of obtaining medical care immediately.	Prompt recognition of symptoms of torsion and rapid surgical correction are necessary to preserve testicular function.
Hyperthermia related to systemic infection	Administer (or teach patient to self-administer) antipyretic medications for fever.	Antipyretic medications temporarily reduce fever.

→ > >

NURSING DIAGNOSIS	NURSING INTERVENTIONS	RATIONALE
	Administer parenteral or oral antiinfective agents as prescribed; teach patient to self-administer these medications when feasible.	Antiinfective medications reduce fever by eradicating bacteria producing infection.
Potential fluid volume deficit related to nausea and vomiting	Evaluate for signs of dehydration and history of vomiting with inability to tolerate oral fluids.	Prolonged vomiting rids the body of needed fluid and associated electrolytes, producing clinically significant dehydration.
	Discontinue oral intake of food and beverages when nausea and vomiting are severe.	Food and beverages only intensify nausea and vomiting when scrotal and associated systemic infection are severe.
	Administer intravenous fluids as prescribed.	Parenteral fluid and nutrients replenish those depleted by vomiting until oral beverages and foods can be tolerated.
Altered patterns of urinary elimination related to lower urinary tract infection	Enable patient to obtain adequate fluid intake (at least 1,500 ml/day).	Fluid intake helps urinary tract flush pathogens from system.
	Administer (or teach patient to self-administer) antiinfective medications as prescribed.	Antiinfective medications help the body to eradicate urinary system infection.
Sexual dysfunction (potential for infertility) related to ischemia of torsion or inflammation of epididymitis or orchitis	Advise patient that ischemia of torsion or inflammation of orchitis or epididymitis may affect testicular function.	Tissue infarction caused by torsion is likely to adversely affect spermiogenesis of the affected testis; infection and inflammation also may compromise testicular function; when contralateral testis is normal, sperm count should be adequate for fertilization; if function of contralateral testis is compromised, infertility may result.
	Advise patient to consult a urologist and obtain results of a sperm analysis as part of a fertility counseling program if necessary.	Sperm analysis and expert counseling are the first steps to a successful program for family planning when infertility is suspected.
	Reassure patient that infertility problems are uncommon following torsion of a single testis and that problems that occasionally arise are amenable to treatment.	Accurate information, gently presented, enables patient to make informed decisions and to seek appropriate care for altered fertility function when indicated.
Knowledge deficit	See Patient Teaching.	

5   EVALUATE

PATIENT OUTCOME	DATA INDICATING THAT OUTCOME IS REACHED
Scrotal (testicular or epididymal) pain has resolved.	The patient states that scrotal pain has dissipated.
Ischemia caused by torsion has been reversed.	Ultrasonography and radionuclide studies demonstrate normal perfusion of affected testis.
Inflammation caused by epididymal or testicular infection has resolved.	Signs of scrotal inflammation have resolved; scrotal skin returns to normal appearance; testicular palpation reveals normal contour and size of organ.
Fever related to epididymitis, orchitis, or systemic infection has disappeared.	Body temperature returns to premorbid level.
Fluid volume deficits have been avoided or reversed.	Clinical signs of dehydration are absent or have been alleviated; laboratory studies show normal serum sodium, potassium, and other electrolyte levels.
Irritative voiding symptoms have resolved.	Voiding diary shows return to premorbid values of functional capacity, diurnal frequency, and nocturia.
Infertility potential related to testicular damage has been avoided or successfully managed.	Sperm analysis demonstrates normal sperm count, morphology, and motility; or patient is knowledgeable about strategies to manage infertility problems should they arise.

PATIENT TEACHING

1. Teach the patient about the potential association between sexually transmitted urethritis and epididymitis. Use this as an opportunity to teach the principles of safe sexual behavior.
2. Teach the patient about the connection between testicular function, epididymitis, orchitis, and torsion.
3. Teach the patient the dosage, schedule, and potential side effects of analgesic, antiinfective, antiemetic, or antiinflammatory drugs he is taking.
4. Teach the patient strategies to manage potential recurrent episodes of orchitis, epididymitis, or torsion.

CHAPTER 5

Urinary Incontinence/Voiding Dysfunction

Voiding dysfunction is a broad term used to describe any change in urinary elimination patterns. Dysfunctional voiding conditions include urinary incontinence, urinary retention, and sensory disorders of the bladder. **Urinary incontinence** is defined as the uncontrolled loss of urine of sufficient amount and frequency to cause a social or hygienic problem for the patient or his family.[62] **Urinary retention** is the inability to evacuate the bladder completely during micturition. This chapter focuses on the various types of incontinence and urinary retention. Chapter 3, "Inflammations of the Genitourinary System," contains information on common sensory disorders of the urinary system.

Urinary incontinence is a symptom rather than a disease. In some cases it represents a simple mechanical disorder of the urinary system; in other cases it is the presenting sign of a serious urologic, neurologic, or related-system disorder. The diagnosis and management of urinary incontinence are based on knowledge of the types of urinary leakage, its underlying cause, and its potential to produce urinary system distress.

Urinary incontinence can be divided into transient and chronic cases. Transient incontinence occurs as the result of immobility, infection, or acute disease. Resolving the underlying infection or disease resolves the incontinence. Chronic incontinence is an ongoing condition that represents a dysfunctional state of the lower urinary tract. There are several classification systems for chronic urinary incontinence/voiding dysfunction. Gray and Dougherty[79] identified four types of incontinence based on the system described by Wheatley.[93] **Stress incontinence** is the leakage of urine with physical exertion but without detrusor contraction. **Instability incontinence** is the leakage of urine caused by unstable or hyperreflexic detrusor contractions. Urge incontinence is the presenting symptom with uncontrolled or unstable detrusor contractions and normal bladder sensations; and reflex incontinence is the presenting symptom with unstable contractions without normal bladder sensations. **Overflow incontinence** is the presenting symptom of **urinary retention,** the inability to completely empty the bladder by voiding. **Extraurethral incontinence** occurs when ectopia, fistula, or surgical diversion produces leakage by some route that bypasses the normal sphincter mechanism.

The North American Nursing Diagnosis Association (NANDA) uses a system of six diagnoses for incontinence.[80] **Altered patterns of urinary elimination** is a broad diagnosis intended to describe any dysfunctional voiding state. **Stress incontinence** describes milder cases of sphincter dysfunction, whereas a more vague diagnosis, **total incontinence,** is used for both severe stress incontinence caused by sphincter incompetence and extraurethral leakage. NANDA labels instability leakage by its presenting symptoms, **urge incontinence or reflex incontinence. Urinary retention** corresponds to the diagnosis "overflow incontinence," and **functional incontinence** refers to urinary leakage caused by or associated with altered mobility, dexterity, or cognition.

Table 5-1 _____

CLASSIFICATION SYSTEMS FOR URINARY INCONTINENCE

Gray/Dougherty[79]	North American Nursing Diagnosis Association (NANDA)[80]	Urodynamic classification[60]
Stress incontinence	Stress incontinence Total incontinence (severe cases with sphincter incompetence)	Failure to store because of the outlet
Instability incontinence	Urge incontinence Reflex incontinence	Failure to store because of the detrusor
Overflow incontinence (urinary retention)	Urinary retention	Failure to empty because of the outlet; failure to empty because of the detrusor
All leakage with functional aspects	Functional incontinence	

A urodynamic classification system describes urinary incontinence by the underlying urinary system dysfunction.[60] **Failure to store** implies urinary leakage, and **failure to empty** implies urinary retention. The underlying reason for leakage or retention is explained by the phrases **because of the detrusor** and **because of the outlet.** Thus stress incontinence is the **failure to store because of the outlet,** and instability incontinence is the **failure to store because of the detrusor.** Urinary retention is the **failure to empty because of the detrusor** or the **failure to empty because of the outlet.**

Each classification system has strengths and weaknesses. It is more important for the nurse to understand the underlying concepts of these classification systems and to choose the system that best suits her clinical needs (Table 5-1).

The absolute incidence of incontinence among individuals in the United States remains unknown. Urinary incontinence is an underreported problem, probably because of its social connotations. The National Institutes of Health estimates that at least 10 million adults experience urinary incontinence, creating an annual cost exceeding $10.3 billion.[87a] As many as 50% of elderly adults who are institutionalized are incontinent, and 70% suffer from at least occasional urinary leakage.[65] Among the elderly in the community, approximately 15% to 30% experience urinary incontinence.[87a] Many cases of urinary incontinence are transient, brought on by infection, immobility, or acute disease. Nonetheless, many others represent a chronic condition that persists until proper treatment and bladder management strategies are instituted.

Stress Incontinence (Pelvic Descent)

Stress urinary incontinence (SUI) is a sign, a symptom, and a urinary diagnosis. "Genuine stress urinary incontinence" is a term used to describe sphincter leakage as an isolated finding. Mixed incontinence (stress urinary incontinence coexisting with instability incontinence) is also common.

Stress urinary incontinence is further conceptualized as a symptom, sign, or urodynamic diagnosis. The symptom of stress urinary incontinence is the patient's subjective report or perception that physical exertion causes urinary leakage. Clinicians elicit the sign by observing leakage in response to physical exertion such as coughing, jumping, or other provocative maneuvers. The urodynamic diagnosis is the demonstration of leakage caused by increased intravesical pressure driving urine across the bladder outlet.[62]

The normal sphincter mechanism resists leakage through two types of action, compression and tension. Elements of compression include the pliable, soft epithelium of the urethra, mucous secretions, and the submucosal vascular cushion. Elements of active tone, or tension, include the smooth and skeletal muscle of the proximal urethra, the pelvic floor muscles, and pelvic support structures. Two clinically demonstrable conditions, pelvic descent and sphincter incompetence (see Figures 5-1 and 5-2), cause stress urinary incontinence.

PATHOPHYSIOLOGY

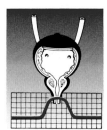

Pelvic descent is caused by weakness of the pelvic floor support structures. The principal support structures of the lower urinary tract are the pelvic floor muscles and ligaments. A variety of factors may contribute to the weakening of these supportive structures in women (box). In many women, pelvic descent is associated with stress urinary incontinence; other women have pelvic descent but no urinary leakage. The occurrence of stress incontinence with pelvic descent is attributed to distortion of the urethrovesical anatomy and loss of normal pressure transmission from abdomen to pelvis (Figure 5-1).

Distortion of the urethrovesical anatomy adversely affects sphincter muscle tone, which is crucial for efficient closure of the urethral sphincter. Normally, the urethra exits the bladder at a 16-degree angle and follows a relatively straight course to the meatus superior to the vaginal introitus. This course provides the circular and longitudinal muscle of the urethra with an ideal position and support, effectively sealing the urethra to prevent leakage, particularly when the bladder is stressed by physical exertion. Pelvic descent allows urethral excursion (movement) with abdominal pressure increases; this interferes with the sphincter's ability to seal the urethra and maintain urinary continence.

Pelvic descent also affects the transmission of abdominal pressure to the urethra. In a continent individual, the urethrovesical unit remains in an intraabdominal position. When a woman coughs, sneezes, or physically exerts herself, pressure is transmitted equally to the bladder and the urethra. This transmission of pressure to the urethra is assisted by active muscle tone of the urethral sphincter mechanism, maintaining urethral closure pressure that exceeds intravesical pressure and thus maintaining continence. In contrast, pelvic descent causes less effective pressure transmission to the urethra, and hypermobility and anatomic distortion lessen the sphincter's ability to exert active tone to the urethral lumen. As a result, intravesical pressure is more likely to exceed urethral closure pressure, resulting in stress leakage.

The role of estrogens in the pathophysiology of pelvic descent and loss of effective urethral compression remains unclear.[64] It is certain that stress urinary in-

For videourodynamic image of stress incontinence (pelvic descent), see Color Plate 1, page x.

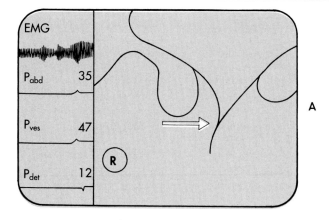

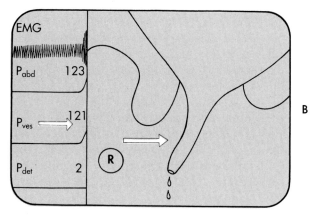

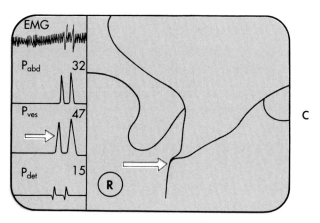

FIGURE 5-1

Diagrams of stress urinary incontinence. **A,** Pelvic descent with closed bladder outlet at rest. Patient is standing. Arrow indicates bladder neck below inferior aspect of symphysis pubis. **B,** Coughing causes urethral descent, transient funneling of bladder outlet with stress urinary leakage. Arrow on right indicates open urethra, and arrow on left shows high intravesical pressure (121 cm H_2O) produced by cough. **C,** After the cough the outlet rapidly closes and leakage is stopped. Arrow on left demonstrates cough occurring several seconds earlier, and arrow on right shows closed bladder outlet.

ETIOLOGY OF PELVIC DESCENT

Childbearing: multiple deliveries, difficult delivery requiring forceps assistance, breech deliveries

Hormonal changes: menopause, hypoestrogenic changes related to aging, hysterectomy, oophorectomy

Pelvic floor denervation: peripheral neuropathy, pudendal nerve damage, sacral spine lesions, cauda equina syndrome

Aggravating factors

  Obesity

  Alpha blockade drugs: phenoxybenzamine, prazosin, terazosin, doxazosin

PATIENT ADVOCACY AND SUPPORT GROUPS FOR INCONTINENCE

Continence Restored, Inc.

Co-directors: Anne Smith-Young, C.U.T.
              Douglas Whitehead, M.D.
Address: 785 Park Avenue
              New York, New York 10021

Help for Incontinent People, Inc. (HIP)

Director: Katherine Jeter, Ed.D., E.T.
Address: P.O. Box 544
              Union, South Carolina 29379

SIMON Foundation for Continence

Director: Cheryl Gartley
Address: P.O. Box 835
              Wilmette, Illinois 60091

continence is more prevalent among postmenopausal women than among women of childbearing age. Estrogens are directly beneficial to the compressive factors of the sphincter mechanism and to pelvic muscle tone. They exert a trophic effect (stimulating cellular growth and development) on the urethral epithelium and increase the volume of mucus produced by these cells. In addition, estrogens encourage the growth and development of the submucosal vascular cushion, which is needed to seal the soft mucosa effectively. Loss of circulating estrogens, resulting from menopause or other factors, causes vaginal and urethral atrophic changes that may contribute to irritative voiding symptoms, stress urinary incontinence, and pelvic descent.

In some cases exogenous estrogens, administered as an intravaginal cream or in oral forms, reverse atrophic vaginitis and may lessen the symptoms of stress urinary incontinence. Unfortunately, some women, particularly elderly women or those who have been hypoestrogenic for a prolonged period, may not respond as expected to exogenous hormone therapy.

COMPLICATIONS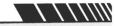

Detrusor instability (urge incontinence)
Cystitis (urinary tract infection)
Altered perineal skin integrity
Odor, shame, humiliation, social isolation
Bladder outlet obstruction

DIAGNOSTIC STUDIES AND FINDINGS

Diagnostic Test	Findings
Voiding diary	Genuine SUI: Functional capacity normal with diurnal frequency q 2 h or less often, no nocturia or one episode per night, leakage provoked by physical exertion or activity with no urge to void Mixed incontinence: Reduced functional capacity, diurnal frequency more often than q 2 h, nocturia once or more per night, leakage with urgency to void on physical exertion
Urodynamics	Genuine SUI: Cystometrogram demonstrates normal capacity, adequate compliance, and normal sensations of filling with stable detrusor; voiding pressure study shows explosive flow pattern with low-pressure contraction characteristic of reduced bladder outlet resistance; urethral pressure study may demonstrate reduced maximum closure pressure (<50 cm H_2O) and reduced functional length (<2.5-3 cm H_2O); provocative urethral pressure study demonstrates negative pressure transmission ratio with intravesical pressure exceeding urethral closure pressure with leakage; leak point pressure exceeds 70 cm H_2O
Videourodynamics	Demonstrates urethral excursion (movement) with or without leakage on provocation; descent below inferior margin of symphysis pubis may be noted even at rest when patient is upright Mixed incontinence: Cystometrogram demonstrates small capacity with unstable detrusor contractions and sensory urgency; other studies comparable to genuine SUI

Continued.

DIAGNOSTIC STUDIES AND FINDINGS—cont'd

Diagnostic Test	Findings
Endoscopy	Normal except for signs of pelvic descent; leakage provoked by coughing and straining
Cystogram/voiding cystourethrogram	Normal bladder contour when patient is supine; bladder descends below inferior margin of symphysis pubis when patient is upright; coughing provokes urethral excursion (movement); leakage may be noted
Intravenous pyelogram/ urogram (IVP/IVU)	Normal; IVP performed only with urinary tract infections or signs of upper tract distress

MEDICAL MANAGEMENT

Surgical repair of anatomic distortion (more than 100 surgical procedures are described in the literature; most use an abdominal, vaginal, or needle technique)

Administration of oral alpha sympathomimetic medications (see box below)

Administration of imipramine for combination of alpha sympathomimetic and antispasmodic effects

Administration of topical or oral estrogens to reverse effects of atrophic vaginitis (see box on next page)

Pelvic floor physiotherapy administered by nurse (electrostimulation may be used to supplement physiotherapy)

Placement of pessary to restore distorted anatomy

DRUGS USED FOR STRESS INCONTINENCE

Alpha sympathomimetics: Ephedrine, pseudoephedrine, phenylpropanolamine

Over-the-counter preparations (preparations with antihistamines are avoided): Sudafed, Sudafed S.A. capsules, Dexatrim without caffeine capsules (generic substitutes are available)

Prescription preparations: Entex L.A., Ornade spansules

Action and administration: Increases tone of urethral smooth muscle and rhabdosphincter; taken only during daytime hours and may be taken before physically demanding activities (exercise, walking) exclusively

Side effects: Tachycardia, hypertension, anxiety, nervousness, insomnia

Tricyclic antidepressant

Prescription preparations (may be used with estrogens): Imipramine

Action: Alpha sympathomimetic action increases tone of urethral smooth muscle and rhabdosphincter; anticholinergic effect relaxes detrusor and increases functional capacity in cases of SUI mixed with unstable detrusor

Administration: 10-25 mg PO, tid to qid; administered over a 24-hour period; individual is gradually withdrawn from drug using tapered doses

Side effects: Drowsiness, urinary retention, dry mouth, constipation, mydriasis (mild), hypertension

ESTROGEN REPLACEMENT THERAPY FOR STRESS INCONTINENCE

Action: Stimulates cellular growth of urethral epithelium, increased production of mucus, and trophic effect of submucosal vascular cushion*

Local (intravaginal) estrogen therapy

   Administration: 0.1 mg/g cream with intravaginal dispenser, 2-4 g/day for 1-2 wk, then 1-2 g for 1-2 wk and maintenance dose of 1-3 g/wk

Oral/parenteral (systemic) estrogen therapy (estradiol, estradiol cypionate, estradiol valerate)

   Administration: *Oral:* 1-2 mg/day with cyclic regimen, dosage titrated to minimal dosage for therapeutic effects; *Transdermal:* 1 patch (0.05 mg) 2 times/week with cyclic regimen, titrated to minimal dosage for therapeutic effects; *IM:* 10-20 mg/4 wk
   Side effects: Nausea (administer after meals), abdominal cramps and discomfort, constipation, headache, migraine, risk of thromboembolic disorders, hypertension

From Govoni L and Hayes J: *Drugs and nursing implications,* Norwalk, Conn, 1988, Appleton & Lange; Benness C et al: Lower urinary tract dysfunction in postmenopausal women: the role of estrogen deficiency, *Neurourology and Urodynamics* 10:24, 1991.

*Effects of exogenous estrogens on SUI remain unclear; response of urethral/vaginal tissues may be affected by time since menopause, age, surgical history.

1   ASSESS

ASSESSMENT	OBSERVATIONS
Stress incontinence	Urinary leakage provoked by physical exertion; patient reports no urgency to void at point of leakage
Altered urinary elimination patterns	Genuine SUI: diurnal frequency q 2 h or less often; nocturia once per night common; no urgency or urge incontinence Mixed incontinence: diurnal frequency more often than q 2 h; nocturia once per night or more often; urgency and urge incontinence
Pelvic descent	Physical examination of pelvic organs reveals cystocele (bulging of bladder into rectal vault), rectocele (bulging of rectum into vaginal vault), or uterine prolapse (migration of cervix and uterus into vaginal vault); patient notes symptoms of suprapubic pressure and lower back pain that is aggravated by standing and walking and alleviated by assuming a supine position
Signs of hypoestrogenic urethra and vagina	Physical examination of pelvic organs reveals dry, tender, nonrugated vaginal mucosa; irritative voiding symptoms may be noted

→ > >

ASSESSMENT	OBSERVATIONS
Altered skin integrity	Physical examination of pelvic organs reveals moist, odorous skin and red, maculopapular rash with satellite lesions characteristic of monilial rash or pale, papillary lesions of ammonia contact dermatitis

2 DIAGNOSE

NURSING DIAGNOSIS	SUBJECTIVE FINDINGS	OBJECTIVE FINDINGS
Stress incontinence related to pelvic descent	Reports leakage on physical exertion without urgency to void	Leakage provoked by physical exertion, coughing, laughing, and sneezing
Altered patterns of urinary elimination related to SUI and coexisting unstable detrusor (certain cases)	Reports symptoms of urgency and urge incontinence	Voiding diary demonstrates diurnal frequency q 2 h or less often with no nocturia or one episode per night; leakage associated with physical exertion Diurnal frequency more often than q 2 h with more than one episode of nocturia per night, urgency, urge incontinence with unstable detrusor
Impaired skin integrity related to prolonged exposure to urinary leakage	Reports that urinary leakage is not adequately contained by collection devices currently used	Moist, odorous perineal skin with monilial rash or ammonia contact dermatitis; collection device and clothing moist or saturated
Social isolation related to urinary leakage and fear of ostracism	Reports limiting social activities or fear of participating in activities	Appears unkempt; poor hygiene; reports limiting activities of daily living (ADLs) or avoiding interaction with others

3 PLAN

Patient goals

1. Stress urinary leakage will be adequately contained until definitive management is completed.
2. Stress urinary leakage will be eradicated or minimized.
3. Patterns of urinary elimination will return to normal.
4. Skin integrity will remain intact (perineal skin rashes will resolve).
5. Social isolation, humiliation, and shame will be reversed.

4 IMPLEMENT

NURSING DIAGNOSIS	NURSING INTERVENTIONS	RATIONALE
Stress incontinence related to pelvic descent	Help patient select an appropriate collection device.	A collection device is not a permanent answer for stress urinary leakage, but it provides temporary relief until definitive management is completed.

NURSING DIAGNOSIS	NURSING INTERVENTIONS	RATIONALE
	Help the patient decide on an appropriate containment system; provide her with the name and address of a local or regional supply house for urinary containment supplies.	Only the more commonly used pads or diapers are available at supermarkets; a local or regional supply house provides a larger variety of products when required, and many such suppliers deliver products by mail or other couriers.
	Consult the patient and physician about definitive interventions to correct stress incontinence.	There are several options for treating stress incontinence related to pelvic descent; an appropriate decision is made by mutual goal-setting involving the physician, nurse, patient, and significant others as appropriate.
	Administer or teach the patient to self-administer alpha sympathomimetic drugs for stress incontinence as prescribed by the physician.	Alpha sympathomimetic agents will palliate or eradicate leakage temporarily; oral alpha sympathomimetics are available over the counter or by prescription (see box on page 94).
	Administer or teach the patient to self-administer oral or topical estrogens as prescribed; advise the patient that long-term therapy is necessary for palliation of symptoms.	Exogenous estrogens may alleviate SUI by promoting compression of urethral tissue (through mucosal reproduction, production of mucus, and vascular cushion growth), leading to effective closure[17] (see box on page 95).
	Administer or teach the patient to self-administer antispasmodic or combination antispasmodic-sympathomimetic agents for mixed incontinence; advise the patient that prolonged administration of medication is expected for relief of symptoms.	Oral antispasmodic agents relieve unstable detrusor contractions of mixed incontinence; combination agents relieve symptoms of both incontinence types (see box on page 94).
	Institute pelvic muscle exercise program based on principles of physiotherapy: help the patient identify the appropriate muscle group using simple or complex biofeedback principles; teach her to avoid contracting and relaxing distant muscle groups. Provide the patient with a schedule of regular home exercise, emphasizing both maximum strength and endurance exercises (see Pelvic Muscle Exercises, page 304) and regular follow-up evaluations; advise the patient that in rare cases, results from a pelvic muscle exercise program may be noted in as little as 1 month but more likely will require 3 to 6 months.	Pelvic muscle exercises alleviate or cure stress incontinence by strengthening periurethral striated muscles that contribute to the sphincter mechanism[71]; exercises may prevent leakage by restoring more nearly normal anatomic relationships of the bladder, urethra, and adjacent pelvic organs.[79a]
	Teach the patient to exercise pelvic muscles three times a week for a maintenance program.	Pelvic muscle exercises produce long-term results *only* when initial and maintenance programs are followed.

→ > >

NURSING DIAGNOSIS	NURSING INTERVENTIONS	RATIONALE
	Begin electrostimulation therapy to supplement pelvic muscle exercises, using transvaginal or transrectal route; consult the physician about the length of stimulation and rest periods, pulse frequency and width, and the duration of each session; teach the patient to use the device daily and to schedule regular follow-up to evaluate progress.	Electrostimulation may supplement pelvic muscle exercises and may alleviate unstable detrusor contractions; it is particularly useful for women with markedly weak pelvic muscles.
	Consult the physician about using a pessary to prevent SUI.	A pessary is inserted into the vagina to mechanically reverse the effects of pelvic descent (Figure 5-1); when inserted correctly, it is worn comfortably and may correct SUI without obstructing urinary flow.
	Advise the patient that the pessary is successful only when cared for meticulously; teach her that complications of infection and erosion are prevented by strict adherence to changing schedules and that follow-up visits are crucial.	The principal complications of a pessary are erosion and local infection resulting from infrequent changes; regular follow-up by experienced clinicians will prevent these complications.
	Advise the patient that sexual intercourse is not feasible when a pessary is in place.	Because the pessary is placed in the vaginal vault, sexual intercourse will displace it.
	In consultation with the physician, prepare the patient for surgical repair of SUI.	Surgery may prevent urinary leakage by restoring more nearly normal urethrovesical anatomy (see pages 101-105).
Altered patterns of urinary elimination related to SUI and coexisting unstable detrusor	Advise the patient to void on a timed schedule based on the results of her voiding diary.	Timed voiding may prevent leakage from detrusor instability by preventing the bladder from reaching sufficient volume to trigger unstable contraction.
	Advise the patient to avoid drinking large amounts of fluids with meals while avoiding fluid intake between meals; instruct the patient to drink no more than 8 ounces of fluid with meals, to sip beverages between meals, and to drink only sips for a 2-h period before sleep (see Fluid Intake: What, When, and How Much, page 303).	Bolus fluid intake is likely to produce unstable detrusor contractions and intensify frequency.
	Advise the patient to drink an adequate volume of fluids each day (approximately 1 to 1½ quarts).	Limiting fluids concentrates urine, exaggerating the symptoms of urgency rather than relieving these sensations; also limiting fluid intake predisposes the urinary system to infection.

NURSING DIAGNOSIS	NURSING INTERVENTIONS	RATIONALE
Impaired skin integrity related to prolonged exposure to urinary leakage	Help the patient choose and obtain an appropriate urinary containment device.	The ideal urinary containment device protects the skin and clothing by completely absorbing leakage, minimizes odor, cannot be detected under clothing, and is affordable.
	Teach the patient the principles of skin care (i.e., regular washing, complete drying, protecting the skin with a moisture barrier or skin sealant, and using the collection device).	Maintaining skin integrity relies on regular cleansing and complete drying; moisture barriers or skin sealants offer some protection from exposure to urinary leakage; collection devices protect skin by minimizing or preventing exposure to urine.
	Administer or teach the patient to self-administer cream or powder for monilial rash as prescribed.	Monilial rashes are managed by routine skin care and local application of a cream or powder containing an antimonilial agent.
	Teach patient with ammonia contact dermatitis to clean skin with soap and water, thoroughly dry skin, and direct warm, dry air to the area for 15 min each day; advise her to use a hand-held hair dryer set at the lowest setting. Teach the patient to apply a skin sealant and moisture barrier and to use an appropriate containment device between treatments.	Ammonia contact dermatitis results from prolonged exposure of the skin to urine; regular, complete drying and using a moisture barrier or skin sealant and collection device minimize exposure.
	Encourage the patient to implement definitive management program for stress urinary leakage.	Definitive management of stress leakage protects the skin, eliminating exposure to urine.
Social isolation related to urinary leakage and fear of ostracism	Encourage the patient to seek definitive management for urinary leakage.	Many patients are advised by families, friends, or even health care professionals to "live with" their condition; treatment and resolution are realistic goals that prevent complications, including social isolation.
	Reassure the elderly patient that urinary leakage is more common among older persons, but leakage *is not* an inevitable part of growing older.	Elderly patients, in particular, are likely to be told that urinary leakage is inevitable and must be "lived with."
	Reassure the patient who has tried one unsuccessful bladder management program that incontinence is likely to respond to one or more alternative treatments.	Several treatments are appropriate for each type of incontinence; failure of one treatment plan does not imply that all strategies will fail.

NURSING DIAGNOSIS	NURSING INTERVENTIONS	RATIONALE
	Help the patient contact an advocacy or support group such as Help for Incontinent People (HIP), the SIMON Foundation for Continence, or Continence Restored, Inc. (see box on page 93).	Patient advocacy groups provide support and help patients obtain appropriate health care for urinary leakage; these groups also help the patient identify strategies for coping with leakage until a definitive management program has been completed.
Knowledge deficit	See Patient Teaching.	

5 EVALUATE

PATIENT OUTCOME	DATA INDICATING THAT OUTCOME IS REACHED
Stress incontinence is adequately contained.	Patient or caregiver demonstrates ability to use appropriate containment device.
Stress urinary leakage has been eradicated or minimized.	Patient has no urinary leakage on physical exertion, or leakage has diminished enough that there are no complications and patient feels no need for further intervention.
Patterns of urinary elimination have returned to normal.	Diurnal voiding frequency returns to q 2 h; nocturia is reduced to one episode or none each night.
Skin integrity remains intact.	Skin is dry and odor free, and no rashes are noted on perineal skin.
Social isolation, humiliation, and shame have been reversed.	Patient is knowledgeable about advocacy and support groups and states that she no longer feels humiliation, shame, or hopelessness; she also identifies specific strategies for seeking care for urinary leakage.

PATIENT TEACHING

1. Teach the patient to select, obtain, and use an appropriate containment or collection device for urinary leakage.
2. Teach the patient to routinely cleanse and dry the skin and to apply a barrier or sealant to prevent skin problems.
3. Teach the patient the names, dosage, administration schedules, and common side effects of medications used to manage stress incontinence. Teach her specific strategies for managing side effects should they occur.
4. Teach the patient to perform pelvic muscle exercises. Discuss the potential preventive value of pelvic muscle exercises during the postpartum period.
5. Teach the patient to perform electrostimulation using a home unit.
6. Teach the patient the common side effects of using a pessary and specific strategies to manage these effects should they occur.

SUPRAPUBIC PROCEDURES TO CORRECT STRESS INCONTINENCE

More than 100 procedures and variations are described in the urologic literature for managing stress urinary incontinence (SUI) associated with pelvic descent. Fixation of the vesicourethral junction in a more anatomically advantageous position often corrects stress-induced leakage. In the **Marshall-Marchetti-Krantz procedure,** the surgeon approximates periurethral fascia to the cartilage of the posterior symphysis pubis; a **retropubic colposuspension** (Burch procedure) involves fixating the vesicourethral junction to Cooper's ligament; and an **anterior urethropexy** involves placing absorbable sutures to anchor the vesicourethral junction to the periosteum of the symphysis pubis bone.[76]

INDICATIONS

Stress urinary incontinence associated with urethral hypermobility

Mixed stress and urge incontinence with detrusor instability

CONTRAINDICATIONS

Stress urinary incontinence related to sphincter incompetence

Detrusor hyperreflexia in neuropathic bladder dysfunction

Detrusor instability without urethral hypermobility or demonstrable SUI

COMPLICATIONS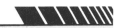

Urinary retention
Wound infection
Hemorrhage
Urinary tract infection

PREPROCEDURAL NURSING CARE

NURSING DIAGNOSIS	NURSING INTERVENTIONS	RATIONALE
Knowledge deficit related to surgical procedure, anesthesia, and potential adverse effects	Reinforce teaching before surgery, focusing on the goals of the procedure, potential adverse effects, and anticipated nursing care.	Anxiety limits the patient's ability to remember teaching before surgery; repeating this information helps reduce her anxiety.
	Prepare the patient for general anesthesia as prescribed, using hospital protocol.	Abdominal urethropexy typically requires general anesthesia.
	Inform the patient that a Foley catheter or suprapubic catheter will be in place for about 5 days after the surgery.	Postoperative edema at the urethrovesical junction may cause urinary retention; straining to urinate aggravates pain and may disrupt healing.
	Advise the patient that she will receive intravenous fluids for a short period after surgery until she can tolerate oral fluids.	Intravenous fluids are administered to avoid dehydration and as access for medications (if needed) until oral liquids can be tolerated.
	Advise the patient that urinary retention may occur following removal of the catheter.	Urinary retention following removal of the catheter is a response to edema and surgical manipulation; spontaneous micturition should occur unless preoperative urodynamic testing raises a suspicion of deficient detrusor muscle contractility.

→ › ›

NURSING DIAGNOSIS	NURSING INTERVENTIONS	RATIONALE
Urinary retention (potential) related to surgical fixation of urethrovesical junction	Teach intermittent catheterization (IC) **before** procedure if it is to be used as bladder management for retention (see Intermittent Self-Catheterization for Women, page 307).	IC is a new skill to most patients that requires coordination of visual, tactile, and cognitive skills; learning is enhanced when IC is taught before urinary retention is noted in the first week after surgery.
	Before surgery, teach the patient self care of an indwelling Foley catheter (see Care of an Indwelling Foley Catheter, page 308) if the catheter is to be used for bladder drainage after surgery.	Instruction is enhanced when the skills of care are reviewed before the first postoperative week.

POSTPROCEDURAL NURSING CARE

NURSING DIAGNOSIS	NURSING INTERVENTIONS	RATIONALE
Altered patterns of urinary elimination related to surgical fixation of urethrovesical junction	Monitor the indwelling catheter for patency.	Occlusion of the catheter intensifies pain and may disrupt surgical repair.
	Remove the indwelling catheter as directed (typically on the fifth day after surgery); monitor the patient closely for ability to urinate and check postvoid residual volumes as directed.	Urinary retention may follow removal of the Foley catheter, possibly because of postoperative edema and discomfort; bladder distention is avoided, because it may damage the surgical repair.
	Reinsert the catheter or institute an IC program if retention occurs; reassure the patient that retention is expected to be temporary.	Spontaneous urination is enhanced by reducing postoperative edema and discomfort and prolonged by overdistention of the bladder; catheter drainage prevents overdistention until spontaneous voiding returns.
	Advise the patient that urge incontinence may be relieved by urethropexy or that these symptoms may persist; reassure her that persistent or new symptoms of urgency and urge incontinence will be managed if they occur.	Detrusor instability may be alleviated by urethropexy; unfortunately, in some cases these symptoms are not relieved and in some cases detrusor instability and urge incontinence may begin after surgical repair.
Pain related to surgical trauma	Assess the character, location, and duration of pain.	Incisional pain typically is perceived as dull, boring, and prolonged, whereas bladder spasms are more transient with a sudden onset and short duration.
	Administer analgesics for incisional pain as prescribed.	Incisional pain responds to narcotic drugs.
	Administer anticholinergic medications for pain related to bladder spasms.	Bladder spasms are caused by unstable detrusor contractions against an occluded (catheterized) outlet; anticholinergic medications relax the detrusor muscle, preventing contractions.

NURSING DIAGNOSIS	NURSING INTERVENTIONS	RATIONALE
	Monitor the catheter for patency.	Incisional and bladder spasm pain are exacerbated by bladder overdistention caused by an occluded or kinked catheter.
	Position the patient on her side or back; splint the incision as needed for turning, coughing, and deep-breathing exercises.	Incisional pain is relieved by proper positioning and by protecting the incision during provocative maneuvers.
	Minimize noise, bright lighting, and environmental distractions during immediate postoperative period.	Environmental factors may intensify postoperative pain.

PATIENT TEACHING

1. Patient teaching before surgery should include a management plan for possible postoperative urinary retention.
2. Teach the patient home management of an indwelling Foley catheter or an intermittent catheterization program before surgery.
3. Teach the patient the signs and symptoms of urinary tract infection and a strategy to manage infection if it occurs.
4. Teach the patient the symptoms of urge incontinence and what to do if symptoms occur.
5. Teach the patient to avoid heavy lifting or strenuous exercise for about 6 weeks after surgery.

NEEDLE PROCEDURES (COMBINED SUPRAPUBIC/VAGINAL APPROACH)

The technique for a needle suspension procedure was described by Pereyra in 1959. A vaginal incision is made, and the vagina and urethra are carefully separated. The urethra is mobilized to an intraabdominal position by ligature carriers; access is gained through two 3 to 5 cm incisions in the abdominal wall. Special needles are used to buttress the mobilized urethra to endocervical and endopelvic fascia. A **Stamey procedure** involves mobilizing the tissue lateral to the urethra to restore the position of the urethrovesical junction.[60] A **Raz procedure** is a vaginal procedure in which sutures are used to mobilize the vaginal wall and endopelvic fascia used for the Stamey technique. Using the ligature carrier, the surgeon transfers these sutures to an intraabdominal position, where they are anchored to rectus fascia. Needle procedures resolve stress urinary incontinence in about 85% to 90% of these cases.[76]

INDICATIONS

Stress incontinence associated with urethral hypermobility

Mixed stress and urge incontinence with detrusor instability

CONTRAINDICATIONS

Stress incontinence related to sphincter incompetence

Detrusor hyperreflexia in neuropathic bladder dysfunction

Urge incontinence with unstable detrusor contractions but without urethral hypermobility or demonstrable SUI

COMPLICATIONS

Urinary retention
Wound infection
Urinary tract infection

PREPROCEDURAL NURSING CARE

NURSING DIAGNOSIS	NURSING INTERVENTIONS	RATIONALE
Knowledge deficit related to surgical procedure, anesthesia, and potential adverse effects	Reinforce teaching **before** surgery, including the goals of the procedure, potential adverse effects, and anticipated nursing care.	Anxiety before surgery may reduce the patient's retention of preoperative instruction; reinforcing teaching increases retention and reduces anxiety.
	Prepare the patient for spinal or general anesthesia as directed, using hospital protocols.	Needle suspension may be performed with either general or spinal anesthesia.
	Advise the patient that she will have a Foley catheter for 24 h after surgery.	Postoperative edema and discomfort cause urinary retention, which is potentially harmful to the urinary system and the surgical repair; catheter drainage prevents these complications.
	Advise the patient that approximately 50% of women who undergo needle surgery may need to perform self intermittent catheterization for a brief period (several weeks to a month) after surgery.[76]	Prolonged urinary retention may occur as a result of increased bladder outlet resistance, which itself may result from the surgical repair or from edema or discomfort; intermittent catheterization provides regular, complete bladder evacuation until spontaneous voiding returns.
	Advise the patient that intravenous fluids will be infused for a brief period after surgery until she can tolerate oral fluids.	Intravenous fluids are administered to prevent dehydration and as an access route for medications until oral liquids can be tolerated.
	Inform the patient that a pack will remain in the vagina for 24 h.	The vaginal pack provides hemostasis and contains drainage from the vaginal incision.
Urinary retention related to surgical repair of urethrovesical junction	Teach intermittent catheterization **before** surgery.	IC is a new skill to most patients that requires coordination of visual, tactile, and cognitive skills; learning is enhanced when IC is taught before postoperative urinary retention is noted.
Potential for infection related to surgical incision and manipulation	Administer or help the patient give herself a Betadine douche the night before surgery.	The Betadine douche eradicates bacteria in preparation for the vaginal incision.
	Administer antiinfective medications before surgery as prescribed.	Antiinfective medications may be given before surgery as prophylaxis against postoperative wound infection.

POSTPROCEDURAL NURSING CARE

NURSING DIAGNOSIS	NURSING INTERVENTIONS	RATIONALE
Altered patterns of urinary elimination (potential for urinary retention) related to surgical repair of urethrovesical junction	Remove the Foley catheter as directed (commonly first postoperative day).	Approximately 50% of women patients can void spontaneously after brief catheter drainage.
	Closely monitor the patient for spontaneous voiding, and check residual urinary volumes as indicated.	When urinary retention occurs, it is quickly managed to avoid pain, infection, and disruption of the surgical fixation.
	Institute intermittent catheterization if urinary retention occurs.	Intermittent catheterization is used to prevent stasis, overdistention, and urinary infection.
Pain related to surgical trauma	Assess character, location, and duration of pain.	Incisional pain typically is perceived as dull, boring, and prolonged, whereas bladder spasms are more transient with a sudden onset and short duration.
	Administer analgesics for incisional pain as prescribed.	Incisional pain responds to narcotic drugs.
	Administer anticholinergic medications for pain related to bladder spasm.	Bladder spasms are caused by unstable detrusor contractions against an occluded (catheterized) outlet; anticholinergic medications relax the detrusor muscle, preventing contractions.
	Monitor catheter for patency.	Incisional and bladder spasm pain are exacerbated by bladder overdistention, which is caused by an occluded or kinked catheter.
	Minimize noise, bright lighting, and environmental distractions during immediate postoperative period.	Environmental factors may intensify postoperative pain.

Stress Incontinence (Sphincter Incompetence)

Stress incontinence also occurs when the urethral sphincter mechanism is damaged and fails to close completely. The resulting leakage is similar to SUI caused by pelvic descent, although the incontinence is often severe. Correct identification of sphincter damage is crucial, since the management is different from maneuvers used to correct pelvic descent (Figure 5-2).

For videourodynamic image of stress incontinence (sphincter incompetence), see Color Plate 2, page x.

PATHOPHYSIOLOGY

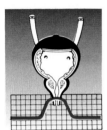 In addition to pelvic descent, sphincter incompetence also causes stress urinary incontinence (SUI). With pelvic descent, the sphincter mechanism is adversely affected by anatomic distortion. With sphincter incompetence, the sphincter mechanism is directly damaged as the result of trauma, surgery, or denervation of its muscular elements.

Iatrogenic sphincter incompetence is a rare complication of transurethral resection of the prostate and an uncommon complication of open or radical prostatectomy procedures.[93] Transurethral resection of the prostate (see Benign Prostatic Hypertrophy [Hyperplasia], Chapter 6) requires endoscopic incision of obstructive prostatic tissue. In rare cases inadvertent incision of the rhabdosphincter causes sphincter incompetence, with resulting stress urinary incontinence. Radical prostatectomy (see Prostate Tumors, Chapter 7) is the surgical resection of the entire prostate and its capsule for treatment of cancer. Because this is a lifesaving procedure, partial resection of the tissues of the sphincter mechanism, with resulting stress urinary incontinence, may be necessary.[67,95]

Other procedures carry some risk of rendering the sphincter mechanism incompetent. Bladder neck incision, Y-V plasty, and implantation of an artificial urinary sphincter, with subsequent deactivation or explantation, alter the sphincter mechanism, increasing the risk of stress urinary incontinence.

Denervation of the pudendal nerve or lesions of the sacral micturition center (particularly sacral spinal levels 1 through 3) increase the risk of primary sphincter incompetence and stress urinary leakage. Spina bifida

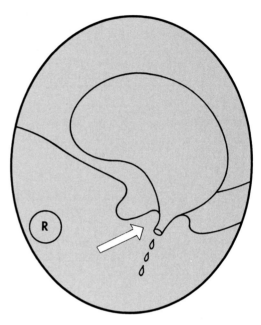

FIGURE 5-2
Cystogram of bladder with sphincter incompetence. Arrow indicates open bladder outlet; patient is standing without coughing or straining. Active leakage is noted.

defects may adversely affect neurologic function of lumbosacral segments, producing denervation of the pelvic floor muscles and intrinsic sphincter mechanism. Cauda equina abnormalities or lower back injuries (affecting bony spinal segments T12 or lower) also denervate the muscular components of the sphincter mechanism.

COMPLICATIONS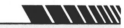

Altered skin integrity
Deficient detrusor contractility
Odor, shame, humiliation, social isolation
Urinary tract infection (rare)

DIAGNOSTIC STUDIES AND FINDINGS

Diagnostic Test	Findings
Voiding diary	Diurnal frequency may be noted with behavioral attempts to minimize leakage; functional capacity is small, with marked stress-related leakage produced by minimal exertion or position change; particularly severe cases may be characterized by failure to store urine (absent voiding) with essentially continuous urinary leakage
Urodynamics	Reduced cystometric capacity with SUI on minimal exertion (occlusion of the bladder outlet is used to evaluate potential capacity after correction of outlet incompetence); detrusor typically is stable; voiding pressure study shows explosive flow with low-pressure contraction characteristic of reduced bladder outlet resistance; urethral pressure shows profoundly low maximum urethral closure pressure (20 cm H_2O or less); pressure transmission ratio demonstrates greater transmission of pressure to bladder as opposed to urethra
Videourodynamics	Shows funneled (open) bladder outlet on upright cystogram with SUI provoked by minimal exertion; leak point pressure 70 cm H_2O or significantly less; pelvic descent and urethral hypermobility often absent
Endoscopy	Bladder neck open without exertion, indicating sphincter muscle incompetence
Cystogram/voiding cystourethrogram	Funneled, open bladder outlet on upright films

MEDICAL MANAGEMENT

GENERAL MANAGEMENT AND DRUG THERAPY

Administration of alpha sympathomimetic drugs

SURGICAL THERAPY

Pubovaginal sling

Artificial urinary sphincter (more successful in men)

Periurethral injection of GAX collagen or polytef paste (under investigation)

1 ASSESS

ASSESSMENT	OBSERVATIONS
Stress incontinence	Leakage caused by mild to minimal physical exertion (walking, lifting, position changes); leakage with movement in bed may be noted in severe cases
Altered urinary elimination patterns	Diurnal frequency greater than q 2 h; nocturia common; enuresis may be noted

ASSESSMENT	OBSERVATIONS
Pelvic descent	Pelvic descent (cystocele, rectocele, uterine prolapse) may be noted in women; descent is not a factor in men and some women with previous surgical repair of pelvic descent
Altered skin integrity	Moist, odorous skin and a red, maculopapular rash with satellite lesions (monilial rash) or pale papillary lesions of ammonia contact dermatitis

2 DIAGNOSE

NURSING DIAGNOSIS	SUBJECTIVE FINDINGS	OBJECTIVE FINDINGS
Stress incontinence related to sphincter incompetence	Complains of leakage with minimal exertion or notes essentially continuous leakage unrelated to detectable physical exertion	Sign of stress incontinence provoked by even minimal exertion
Altered patterns of urinary elimination related to sphincter incompetence and stress incontinence	Reports frequent need to urinate or absence of voiding with continuous leakage into containment device	Diurnal frequency greater than q 2 h, nocturia common; *or* failure to urinate with complete reliance on containment device
Impaired skin integrity related to severe incontinence caused by sphincter incompetence	Reports problems with perineal skin (i.e., redness, rashes, itching, and odor)	Red, maculopapular rash with satellite lesions (monilial rash); pale papillary lesions (ammonia contact dermatitis); moist, odorous skin
Social isolation related to urinary leakage, odor, and fear of embarrassment, discovery	Reports reluctance, inability to participate in activities requiring interaction with others	Appears unkempt; poor hygiene; activities of daily living (ADLs) involve minimal interaction with others

3 PLAN

Patient goals

1. The patient will regain urinary continence.
2. Diurnal frequency and nocturia will return to normal.
3. Perineal skin will be intact.
4. Social isolation will be reversed.

4 IMPLEMENT

NURSING DIAGNOSIS	NURSING INTERVENTIONS	RATIONALE
Stress incontinence related to sphincter incompetence	Help the patient identify, obtain, and use an appropriate containment device (see Choosing a Containment Device for Urinary Leakage, page 300).	A urinary containment device collects urine protecting skin and clothing until a definitive management program has been instituted.

NURSING DIAGNOSIS	NURSING INTERVENTIONS	RATIONALE
	Administer or teach the patient to self-administer alpha sympathomimetic medications to stop or minimize urinary leakage.	Alpha sympathomimetic medications increase sphincter closure by stimulating urethral smooth muscle and the rhabdosphincter; in atypically mild cases, alpha sympathomimetic drugs ablate urinary leakage; more commonly, these drugs reduce the severity of leakage (refer to Table 5-3).
	Consult the physician about pelvic muscle exercises with or without transvaginal or transrectal electrostimulation therapy.	Pelvic muscle exercises alleviate stress incontinence by strengthening pelvic floor and periurethral muscles. Electrostimulation passively exercises the pelvic floor and periurethral muscles. Their effect on stress incontinence related to sphincter incompetence remains unclear. Nonetheless, since these interventions are noninvasive and not associated with serious complications, a trial of therapy may be appropriate for the patient who does not wish to undergo surgical repair or pharmacotherapy.
	Prepare the female patient for pubovaginal sling surgery (see Pubovaginal Sling Procedure, page 112).	A pubovaginal sling surgically fixates the proximal one third of the urethra to correct stress incontinence caused by sphincter incompetence.
	Prepare the patient for implantation of an artificial urinary sphincter prosthesis (see Artificial Urinary Sphincter Implantation, page 114).	An artificial urinary sphincter is a prosthetic device designed to prevent stress incontinence caused by sphincter incompetence.
	Prepare the patient for periurethral injection of GAX collagen or polytef paste as directed (see Periurethral Injection Therapy, page 118).	Urethral bulking minimizes or reverses leakage caused by sphincter incompetence.
Altered patterns of urinary elimination related to sphincter incompetence and stress incontinence	Reassure the patient with urinary frequency that restoring continence improves bladder capacity.	Urinary frequency may be a behavioral attempt to reduce urinary leakage caused by sphincter incompetence; other individuals may have reduced functional capacity because of a compromised ability to store urine in the bladder. Restoration of continence will improve functional bladder capacity.
	Advise the patient with urinary frequency and detrusor instability (noted on urodynamic testing) that urgency to void and urge incontinence may occur after stress urinary leakage is resolved; assure the patient that management of this form of incontinence will be undertaken when stress incontinence has been resolved.	Detrusor instability produces small functional bladder capacity, which is related to inappropriate bladder contractions. Symptoms of instability are masked in cases of severe stress incontinence and will be magnified when SUI is resolved. Detrusor instability is treated as a separate form of incontinence.

NURSING DIAGNOSIS	NURSING INTERVENTIONS	RATIONALE
	Advise the patient with intermittent flow and low-pressure or absent contractions that resolving stress incontinence may cause urinary retention.	Low-pressure contractions are characteristic of individuals with stress incontinence. However, low-pressure contractions associated with intermittent flow and straining raise the suspicion of deficient detrusor contractility. These individuals have a significant risk of temporary or long-term urinary retention following resolution of stress incontinence.
	Teach intermittent catheterization, as directed, to the patient at risk for urinary retention following resolution of stress incontinence.	Intermittent catheterization is a skill requiring integration of cognitive and motor skills; these skills are more easily learned before surgical repair rather than during the first postoperative weeks.
Impaired skin integrity related to severe incontinence caused by sphincter incompetence	Help the patient identify, choose, and obtain an appropriate urinary collection device.	The ideal urinary collection device protects skin by completely absorbing leakage, thus minimizing the time urine is in contact with the skin (see Choosing a Containment Device for Urinary Leakage, page 300).
	Teach the patient the principles of skin care, including regular washing, complete drying, protecting the skin with a moisture barrier or skin sealant, and using a collection device.	Maintaining skin integrity depends on regular cleansing and complete drying; moisture barriers or skin sealants offer some protection from exposure to urinary leakage, and collection devices protect skin by minimizing exposure to urine.
	Administer or teach the patient to self-administer cream or powder for monilial rash as prescribed.	Monilial rashes are managed by routine skin care and local application of an anti-monilial agent.
	Teach the patient with ammonia contact dermatitis to clean the skin with soap and water; thoroughly dry the skin; and direct warm, dry air to the area for 15 min each day; advise her to use a hand-held hair dryer set at lowest setting; between treatments teach the patient to apply a skin sealant or moisture barrier and to use an appropriate containment device.	Ammonia contact dermatitis occurs as a result of prolonged exposure of the skin to urine. Regular, complete drying and using a moisture barrier or skin sealant and collection devices minimize exposure.
	Encourage the patient to implement a definitive management program for SUI.	Definitive management of incontinence protects the skin, eliminating exposure to urine.
Social isolation related to urinary leakage, odor, and fear of embarrassment, discovery	Encourage the patient to seek a definitive management program for urinary leakage.	Many patients are advised by families, friends, or even health care professionals to "live with" their condition; treatment and resolution are realistic goals and prevent complications, including social isolation.

NURSING DIAGNOSIS	NURSING INTERVENTIONS	RATIONALE
	Reassure the elderly patient that urinary leakage is more common among older persons, but leakage *is not* an inevitable part of growing older.	Elderly patients, in particular, are likely to be advised—incorrectly—that urinary leakage is inevitable and best "lived with."
	Reassure the patient who has undergone unsuccessful surgery to correct stress incontinence that alternative methods may be able to stop the leakage.	Several treatments are appropriate for stress incontinence; treatment approaches appropriate for stress incontinence related to pelvic descent may not be ideal for leakage produced by sphincter incompetence.
	Help the patient contact an advocacy or support group such as Help for Incontinent People (HIP), the SIMON Foundation, or Continence Restored, Inc. (see box on page 93).	Patient advocacy groups provide support and help patients obtain appropriate health care for urinary leakage; these groups also help the patient identify strategies for coping with leakage until a definitive management program has been completed.
Knowledge deficit	See Patient Teaching.	

5 EVALUATE

PATIENT OUTCOME	DATA INDICATING THAT OUTCOME IS REACHED
The patient has regained urinary continence.	Stress urinary incontinence has resolved or is controlled to the patient's satisfaction.
Diurnal frequency and nocturia have returned to normal.	Diurnal frequency is q 2 h or less often, and nocturia is one or no episodes per evening.
Perineal skin remains intact.	Skin rashes and lesions have resolved, and physical examination shows the perineal skin is intact.
Social isolation has been reversed.	Patient reports returning to social activities she enjoyed before the onset of incontinence; her appearance and hygiene are improved.

PATIENT TEACHING

1. Explain the pathophysiology of stress incontinence caused by sphincter weakness. Contrast this with commonly held beliefs about stress incontinence and the "dropped bladder."
2. Teach the patient the names, dosage, administration schedules, and potential side effects of alpha sympathomimetic drugs used to reduce or cure stress incontinence.
3. Teach the patient to perform pelvic floor muscle exercises with or without electrostimulation. Explain how they are supposed to help and that the outcome may be positive but that health care professionals have only limited experience in applying these techniques for this condition.
4. Teach the patient the signs and symptoms of urinary tract infections and how to manage an infection should it occur.

PUBOVAGINAL SLING PROCEDURE

The pubovaginal sling procedure is performed through an abdominal incision. First, a strip of anterior rectus fascia or other material is placed around the proximal third of the urethra through a midline vaginal incision. Then the limbs of the sling are pulled through the retropubic space and fixated to the anterior rectus fascia superior to the symphysis pubis. The tension of the sling is adjusted to ensure obstruction during bladder filling and storage while allowing unobstructed micturition.

INDICATIONS

Stress incontinence resulting from sphincter incompetence

Occasionally used with urethral hypermobility and severe stress incontinence

CONTRAINDICATIONS

Stress incontinence resulting from urethral hypermobility with mechanical obstruction

Detrusor instability without demonstrable stress urinary incontinence

Neuropathic bladder dysfunction with poor compliance or detrusor hyperreflexia (*unless* additional surgery is done to alleviate poor compliance or hyperreflexia)

COMPLICATIONS

Urinary retention
Wound infection
Urinary tract infection

PREPROCEDURAL NURSING CARE

NURSING DIAGNOSIS	NURSING INTERVENTIONS	RATIONALE
Knowledge deficit related to procedure, its goals, anesthesia, and potential side effects	Reinforce preoperative teaching, including the procedure, its goals, and potential side effects.	Anxiety is likely to reduce effective learning and retention of preoperative teaching; repeating the instruction enhances retention and reduces anxiety.
	Prepare the patient for general or spinal anesthesia.	General or spinal anesthesia is used for pubovaginal sling surgery.
	Advise the patient that she will have a Foley or suprapubic catheter for about 24 h after surgery.	Catheter drainage prevents overdistention of the bladder and reduces postoperative edema.
	Advise the patient that a vaginal pack will remain in the vagina for 24 h after surgery.	The vaginal packing absorbs exudate from the vaginal incision and provides hemostasis.
	Inform the patient that urinary retention may occur after pubovaginal sling surgery; inform her that an indwelling catheter may be used or that she will be taught intermittent catheterization (IC).	Urinary retention may occur due to inflammation, edema, and surgical manipulation. An indwelling catheter or self IC program is used to drain urine until spontaneous voiding returns.
	Teach IC or care of an indwelling catheter **before** surgery as directed.	IC teaching requires integration of visual tactile and motor skills; learning is enhanced by instruction before the first postoperative week.

NURSING DIAGNOSIS	NURSING INTERVENTIONS	RATIONALE
Potential for infection related to surgical trauma, manipulation	Administer or teach patient to self-administer vaginal douche before surgery as prescribed.	The vaginal douche eradicates flora before surgery.
	Administer preoperative antiinfective drugs as prescribed.	Antiinfective drugs are used to prevent wound or systemic infections.

POSTPROCEDURAL NURSING CARE

NURSING DIAGNOSIS	NURSING INTERVENTIONS	RATIONALE
Altered urinary elimination patterns related to surgical manipulation of bladder outlet	Monitor indwelling catheter for patency.	Acute overdistention increases pain and inflammation and enhances the risk of prolonged retention.
	Remove the indwelling catheter on the first postoperative day as prescribed; carefully monitor the patient for spontaneous voiding and residual volumes.	Urinary retention may occur following surgical manipulation of the bladder outlet because of edema or inflammation or because of the surgical manipulation itself.
	Institute intermittent catheterization or reinsert indwelling catheter if necessary.	Temporary drainage of the bladder may be necessary to prevent overdistention and infection, which prolong retention.
	Advise the patient that detrusor instability and urge incontinence may be noted after surgery; reassure her that the symptoms of urge incontinence will be managed.	Unstable detrusor contractions and urge incontinence may occur after surgical manipulation of the bladder outlet.
Pain related to surgical trauma	Assess the character, location, and duration of pain.	Incisional pain typically is perceived as dull, boring, and prolonged, whereas bladder spasms produce a transient, cramping pain that may be associated with urinary leakage.
	Administer analgesics for incisional pain as prescribed.	Incisional pain responds to narcotic drugs.
	Administer anticholinergic medications for pain related to bladder spasms.	Bladder spasms are caused by unstable detrusor contractions against an occluded (catheterized) outlet; anticholinergic medications relax the detrusor muscle, preventing contractions.
	Monitor the indwelling catheter for patency.	Incisional and bladder spasm pain is exacerbated by bladder overdistention, which can be caused by an occluded or kinked catheter.

NURSING DIAGNOSIS	NURSING INTERVENTIONS	RATIONALE
	Position the patient on her side or back; splint the incision as needed for turning, coughing, and deep-breathing exercises.	Pain from the incision is relieved by position and protection during provocative maneuvers.
	Minimize noise, bright lights, and environmental distractions during the immediate postoperative period.	Environmental factors may intensify postoperative pain.

PATIENT TEACHING ▪▪▪▪▪▪▪▪▪▪▪▪▪▪▪▪▪▪▪▪▪▪▪▪▪▪▪▪▪▪▪▪▪▪▪▪▪▪▪

1. Explain the cause of stress incontinence resulting from sphincter incompetence; compare it with incontinence caused by pelvic descent.
2. Explain that temporary or long-term urinary retention may follow pubovaginal sling surgery. Teach the patient how to do intermittent catheterization when indicated, preferably before surgery.
3. Instruct the patient to avoid lifting heavy objects or strenuous exercise for 6 weeks after surgery.

ARTIFICIAL URINARY SPHINCTER IMPLANTATION

An artificial urinary sphincter (AUS) is a urologic prosthetic device with three principal components: an abdominal reservoir, a periurethral cuff, and a pump mechanism (Figure 5-3). The device is operated by movement of fluid through a tubing network from the cuff to the abdominal reservoir. The cuff is placed near the bladder neck or bulbous urethra in men and near the bladder neck in women. A range of cuff sizes is available, allowing custom fitting for each patient.

A balloon that regulates the pressure exerted by the periurethral cuff is placed in the prevesical space in the abdomen. The choice of balloon size and the amount of pressure to be exerted on the urethra are influenced by the size of the cuff and the characteristics of the urethral tissue. It is important to remember that the higher the cuff pressure, the greater the likelihood of effective urethral closure; but also, the greater the risk of urethral ischemia or erosion.

The pump mechanism of the artificial sphincter is placed in the scrotum in men or underneath the labia in women. The mechanism consists of a baffling device capable of transferring fluid from the balloon reservoir to the cuff. The mechanism also houses a deactivation button, located immediately above the baffling device.

Deactivating the pump traps fluid in the abdominal reservoir so that the pump remains in the open position.

The artificial sphincter operates by mechanical compression of the urethra. It is meant to serve as a zone of tension or active compression, substituting for the muscular elements of a normal urethra. An artificial urinary sphincter operates with the cuff inflated during bladder filling and storage. Before bladder evacuation, the individual firmly compresses the pump mechanism to baffle fluid from the pump to the abdominal reservoir, relieving urethral pressure. Bladder evacuation is accomplished by spontaneous voiding or by catheterization. After decompression fluid slowly returns to the cuff, restoring continence in 1 to 3 minutes.

INDICATIONS

Stress incontinence caused by sphincter incompetence

CONTRAINDICATIONS

Patient or caregivers lack dexterity or motivation to operate pump mechanism
Uncontrolled detrusor hyperreflexia or compromised bladder wall compliance
Vesicoureteral reflux or progressive renal deterioration

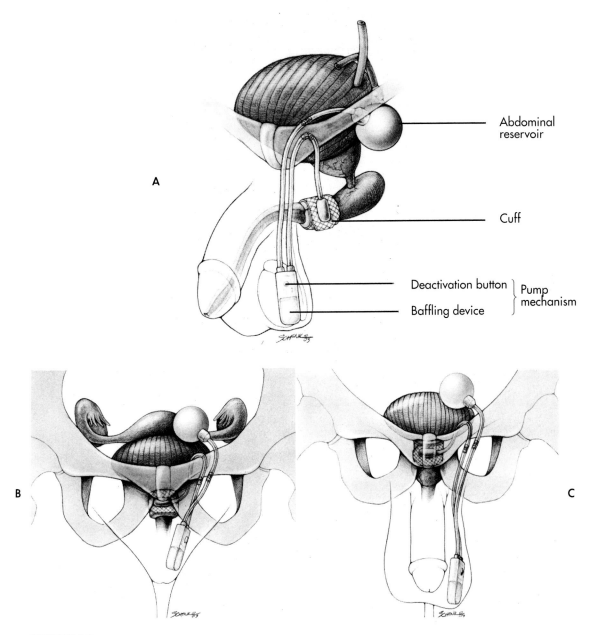

FIGURE 5-3
A, Placement of AUS cuff around bulbous urethra in male. **B,** Placement of AUS in female. Cuff is placed around bladder neck, balloon is placed in prevesical space, and pump is placed in labia. **C,** Placement of AUS in male. Cuff is placed around bladder neck, bolloon is placed in prevesical space and pump is placed in scrotum. (Courtesy American Medical Systems, Inc., Minnetonka, Minn.) (From Doughty D: *Urinary and fecal incontinence,* St Louis, 1991, Mosby–Year Book.)

PREPROCEDURAL NURSING CARE

NURSING DIAGNOSIS	NURSING INTERVENTIONS	RATIONALE
Knowledge deficit related to surgical procedure, its goals, and potential complications	Reinforce preoperative instruction, including the procedure, its goals, and potential adverse effects.	Anxiety is likely to reduce effective learning and retention of preoperative teaching; repeating the instruction enhances retention and reduces anxiety.
	Teach the patient to manipulate the artificial urinary sphincter, using an air-filled model, **before** surgery.	Manipulating the device requires integration of tactile, visual, and cognitive skills; preoperative instruction helps the patient successfully activate and operate the implanted prosthesis.
	Advise the patient that he will have an indwelling catheter for 6 to 8 days.	The catheter provides urinary drainage and allows monitoring of urine output.
	A small drain may be left in place for several days after surgery.	A closed-system drain is used to promote evacuation of exudate and prevent infection.
	Advise the patient that the sphincter will remain unused for about 6 weeks after surgery.	Manipulation of the device is limited until the incision has healed.
Potential for infection related to surgical implantation of prosthetic device	Obtain a urine culture before surgery; administer antiinfective agents for bacteriuria as directed based on laboratory-guided sensitivities.	Infection of the prosthesis is a leading complication that may necessitate explanation; aggressive eradication of bacteria in the urine lowers the risk of prosthetic infection.
	Administer prophylactic antiinfective medications as directed.	Antiinfective medications reduce the risk of infection of the prosthetic device.

POSTPROCEDURAL NURSING CARE

NURSING DIAGNOSIS	NURSING INTERVENTIONS	RATIONALE
Potential for infection related to surgical implantation of prosthetic device	Administer antiinfective medications as directed.	Parenteral antiinfective medications are administered for 4 days after surgery; oral suppressive medications are then given for an additional 14 days.
	Monitor drainage from the wound drain; maintain a closed system.	A wound drain is used to evacuate excessive exudate; a closed system further reduces the risk of infection.
	Maintain urinary drainage by means of an external collection device or containment device.	Because of the risk of bacteriuria, drainage by indwelling catheter is avoided until initial activation has been completed.
	Obtain a urine culture, and administer antiinfective medications as prescribed before initial activation.	Sterile urine and aggressive prophylaxis against implant infection are required for initial activation.

NURSING DIAGNOSIS	NURSING INTERVENTIONS	RATIONALE
Altered patterns of urinary elimination related to surgical implantation of prosthesis	Maintain urinary collection device or containment system during postoperative period before initial pump activation.	Stress incontinence will persist until the prosthesis is activated.
	Maintain deactivation of the cuff as directed.	Initially the periurethral cuff is left deactivated to allow revascularization under the cuff as the surgical site heals.
	Prepare the patient for initial activation; brief surgical manipulation is recommended.	Following adequate healing, cuff activation is completed to restore sphincter function.
	Teach the patient to place gentle downward traction on the pump device.	A dependent position is required to manipulate the AUS; scarring may cause upward migration of the pump.
	After initial activation, help the patient deflate and reinflate the AUS q 3 h.	Repeated inflation and deflation of the AUS assists in formation of a fibrous capsule around the device and helps the patient sharpen his skill in manipulating the device.
	Teach the patient to manipulate the pump mechanism. A man grasps the pump under the loose skin under the scrotum and squeezes the lower portion of the pump three to five times until it is soft and slightly collapsed. A woman is taught to work the pump in a similar manner by manipulating it under the labial skin. The pump passively refills over 1 to 3 minutes. Teach the patient to recognize the difference in the pump when the cuff is inflated and deflated.	The AUS substitutes for the normal sphincter mechanism; the patient must learn the function of the normal sphincter and proper manipulation of the AUS to maintain continence and to avoid complications from misuse of the device.
	Teach the patient who spontaneously voids or strain voids to deflate the cuff just before urination.	The inflated cuff produces continence by obstructing the urethra; deflating the cuff reverses this obstruction, allowing effective emptying.
	Teach the patient who self-catheterizes to deflate the cuff before inserting the catheter.	Inserting the catheter through the inflated cuff increases the risk of trauma to the urethra and subsequent infection of the AUS.
	Advise the patient that limited-volume stress incontinence may occur after successful AUS implantation, particularly with vigorous physical exertion; advise the patient to use a pad or dribble pouch if needed.	Even with successful AUS implantation, stress leakage may result from excessive bladder filling or with vigorous exertion; because excessive pressures are likely to produce cuff erosion or infection, small-volume stress leakage is an unavoidable outcome.

NURSING DIAGNOSIS	NURSING INTERVENTIONS	RATIONALE
	Advise the patient to obtain a medical alert bracelet that lists the AUS.	The presence of an AUS affects proper urinary drainage and urethral instrumentation; the medical alert bracelet will identify the patient's device if she or he is injured and unable to provide a medical history.

PATIENT TEACHING

1. Teach the patient to manipulate the artificial urinary sphincter, using a demonstration device, before surgery. Give careful, repeated instructions after the surgical implantation.
2. Teach the patient how a normal urinary sphincter functions, and explain how the artificial device reproduces this function.
3. Explain the possible complications associated with the artificial urinary sphincter. Teach the patient the signs of device infection and cuff erosion, and help him formulate a strategy to manage infection aggressively, thus minimizing the likelihood of explanation.
4. Teach the patient to consult the physician before invasive procedures are done. Explain that urologic instrumentation and other procedures may be preceded by antibiotic prophylaxis when an artificial urinary sphincter is in place.
5. Teach the patient to deactivate the pump, baffling fluid into the abdominal reservoir if indicated.

PERIURETHRAL INJECTION THERAPY

Periurethral injection therapy uses a bulking substance to reduce urethral caliber and prevent leakage (Figure 5-4). Two substances, GAX collagen and polytef paste, have been used in clinical trials. They are injected transurethrally or transperineally using local anesthesia with or without systemic sedation. The surgeon passes a special needle delivery system through the working port of a cystoscope. The needle is inserted just under the urethral mucosa, and the substance is injected until the urethral lumen is occluded (closed). A video monitoring system is helpful in the injection of periurethral collagen or polytef paste.

Periurethral injection offers several possible advantages over surgical procedures. These substances are injected via an endoscopic route so that no incision is needed. The procedures are completed on an outpatient basis, and a repeat injection can be done within 30 days if initial treatment does not restore continence. However, periurethral injection therapy also has certain potential disadvantages. Collagen is reabsorbed, and reinjection may be required after 2 to 5 years. In addition, polytef paste is known to migrate,[83] and the risks associated with this process remain unclear for

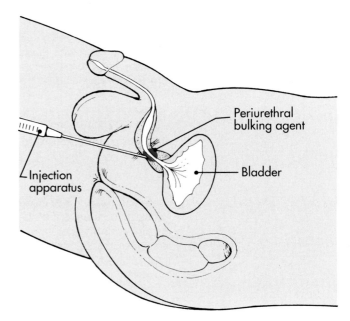

FIGURE 5-4
Transperineal injection of a urethral bulking agent in a male.

young adults or children, although short-term complications associated with migration of Teflon particles have not proved problematic. Polytef paste has been approved by the U.S. Food and Drug Administration for use in stress incontinence in men. No final decision has been made on the use of GAX collagen.

INDICATIONS

Stress incontinence stemming from sphincter incompetence

CONTRAINDICATIONS

Stress incontinence resulting from urethral hypermobility with mechanical obstruction

Detrusor instability without demonstrable stress urinary incontinence

Neuropathic bladder dysfunction with poor compliance or detrusor hyperreflexia (*unless* additional surgery is done to alleviate poor compliance or hyperreflexia)

Hypersensitivity to injection substance

COMPLICATIONS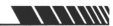

Persistent stress urinary incontinence (SUI)
Urinary retention (typically transient)
Recurrence of stress urinary incontinence

PREPROCEDURAL NURSING CARE

NURSING DIAGNOSIS	NURSING INTERVENTIONS	RATIONALE
Knowledge deficit related to procedure, its goals, and potential side effects	Reinforce preprocedural instruction, including the procedure, its goals, and potential side effects.	Anxiety before periurethral injection is likely to reduce learning and retention of knowledge; reinforcing preoperative teaching increases retention and reduces anxiety.
	Advise the patient that periurethral injection is not an open surgical procedure; local anesthesia, with or without systemic sedation, is used to prevent pain.	Periurethral injection is completed under endoscopic control; general or spinal anesthesia is not required, although local anesthesia and sedation are used for the discomfort caused by endoscopy and injection.
	Advise the patient that repeated injections may be required.	Repeat injections often are required, perhaps because of reabsorption of the substance or incomplete coaptation despite gross endoscopic appearance.
	Advise the patient that transient urinary retention may occur after periurethral injection.	The increased bladder outlet resistance produced by injection may cause transient urinary retention.
	Advise the patient with urinary residual caused by deficient detrusor contractility (noted on urodynamics) that urinary retention after injection may be long term, requiring intermittent catheterization for bladder evacuation.	The increased urethral resistance produced by injection may produce chronic urinary retention in an individual with compromised detrusor contractility.

➔ ❯ ❯ ❯

NURSING DIAGNOSIS	NURSING INTERVENTIONS	RATIONALE
Hypersensitivity response (potential) related to sensitivity to collagen substance	Administer collagen skin test via intradermal injection as directed.	Because of the potential for a hypersensitivity response to a semisynthetic collagen substance, a skin test is given before periurethral injection.
	Teach the patient to recognize a positive response to the skin test (redness, edema of the test site, itching, and discomfort are common) and to contact the physician or nurse promptly if a response is noted.	A positive skin test result indicates hypersensitivity to the collagen substance; the test site may require treatment.
Pain related to periurethral injection procedure	Administer or help physician administer oral or parenteral anxiolytic drugs.	Anxiolytics reduce pain associated with the procedure by their anxiolytic properties and by reducing skeletal muscle tone.
	Administer or help the physician administer a local anesthetic to the periurethral area.	Short-term anesthesia blocks the pain of endoscopy and injection.

POSTPROCEDURAL NURSING CARE

NURSING DIAGNOSIS	NURSING INTERVENTIONS	RATIONALE
Altered patterns of urinary elimination related to periurethral injection of GAX collagen or polytef paste	Monitor catheter for patency and urinary output.	A catheter may be left in place for several hours after the periurethral injection; occlusion of the catheter and retention cause pain and increase the risk of transient retention and urinary tract infection.
	Remove the catheter as directed and closely monitor the patient for spontaneous urination; obtain a urinary residual volume as directed.	Transient retention may occur after periurethral injection.
	Institute an intermittent catheterization program if the patient is unable to void spontaneously after periurethral injection.	Urinary retention is best managed by intermittent catheterization before spontaneous urination returns.
	Advise the patient that stress incontinence may persist or return after periurethral injection; arrange for follow-up evaluation, and reassure the individual that reinjection may be undertaken if leakage recurs or persists.	Stress incontinence may recur or persist after periurethral injection because of absorption of the substance or incomplete urethral occlusion; reinjection overcomes this problem.
	Advise the patient that stress incontinence may recur 2 to 5 years after injection; reassure the patient that reinjection would be expected to restore continence.	Reabsorption of collagen may occur after successful initial treatment; leakage may recur but is expected to respond to reinjection.

NURSING DIAGNOSIS	NURSING INTERVENTIONS	RATIONALE
	Advise the patient that he may note signs of instability (urge) incontinence after periurethral injection, particularly if instability is noted on urodynamic evaluation before injection; advise the patient to consult his physician for management of urge incontinence.	Instability incontinence may be intensified after correction of stress incontinence; it is a distinctive form of leakage from stress incontinence requiring different management strategies.

PATIENT TEACHING

1. Explain to the patient that periurethral injection is not an open surgical procedure. Reassure the patient that the procedure is done on an outpatient basis and that general anesthesia is not required.
2. Explain that GAX collagen is similar but not identical to collagen found in humans. Skin testing is crucial before testing to prevent potential hypersensitive or allergic responses.

3. Explain that incontinence may recur. Teach the patient to recognize the signs and symptoms of stress incontinence and to contact the physician for retreatment should leakage recur.
4. Teach the patient to recognize the distinctive signs of stress versus urge incontinence and to obtain treatment for urge leakage should it occur.

Instability (Urge) Incontinence

For videourodynamic image of instability (urge) incontinence, see Color Plate 3, page x.

Filling contractions occur in a significant portion of normal, adult women and among individuals with urge incontinence. A contraction is unstable when it compromises bladder capacity or produces leakage regardless of its maximum pressure.[77] Instability incontinence is leakage with unstable contractions (Figure 5-5).

PATHOPHYSIOLOGY

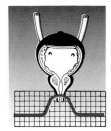

In a normal individual, sensations of urgency signal bladder filling. Nonetheless, bladder contractions are inhibited so that the desire to urinate can be postponed until the individual decides to empty the bladder. In an unstable bladder, however, bladder filling leads to hyperactive contractions that produce leakage unless voiding occurs within a few seconds or minutes. In addi-

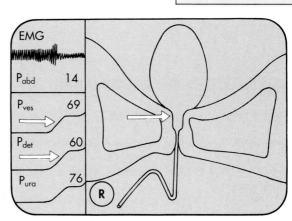

FIGURE 5-5
Diagram of instability (urge) incontinence. Arrows on left show the contraction noted in intravesical and detrusor pressure channels. Arrow on right shows open bladder outlet caused by contraction.

tion, other stimuli (e.g., placing the hands in warm water, anxiety, and physical exertion) also produce unstable detrusor contractions. Instability (urge) incontinence occurs when an individual is unable to gain sufficiently rapid access to a bathroom to relieve the contracting bladder. Instability (reflex) incontinence is leakage associated with bladder contraction without a sensation of urgency. Individuals with instability (reflex) incontinence are commonly alerted to the leakage when they see or feel their clothing absorbing urine.

Several conditions may cause or coexist with instability incontinence. Disorders of the brain may interfere with the inhibitory function of brain centers in the cerebral cortex, thalamus, cerebellum, basal ganglia, or other modulatory centers. Cerebrovascular accident (stroke) is the result of a hemorrhage or thrombus causing ischemia and damage to a portion of the brain. In the United States the middle cerebral and anterior cerebral arteries are most susceptible to stroke.[81] These arteries also supply the detrusor motor area, predisposing the affected individual to instability incontinence. Other brain disorders affecting continence include tumors, hydrocephalus, and certain seizure disorders. Because these disorders affect the central nervous system above the level of the pontine micturition center, bladder sensations remain intact and the striated sphincter remains coordinated with detrusor contractions.[63]

Stress incontinence is **associated** with instability incontinence, although a causal connection between these conditions has not been demonstrated.[85] In some cases instability incontinence resolves when stress incontinence is successfully abolished, whereas in other cases persistent or even more pronounced symptoms of urge leakage follow successful repair of stress leakage.

Bladder outlet obstruction is associated with detrusor instability, and there is some evidence of a causal relationship.[66,69] Obstruction of the bladder causes neurologic disruption of detrusor muscle cells and the nerves of the bladder wall. The greater the magnitude of obstruction, the greater the likelihood of instability with incontinence.

Irritative disorders of the bladder are associated with instability incontinence.[93] Bacterial, viral, fungal, or parasitic cystitis is likely to intensify preexisting instability leakage and irritative voiding symptoms but is not likely to produce incontinence in otherwise normal bladders. Calculi or tumors of the bladder provide a specific irritable focus in the bladder and cause irritative symptoms and instability leakage. Interstitial cystitis causes irritative symptoms and pain but is not likely to cause detrusor instability (see Interstitial Cystitis, page 63).

In many instances the cause of detrusor instability remains unknown. Instability (urge) incontinence is noted among children, elderly adults, and young adults who have no apparent neurologic, urologic, or other coexisting condition. Whether these individuals develop instability incontinence as a result of subtle neuropathy, local irritative foci, or other causes remains uncertain.

COMPLICATIONS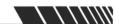

Urinary tract infection
Dyssynergia with urinary retention (principally noted in children)

DIAGNOSTIC STUDIES AND FINDINGS

Diagnostic test	Findings
Urodynamics	Small cystometric capacity with sensory urgency; contractions noted during filling cystometrogram compromise capacity and/or produce leakage; striated sphincter typically coordinated with detrusor contraction
Voiding diary	Small functional bladder capacity; frequent diurnal voiding (q 2 h or more often); patient notes urgency to void and associates leakage with strong urge to urinate; nocturia more often than one episode per night is common
Intravenous pyelogram/ urogram (IVP/IVU)	Dilation of upper tracts and bladder trabeculation with instability incontinence associated with obstruction (IVP/IVU is indicated only in cases where obstructive uropathy or anatomic defects are suspected)

MEDICAL MANAGEMENT

GENERAL MANAGEMENT AND DRUG THERAPY

Administration of antispasmodic/anticholinergic drugs (see box below)

Electrostimulation therapy

Bladder drill therapy

Pharmacotherapy or chemotherapy for underlying irritative or inflammatory bladder disorders

SURGICAL THERAPY

Surgical resection of obstructive lesion

Surgical repair of stress incontinence

Bladder denervation procedures

Surgical implantation of electrostimulation device

PHARMACOTHERAPY FOR INSTABILITY INCONTINENCE

Anticholinergic/antispasmodic drugs: propantheline, dicyclomine, oxybutynin, hyoscyamine, flavoxate

Action and administration: Unstable detrusor contractions are inhibited by anticholinergic or postganglionic inhibition of smooth muscle; functional capacity is enhanced and sensory urgency reduced; all antispasmodic drugs are administered over a 24-hour period

Dosages: *Propantheline:* 15-30 mg tid; *Dicyclomine:* 10-20 tid; *Oxybutynin:* 2.5 mg bid, then titrated to 5 mg bid-qid; *Hyoscyamine:* 0.125-0.25 mg bid-tid; *Flavoxate:* 100-200 mg tid-qid

Side effects: Dry mouth, constipation, transient mydriasis, flushing or heat intolerance

Combination antispasmodic/alpha sympathomimetic drug: imipramine

Action and administration: Tricyclic antidepressant with antispasmodic and alpha sympathomimetic actions administered over a 24-hour period

Dosage: 10-25 mg tid-qid

Note: Drug is withdrawn in tapered dosage to prevent untoward psychotropic effects

Side effects: Drowsiness, dry mouth, constipation, hypertension, mydriasis (mild)

Calcium channel blockers

Action and administration: Act at smooth muscle cell to block calcium efflux needed for depolarization and contraction; administered in combination with antispasmodic drug

Dosage: 80 mg tid-qid

Side effects: Dizziness, hypotension, mydriasis, fatigue

1 ASSESS

ASSESSMENT	OBSERVATIONS
Instability (urge) incontinence	Patient associates leakage with profound urgency to void; often reports inability to reach toilet in time to avert leakage
Coexisting stress urinary incontinence	Patient also has leakage with coughing, laughing, exercise, or physical exertion
Neurologic disorder	Altered mobility, cognition, and dexterity caused by lesion of the brain; hemiparesis related to cerebrovascular accident
Inflammatory lesion of bladder	Irritative voiding symptoms (urgency, diurnal frequency, nocturia) with cloudy, foul-smelling urine, hematuria, or other evidence of inflammation of urinary system
Bladder outlet obstruction	Poor force of stream with urinary residual in addition to symptoms of urge incontinence
Patterns of urinary elimination	Diurnal frequency, nocturia noted on voiding diary
Altered skin integrity	Perineal skin moist and odorous with red, maculopapular rash with satellite lesions (monilial rash) or pale raised lesions of ammonia contact dermatitis
Social isolation	Patient reports loneliness or fear of social contact
Altered mobility and dexterity	Assistance with walking required; patient requires assistance removing clothing, is unable to manipulate zippers, buttons, and undergarments
Environmental barriers to bathroom	Barriers to toilet access (stairs, excessive distance, doorframe inappropriate for wheelchair access) are noted; patient cannot transfer to toilet seat that lacks appropriate hand rails or is set too low

2 DIAGNOSE

NURSING DIAGNOSIS	SUBJECTIVE FINDINGS	OBJECTIVE FINDINGS
Urge incontinence related to unstable detrusor contractions	Complains of leakage with urge to urinate	Unstable detrusor, small capacity noted on urodynamics
Impaired skin integrity related to instability (urge) incontinence	Reports skin rashes, lesions	Irritation of perineal skin

NURSING DIAGNOSIS	SUBJECTIVE FINDINGS	OBJECTIVE FINDINGS
Social isolation related to urinary leakage, odor, and fear of embarrassment and discovery	Reports decrease in ability to participate in social activities	Appearance unkempt; poor hygiene; activities of daily living (ADLs) involve minimal contact with others
Impaired physical mobility (dexterity) related to neurologic or other deficits	Reports difficulty ambulating, inability to walk, and/or difficulty manipulating clothing	Mobility is slowed; patient uses a cane or other assistive device; patient has difficulty manipulating buttons and zippers

3 PLAN

Patient goals

1. Symptoms of urge incontinence will be resolved or controlled by a bladder management program.
2. Patterns of urinary elimination will return to normal.
3. Skin integrity will be restored and maintained.
4. The patient will have adequate access to a toilet facility and will be able to maneuver onto the toilet seat independently or with minimal assistance.

4 IMPLEMENT

NURSING DIAGNOSIS	NURSING INTERVENTIONS	RATIONALE
Urge incontinence related to unstable detrusor contractions	Consult the patient and physician about definitive interventions to manage instability incontinence.	Several viable options exist for treatment of instability (urge) incontinence; an appropriate decision is made by mutual goal-setting involving the physician, nurse, patient, and significant others as indicated.
	Institute a timed voiding schedule based on the results of the voiding diary.	Unstable detrusor contractions are triggered by bladder filling as well as by other provocative stimuli; a timed voiding schedule is designed to evacuate the bladder before these contractions occur.
	Institute a fluid management program. Advise the patient to avoid a large intake of fluid over a brief period; instead, teach the person to sip beverages throughout the day and to limit fluids to 8 ounces with meals. Liquids are restricted to sips starting several hours before sleep.	The goal of a fluid management program is to avoid a large intake of fluid that provokes instability incontinence while ensuring an adequate fluid intake to minimize the risk of urinary tract infection.
	Administer or teach the patient to self-administer antispasmodic/anticholinergic medications as directed (see box on page 123).	Antispasmodic medications reduce detrusor contractility and irritative voiding symptoms and increase bladder capacity.

→ → →

NURSING DIAGNOSIS	NURSING INTERVENTIONS	RATIONALE
	Administer or teach the patient to self-administer tricyclic antidepressant or calcium channel blocking drugs in combination with antispasmodic agents.	Calcium channel blockers or tricyclic antidepressants inhibit detrusor contractility by postganglionic or central effects; thus they may act synergistically when administered with antispasmodics.
	Teach the patient to avoid excessively restricting daily fluids in an attempt to minimize urinary leakage.	Patients may incorrectly assume that avoiding fluids prevents instability incontinence and urinary frequency; ironically, marked limitation of fluids only concentrates urine, intensifying irritative voiding symptoms and predisposing the system to bacterial infection.
	Inform the patient that particular beverages or other substances may irritate the bladder mucosa; advise him to eliminate substances one at a time and evaluate results.	Caffeinic beverages, citrus juices, carbonated drinks, cigarette smoke, and certain spicy foods may cause mild bladder irritation, intensifying symptoms of instability incontinence.
	Teach the patient to identify stimuli other than urine volume that are likely to cause instability leakage; advise him to empty his bladder before engaging in these activities whenever possible.	Stimuli other than bladder filling may cause unstable contractions. Placing the hands in warm water, entering a cool room or stepping into cold air, coughing, or other events may provoke unstable contractions. Emptying the bladder before engaging in these activities may prevent leakage.
	Institute a bladder drill program in consultation with the physician and patient. Instruct the patient to void every hour while awake regardless of desire to urinate or occurrence of instability incontinence. After the individual achieves success with this interval, the interval is increased by ½ h increments to a goal of 3 h.	A bladder drill program is a behavioral management strategy that reduces symptoms of instability incontinence by increasing functional capacity. The success of the program relies on the patient's motivation and ability to tolerate the program for several weeks. Bladder drill represents an alternative to pharmacologic management that has proven successful among individuals with detrusor instability.
	Institute electrostimulation therapy in consultation with the patient and physician. Teach the patient to self-administer therapy daily at home. Determine the duration of daily therapy and pulse frequency and width in consultation with the physician. Teach the patient to adjust the current at home by slowly increasing the intensity until mild discomfort is perceived. The home unit is reduced to just below this point for best benefit.	Electrostimulation therapy uses transcutaneous, transvaginal, or transrectal probes or an implanted device to stimulate pelvic and pudendal nerves. Therapy works by inhibiting pelvic nerves, enhancing bladder capacity, and reducing sensory urgency.

NURSING DIAGNOSIS	NURSING INTERVENTIONS	RATIONALE
	Combine electrostimulation with bladder drill therapy for best results.	Bladder drill therapy and electrostimulation reduce instability incontinence by enhancing functional capacity; combining these therapies is expected to enhance results.
	Administer or teach the patient to self-administer antispasmodic agents as directed to "paralyze" the detrusor, and institute an intermittent catheterization program.	Antispasmodic drugs may be used to pharmacologically paralyze the detrusor muscle. Bladder evacuation is then accomplished via clean intermittent catheterization. Acceptance of the program is limited by the increased incidence of drug side effects related to greater dosages and intolerance of intermittent catheterization. Therapy typically is reserved for individuals with instability and urinary retention.
Impaired skin integrity related to instability (urge) incontinence	Help the patient identify, choose, and obtain an appropriate urinary collection device.	The ideal urinary collection device protects the skin by completely absorbing leakage, thus minimizing the amount of time urine is in contact with the skin.
	Teach the patient the principles of a skin care program (i.e., regular washing, complete drying, applying a moisture barrier or skin sealant, and using a collection device).	Maintaining healthy skin depends on regular cleansing and complete drying; moisture barriers or skin sealants offer some protection from exposure to urinary leakage, and collection devices protect skin by minimizing exposure to urine.
	Administer or teach the patient to self-administer an antifungal cream or powder as directed for monilial rash.	Monilial rashes are managed by routine skin care and local application of an antifungal cream or powder.
	Teach the patient with ammonia contact dermatitis to clean the skin with soap and water; thoroughly dry the skin; and direct warm, dry air at the area for 15 minutes daily; advise him to use a hand-held hair dryer set at lowest setting. Between treatments teach the patient to apply a skin sealant or moisture barrier and to use an appropriate containment device.	Ammonia contact dermatitis occurs as a result of prolonged exposure of the skin to urine. Regular, complete drying and using a moisture barrier or skin sealant and collection device minimizes exposure.
	Encourage the patient to implement a definitive management program for instability (urge) incontinence.	Definitive management of incontinence protects the skin, eliminating exposure to urine.
Social isolation related to urinary leakage, odor, and fear of embarrassment and discovery	Encourage the patient to seek a definitive management program for instability incontinence.	Many patients are advised by families, friends, or even health care professionals to "live with" their condition; treatment and resolution are realistic goals that can prevent complications such as social isolation.

NURSING DIAGNOSIS	NURSING INTERVENTIONS	RATIONALE
	Reassure the elderly patient that urinary leakage is more common among older persons, but *is not* an inevitable part of growing older.	Elderly patients, in particular, are likely to receive incorrect advice that urinary leakage is an inevitable part of aging.
	Help the patient to contact an advocacy or support group such as Help for Incontinent People (HIP), the SIMON Foundation, or Continence Restored, Inc. (see box on page 93).	Patient advocacy groups provide support and help participants obtain health care for urinary leakage; advocacy groups also help the patient identify strategies for coping with leakage until a definitive management program has been completed.
Impaired physical mobility (dexterity) related to neurologic or other deficits	Remove or reduce barriers to toilet access; install appropriate lighting, remove loose rugs as indicated; install assistive devices, including hand rails and raised toilet seats, as indicated.	Environmental barriers reduce access to the toilet and increase the likelihood of incontinence.
	Help the patient maximize his mobility by obtaining appropriate assistive devices; replace slick-soled shoes with nonskid tennis shoes; consult physical therapist for walker, wheelchair, or cane as indicated.	Immobility reduces access to the toilet and increases the risk of leakage; assistive devices maximize mobility and reduce the incidence of leakage.
	Help the patient alter clothing to maximize compromised dexterity; replace zippers and buttons with Velcro, and eliminate unnecessary undergarments.	Compromised dexterity slows the removal of clothing for urinating; reducing the time required to remove clothing reduces the risk of leakage.
Knowledge deficit	See Patient Teaching.	

5   EVALUATE

PATIENT OUTCOME	DATA INDICATING THAT OUTCOME IS REACHED
Symptoms of urge incontinence have resolved or are controlled by a bladder management program.	Incontinent episodes are avoided, and symptoms of urgency to urinate do not inevitably lead to leakage.
Patterns of urinary elimination have returned to normal.	Diurnal frequency occurs q 2 h or less often; nocturia occurs once per night or not at all.
Skin integrity has been restored and is maintained.	Examination of perineal skin reveals no lesions or rashes; the patient accurately describes a skin care program and use of a collection device.

PATIENT OUTCOME	DATA INDICATING THAT OUTCOME IS REACHED
Patient has adequate access to a toilet facility and can maneuver onto the seat with minimal assistance.	Patient demonstrates ability to reach toilet and manipulate clothing for bladder evacuation; environmental barriers have been removed or circumvented.

PATIENT TEACHING

1. Teach the patient the cause of instability leakage and the stimuli likely to produce leakage.

2. Teach the patient the signs and symptoms of urinary tract infection and a strategy to manage infection should it occur.

Instability (Reflex) Incontinence

Detrusor instability without normal bladder sensations produces leakage without warning signals of sensory urgency. Thus bladder evacuation occurs at unpredictable times and in response to volume or other stimuli such as exposure to cool air or stroking the perineal skin (Figure 5-6).

PATHOPHYSIOLOGY

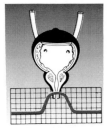

Disease or trauma affecting the spinal cord above the sacral micturition center (S2-4) produces instability (reflex) incontinence. Spinal injury, lesions of multiple sclerosis, spinovascular disease, spinal stenosis, spina bifida defects, transverse myelitis, and related conditions also produce detrusor instability without sensations of bladder filling. Because these lesions occur below the pontine micturition center, detrusor instability coexists with vesicosphincter dyssynergia.

Vesicosphincter dyssynergia is the loss of coordination between striated muscle of the sphincter mechanism and the detrusor muscle. Normally the sphincter mechanism acts as a door between the bladder and the outside world. During bladder filling, the door remains closed, preventing urine from escaping. During micturition, however, the door swings open to allow the passage of urine for effective emptying. The dyssyner-

gic sphincter, in contrast, fails to relax during micturition, causing bladder outlet obstruction and urinary retention.

> For videourodynamic image of instability (reflex) incontinence, see Color Plate 4, page xi.

Because instability (reflex) incontinence is associated with vesicosphincter dyssynergia and obstruction, there is a significant risk of upper urinary tract distress. Specifically, febrile urinary tract infection (pyelonephritis), upper urinary tract dilation (hydronephrosis), vesicoureteral reflux, and compromised renal function may occur as a result of dyssynergia and instability incontinence.

Autonomic dysreflexia also complicates certain cases of instability (reflex) incontinence.[86] Dysreflexia is massive sympathetic firing in response to a noxious stimulus. This neural discharge causes the blood pressure to rise precipitously to potentially dangerous levels. The patient has a pounding headache, tachycardia with palpitations, dilation of the pupils, and a feeling of anxiety. Bladder distention and high-pressure detrusor contractions are the most common source of dysreflexia. Less commonly, bowel distention, digital evacuation maneuvers, and infection of pressure sores or other foci of infection may cause autonomic dysreflexia.

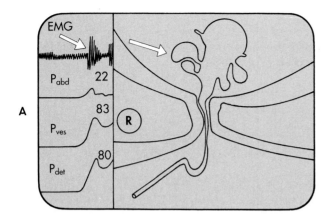

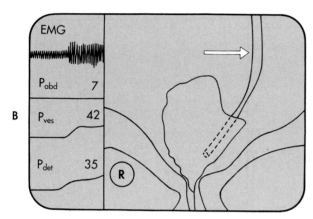

FIGURE 5-6
A, Diagram of reflex incontinence with trabeculation caused by vesicosphincter dyssynergia. Arrow on the left indicates sphincter EMG activity of dyssynergia, and arrow on the right shows severe trabeculation with diverticula. **B,** Diagram of instability (reflex) incontinence with vesicoureteral reflux. Arrow indicates left reflux caused by dyssynergia.

COMPLICATIONS

Urinary tract infection
Pyelonephritis
Vesicoureteral reflux
Compromised renal function
Altered skin integrity
Shame, humiliation, social isolation

PHARMACOTHERAPY FOR VESICOSPHINCTER DYSSYNERGIA

Alpha blocking drugs: phenoxybenzamine, prazosin, terazosin

Action and administration: Selectively blocks alpha-1 adrenergic receptors of bladder neck, prostatic urethra, and rhabdosphincter; used to reduce obstruction produced by vesicosphincter dyssynergia; titration and hs administration to avert side effects of fatigue and postural hypotension

Dosage: *Phenoxybenzamine:* 10 mg at hs, titrated to 20 mg at hs; *Prazosin:* 1 mg at hs, titrated to 10 mg at hs; *Terazosin:* 1 mg at hs, titrated to 10 mg at hs

Side effects: Postural hypotension, fatigue, rhinitis

From Govoni L and Hayes J: *Drugs and nursing implications,* Norwalk, Conn, 1988, Appleton & Lange.

DIAGNOSTIC STUDIES AND FINDINGS

Diagnostic Test	Findings
Voiding diary	Diurnal frequency more often than q 2 h; enuresis
Videourodynamics	Small cystometric capacity; high-pressure, unstable detrusor contractions with dyssynergia on sphincter EMG; fluoroscopy demonstrates funneling of bladder neck with narrowing of membranous urethra in men and midurethra in women, bladder trabeculation; diverticula (herniation of bladder mucosa through muscular wall) and vesicoureteral reflux (retrograde movement of contrast from bladder to kidney) may be present
Intravenous pyelogram/ urogram (IVP/IVU)	Hydronephrosis, caliectasis, and ureteral dilation of one or both collecting systems may be present
Dimercaptosuccinic acid (DMSA) radionuclide scan	Renal scarring of one or both kidneys resulting from pyelonephritis; differential renal function may be asymmetric because of focal scarring
Diethylenetriamine penta-acetic acid (DTPA) radionuclide scan	Obstruction of kidneys usually absent (obstruction arises from dyssynergic sphincter mechanism)

MEDICAL MANAGEMENT

GENERAL MANAGEMENT AND DRUG THERAPY

Administration of antispasmodic agents and an intermittent catheterization program

In men, condom catheter drainage with pharmacologic sphincterotomy

Routine evaluation of upper urinary tract function

Indwelling urinary catheter (suprapubic or urethral)

SURGICAL THERAPY

Surgical sphincterotomy with condom catheter containment

Augmentation enterocystoplasty and an intermittent catheterization program

Continent or incontinent urinary diversion and an intermittent catheterization program or pouch containment device

1 ASSESS

ASSESSMENT	OBSERVATIONS
Reflex incontinence	Voiding with intermittent stream and no control; patient notes no urgency before leakage; incontinence not evoked by physical exertion
Altered patterns of urinary elimination	Voiding diary shows diurnal frequency more often than q 2 h; enuresis
Autonomic dysreflexia	Micturition associated with diaphoresis; a pounding headache; acute, transient hypertension; and tachycardia
Social isolation	Patient reports avoiding activities requiring interaction with those other than family or caregivers
Urinary tract infection	Foul-smelling urine with bacteriuria or pyuria (fever may be present)
Urinary tract distress	Imaging studies of upper urinary tract demonstrate ureterohydronephrosis; radionuclide studies demonstrate focal renal scarring; serum laboratory studies demonstrate abnormal blood urea nitrogen (BUN), creatinine

→ > >

2   DIAGNOSE

NURSING DIAGNOSIS	SUBJECTIVE FINDINGS	OBJECTIVE FINDINGS
Reflex incontinence related to spinal lesion or disease	Reports uncontrolled bladder evacuation without sensations of urgency or physical exertion	Detrusor hyperreflexia, vesicosphincter dyssynergia, and no sensations of bladder filling are noted on urodynamic testing
Potential for infection (urinary) related to urinary retention and obstruction	Reports signs and symptoms of urinary tract infection	Urine culture reveals >100,000 colony-forming units (CFU)/ml of urine
Impaired skin integrity related to chronic exposure to urine	Reports rashes and lesions on perineal skin	Moist, odorous perineal skin with compromised integrity
Autonomic dysreflexia (potential) related to instability (reflex) incontinence	Reports a pounding headache and rapid, pounding pulse of sudden onset	Severe hypertension, diaphoresis above the level of the injury, and tachycardia
Social isolation related to urinary leakage, odor, and fear of embarrassment and discovery	Reports less participation in activities that require interaction with others	Unkempt appearance; poor hygiene; reports that activities of daily living (ADLs) involve minimal interaction with others
Impaired physical mobility (dexterity) related to neurologic or other deficits	Reports difficulty ambulating, inability to walk, and difficulty manipulating clothing	Mobility is slowed; uses wheelchair or assistive device; has difficulty manipulating buttons and zippers

3   PLAN

Patient goals

1. Instability (reflex) incontinence will be prevented, and the patient will evacuate his bladder by intermittent catheterization or will contain urine by using a condom device.
2. Urinary tract infections will be avoided or promptly managed; febrile urinary tract infections will be avoided.
3. Skin integrity will be restored and maintained.
4. Autonomic dysreflexia will be avoided or promptly managed.
5. Social isolation will be avoided.
6. Impaired mobility will be minimized by appropriate assistive devices and rehabilitation.

4 IMPLEMENT

NURSING DIAGNOSIS	NURSING INTERVENTIONS	RATIONALE
Reflex incontinence related to spinal lesion or disease	Determine a bladder management program in consultation with the patient, family, and other members of the health care team.	Reflex incontinence usually occurs with a spinal injury or disease that affects mobility and bladder function; incontinence management is ideally is done in a rehabilitation institution.
	Maintain an indwelling Foley catheter in a patient with an acute spinal injury.	An acute spinal injury produces a period of transient spinal shock during which the bladder is acontractile; an indwelling Foley catheter provides temporary drainage until this phase has passed.
	Administer or teach the patient to self-administer antispasmodic medications as directed. Institute an intermittent catheterization program with pharmacotherapy, and begin teaching the patient and family how to perform clean intermittent catheterization at home.	Antispasmodic medications are used to "paralyze" the detrusor, preventing all contractions (refer to box, page 123). The intermittent catheterization program ensures complete, regular bladder evacuation.
	Administer or teach the patient to self-administer calcium channel blocking drugs or tricyclic antidepressants in combination with antispasmodic drugs.	Calcium channel blocking drugs and tricyclic antidepressants act synergistically with antispasmodics to inhibit unstable contractions.
	Institute a reflex voiding program with a condom collection device as directed; select an appropriate leg bag and show the patient how to use it.	A reflex voiding program ideally is used for men who lack motivation or adequate dexterity to perform intermittent catheterization; this program typically requires reducing the obstruction caused by dyssynergia.
	Administer or teach the patient to self-administer an alpha sympathomimetic antagonist as directed (see box, page 130).	Alpha sympathomimetic antagonists reduce obstruction caused by vesicosphincter dyssynergia by decreasing smooth muscle tone in the bladder neck and proximal urethra; they also may reduce tone at the level of the rhabdosphincter (see box on page 130).
	Prepare the patient for insertion of a urethral stent as directed.	The Uro-Lume urethral stent and Intraprostatic stent have the potential to reduce obstruction from vesicosphincter dyssynergia mechanically by preventing complete closure of the membranous urethra (these devices currently are undergoing clinical trials in the United States and are not approved for this use by the FDA).

→ › ›

NURSING DIAGNOSIS	NURSING INTERVENTIONS	RATIONALE
	Prepare the patient for surgical sphincterotomy as directed.	Surgical sphincterotomy uses a transurethral approach to incise the membranous urethra, reducing obstruction caused by vesicosphincter dyssynergia (see Transurethral Sphincterotomy, page 138).
	Prepare the patient for augmentation enterocystoplasty with a subsequent intermittent catheterization program as directed.	Augmentation enterocystoplasty is the surgical reconstruction of the bladder using a segment of the small or large bowel or stomach (see Augmentation Enterocystoplasty, page 140).
	Prepare the patient for continent or incontinent urinary diversion as directed (see pages 221 and 227).	Creation of a continent or incontinent diversion for individuals with instability (reflex) incontinence is reserved for those with bladders that are not amenable to augmentation procedures or more conservative management options.
Potential for infection (urinary) related to urinary retention and obstruction	Teach the patient to recognize the signs of significant urinary infection: foul-smelling urine with hematuria, fever, chills or acute onset of previously controlled instability (reflex) incontinence.	Significant urinary infection may involve the kidneys and may lead to systemic sepsis unless antiinfective treatment is begun promptly.
	Teach the patient how to obtain a urine specimen for culture, and instruct him to obtain treatment promptly for significant urinary infection; advise him that febrile patients usually are treated empirically before a final culture and sensitivity report is done and that other infections are managed after the final laboratory reports have arrived.	Significant urinary infection may lead to pyelonephritis and sepsis if left untreated.
	Reassure the patient with instability (reflex) incontinence that the presence of bacteriuria does not imply significant urinary infection.	Bacteriuria often is detected among individuals with instability (reflex) incontinence managed by intermittent catheterization or a reflex voiding program. Because attempts to maintain a continuously sterile urine only lead to colonization of the bladder with resistant organisms, asymptomatic bacteriuria is tolerated among these patients.
	Consult the physician about prophylactic antiinfective therapy for bacteriuria.	Suppressive or prophylactic antiinfective drug therapy is used sparingly among individuals with instability (reflex) incontinence because of the danger of creating resistant organisms in the urine.

NURSING DIAGNOSIS	NURSING INTERVENTIONS	RATIONALE
	Instruct the patient to drink adequate fluids (at least 1,500 ml, or about six 8-ounce glasses, for adults each day).	The antegrade movement of urine through the kidneys and ureter and into the bladder is an important defense mechanism against bacterial infection; adequate fluid intake flushes the urinary system, promoting mechanical movement of bacteria away from the kidneys.
	Advise the patient to use clean, dry catheters for intermittent catheterization, to practice good hygiene of the perineal area, and to routinely clean bedside and leg urine collection bags.	Ascending infection from the urethra is the most common cause of cystitis; clean catheters and collection bags and good perineal hygiene reduce the number of bacteria available to invade the reflex neurogenic bladder.
Impaired skin integrity related to chronic exposure to urine	Help the patient identify, choose, and obtain an appropriate urinary collection device.	The ideal urinary collection device protects the skin by completely absorbing leakage, thus minimizing the time urine is in contact with the skin.
	Help the patient managed by a reflex voiding program to obtain and use an appropriate condom device.	The ideal condom device is relatively easy to put on the penis, forms a watertight seal, and readily drains without kinking or twisting at its distal end; the condom should remain in place for 24 h.
	Inspect and teach the patient to inspect the penile skin each time the condom is changed.	The penile skin is visible only with condom catheter changes; regular inspection ensures early detection of lesions and prevents serious complications such as erosion or pressure sores.
	Consult the physician about a temporary indwelling catheter when skin integrity is compromised.	A temporary indwelling catheter hastens healing by allowing the skin to remain dry and free of exposure to urine.
	Teach the patient the principles of skin care (i.e., regular washing, complete drying, applying a moisture barrier or skin sealant, and using a collection device).	Maintenance of skin integrity relies on regular cleansing and complete drying. Moisture barriers or skin sealants offer some protection from exposure to urinary leakage. Collection devices protect skin by minimizing exposure to urine.
	Administer or teach the patient to self-administer an antifungal cream or powder for monilial rash as prescribed.	Monilial rashes are managed by routine skin care and local application of an antifungal cream or powder.

NURSING DIAGNOSIS	NURSING INTERVENTIONS	RATIONALE
	Teach the patient with ammonia contact dermatitis to clean the skin with soap and water; thoroughly dry skin; and direct warm, dry air to the area for 15 min daily. Advise him to use a hand-held hair dryer set at lowest setting. Between treatments teach the patient to apply a skin sealant or moisture barrier and to use an appropriate containment device.	Ammonia contact dermatitis occurs as a result of prolonged exposure of the skin to urine; regular, complete drying and using a moisture barrier or skin sealant and collection devices minimize exposure.
	Encourage the patient to implement a definitive management program for instability (reflex) incontinence.	Definitive management of incontinence protects the skin by eliminating exposure to urine.
Autonomic dysreflexia (potential) related to instability (reflex) incontinence	Teach the patient the signs and symptoms of autonomic dysreflexia (pounding headache, diaphoresis, palpitations, and rapid pulse).	Autonomic dysreflexia is a massive discharge of the sympathetic nervous system, producing transient hypertension, headache, diaphoresis, and tachycardia; rapid management is indicated.
	Quickly move the patient to an upright position as indicated.	Assuming an upright position may temporarily reduce blood pressure.
	Assess the individual for an irritative source producing autonomic dysreflexia; catheterize the bladder, discontinue digital bowel elimination maneuvers, and check for pressure sores and other sources of irritation.	Autonomic dysreflexia is triggered by noxious stimuli. Bladder contractions or distention and manipulation of the bowel for evacuation are common, readily reversible causes of dysreflexia. Other sources of infection occasionally cause dysreflexia.
	Administer antihypertensive drugs as directed.	Antihypertensive drugs temporarily relieve hypertension associated with autonomic dysreflexia.
Social isolation related to urinary leakage, odor, and fear of embarrassment and discovery	Reassure the patient that urinary incontinence will be controlled despite the spinal injury or disease affecting bladder control.	Spinal disease or injury results in complete loss of bladder control, including impaired motor and sensory function. Instituting a bladder management program will not restore normal function but will provide an acceptable level of continence or urinary containment for continued social interaction.
	Encourage and assist the patient to participate in support groups for persons with spinal disease or spinal cord injury.	Patient support groups provide advocacy for members and help participants to identify strategies for coping with the changes in health and life-style caused by spinal injury or disease.

NURSING DIAGNOSIS	NURSING INTERVENTIONS	RATIONALE
	Encourage and assist the patient to participate in outings when participating in a rehabilitation program.	Field trips and outings are an important component of learning to cope with altered bladder function and spinal injury or disease; participation in these outings lessens social isolation during a rehabilitation program and prepares the individual to follow a bladder management program while participating in other social activities.
Impaired physical mobility (dexterity) related to neurologic or other deficits	Select a bladder management program appropriate for the patient's functional abilities and wishes.	The success of any bladder management program depends on the patient's motivation and desires, physical abilities, urologic status, and available in-home support systems.
	Remove or minimize environmental barriers to the bathroom, including wheelchair-inaccessible doorways, low toilet seats, and narrow stalls whenever feasible; provide a bedside urinal, raised toilet seat, and hand rails as appropriate.	Environmental barriers increase the incidence of reflex incontinence by hampering the individual's attempts to execute an appropriate bladder management program; removing these barriers decreases the incidence of leakage.
	Consult occupational and physical therapists for assistive devices and products specifically designed for individuals with compromised manual dexterity.	Manipulation of clothing, catheters, leg bags, and related products requires varying levels of manual dexterity; assistive devices and specially designed products increase self-reliance by minimizing the degree of fine motor movement needed to use a product or device.
Knowledge deficit	See Patient Teaching.	

5 EVALUATE

PATIENT OUTCOME	DATA INDICATING THAT OUTCOME IS REACHED
Instability (reflex) incontinence has been prevented; patient evacuates bladder by intermittent catheterization or contains urine by condom device.	Patient catheterizes q 4-6 h, and no leakage occurs between catheterizations; reflex voiding program is managed successfully, and the condom catheter and collection bag contain all urine output.
Urinary tract infections have been avoided or are promptly managed; febrile urinary tract infections have been avoided.	Symptomatic urinary infection is avoided regardless of presence of bacteriuria.

→ > >

PATIENT OUTCOME	DATA INDICATING THAT OUTCOME IS REACHED
Skin integrity has been restored and is maintained.	Examination of perineal skin reveals no lesions or rashes; the patient accurately describes a skin management program.
Autonomic dysreflexia has been avoided or is promptly managed.	Blood pressure remains within normal range; acute episodes of dysreflexia are rapidly managed, and the source of dysreflexia is identified and treated.
Social isolation has been avoided.	The patient routinely engages in social activities.
Impaired mobility has been minimized by appropriate assistive devices and rehabilitation.	A goal-oriented rehabilitation program has been successfully completed; the patient demonstrates the ability to manage his bladder independently to the extent possible.

PATIENT TEACHING

1. Teach the patient the pathophysiology of reflex incontinence and the roles of the spine and brain in normal bladder function.
2. Teach the patient that a bladder management program will establish an acceptable level of continence or urinary containment but will not cure leakage or restore normal bladder function.
3. Explain the signs and symptoms of cystitis and febrile urinary infections and the importance of prompt management of symptomatic bacteriuria.
4. Teach the patient the names, action, dosage, and potential side effects of medications used to inhibit detrusor instability or reduce outlet obstruction.

TRANSURETHRAL SPHINCTEROTOMY

Sphincterotomy is the surgical incision of the urethral sphincter using a transurethral approach. The membranous urethra is visualized endoscopically, and a 12 o'clock incision is made. A three-way catheter with bladder irrigation is left in place to provide hemostasis and to prevent or evacuate clots from the bladder.

INDICATIONS

Instability (reflex) incontinence with vesicosphincter dyssynergia that does not respond to conservative management

CONTRAINDICATIONS

Bladder wall hypocompliance
Urinary retention with detrusor decompensation

COMPLICATIONS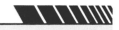

Postoperative hemorrhage
Acute postoperative urinary retention
Persistent urinary retention

PREPROCEDURAL NURSING CARE

NURSING DIAGNOSIS	NURSING INTERVENTIONS	RATIONALE
Knowledge deficit related to procedure, its goals, and potential side effects	Reinforce preoperative instruction, including a description of the procedure, its goals, and potential side effects.	Preoperative learning and retention are reduced by anxiety; reinforcing this teaching enhances learning and retention.
	Prepare the patient for spinal or general anesthesia.	Spinal or general anesthesia may be used for this relatively brief procedure.
	Advise the patient that she will have an indwelling catheter in the urethra for 5 to 7 days after the surgery.	The catheter provides hemostasis and irrigation to prevent clot formation and obstruction in the urethra.
Potential for infection related to surgical trauma of the urethra	Obtain urine cultures as directed.	Bacteriuria is eradicated before sphincterotomy to prevent systemic spread.
	Administer antiinfective medications as directed.	Bacteriuria exposes the blood to urinary bacteria during urethral incision.

POSTPROCEDURAL NURSING CARE

NURSING DIAGNOSIS	NURSING INTERVENTIONS	RATIONALE
Altered tissue perfusion (urethral vascular bed) related to surgical trauma	Maintain the three-way urethral catheter with mild traction.	The relatively large catheter and traction provide hemostasis to the urethra.
	Monitor the urine for bleeding and clots.	Bright red blood and clots indicate active bleeding; pink urine is expected.
	Monitor the vital signs for evidence of significant hemorrhage.	Because of the rich vascular bed of the urethra, uncontrolled bleeding may result in significant blood loss and shock.
Urinary retention (potential) related to surgical trauma	Monitor urinary output; observe urine for clots.	Clots in the urine may obstruct the catheter, resulting in acute retention.
	Administer bladder irrigation as directed; set irrigation rate so that urine is light pink; maintain brisk rate for at least 24 h.	Mechanical irrigation prevents clot formation and urinary retention.
	Irrigate the bladder as directed if clots cause an obstruction.	Irrigation mechanically disrupts and removes blood clots.
	Monitor the urine for bleeding and clots after removing the catheter.	Bleeding occasionally may occur following catheter removal, possibly as a result of disruption of healing scabs in the urethra.

PATIENT TEACHING ▪▪▪▪▪▪▪▪▪▪▪▪▪▪▪▪▪▪▪▪▪▪▪▪▪▪▪▪▪▪▪

1. Before the procedure, teach the patient or family how to perform intermittent catheterization.

2. Teach the patient to recognize the signs and symptoms of serious urinary hemorrhage and how to cope with bleeding should it arise.

Augmentation Enterocystoplasty

Augmentation enterocystoplasty is the surgical reconstruction of the urinary bladder using a segment of the gastrointestinal system (Figure 5-7). A section of small or large bowel or stomach may be used to augment the bladder. The surgeon isolates the bowel from the fecal stream, which is reanastomosed. The segment of bowel is detubularized (formed into a semispherical configuration) to prevent or minimize bolus contractions. The bladder dome is incised, forming a clam cystoplasty, and anastomosed to the bowel segment. The resulting augmented bladder should improve capacity and compliance. The gastrocystoplasty is formed by a segment of the fundus of the stomach. It offers the potential advantage of reducing the risk of infection, since it produces bacteriostatic acid.

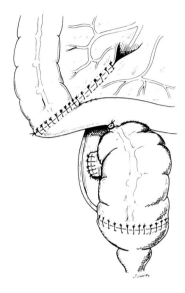

FIGURE 5-7
Augmentation enterocystoplasty. (From Novick A: Augmentation cystoplasty. In Novick A et al, editors: *Stewart's operative urology,* ed 2, vol 2, Baltimore, 1989, Williams & Wilkins.)

INDICATIONS

Instability (reflex) incontinence that does not respond
to conservative management
Hostile neuropathic bladder (poor compliance with febrile urinary tract infections or compromised renal function)

CONTRAINDICATIONS

Inability or unwillingness to perform intermittent catheterization

COMPLICATIONS

Metabolic disorders
Hyperchloremic acidosis
Vitamin B_{12} deficiency
Copious mucus production (may block catheter)
Bladder rupture

PREPROCEDURAL NURSING CARE

NURSING DIAGNOSIS	NURSING INTERVENTIONS	RATIONALE
Knowledge deficit related to procedure, its goals, and potential side effects	Reinforce preoperative instruction, including description of procedure, its goals, and potential side effects.	Preoperative learning and retention are reduced by anxiety; reinforcing this teaching enhances learning and retention.
	Advise the patient that general anesthesia is required.	Augmentation enterocystoplasty requires significant urologic reconstruction and general anesthesia.
	Advise the patient that he will have a nasogastric tube for 3 to 5 days after surgery.	Bowel manipulation produces a temporary ileus; a nasogastric tube connected to suction is used to decompress the gastrointestinal system and prevent vomiting.

NURSING DIAGNOSIS	NURSING INTERVENTIONS	RATIONALE
	Advise the patient that he will have an indwelling catheter 10 to 30 days after surgery.	Catheter drainage is used for overdistention until the anastomosis has healed completely.
	Before the surgery, teach the patient to perform intermittent catheterization (see pages 306 and 307).	Intermittent catheterization is used to evacuate the bladder after bladder augmentation.
	Teach the patient to irrigate the bladder with sterile saline.	Saline irrigation breaks up and removes excessive mucus in the urine.

POSTPROCEDURAL NURSING CARE

NURSING DIAGNOSIS	NURSING INTERVENTIONS	RATIONALE
Altered patterns of urinary elimination related to bladder augmentation surgery	Monitor the indwelling catheter for urinary output.	Urine is evacuated via the indwelling catheter (urethral or ostomy catheter) until wound healing is completed.
	Observe the urine for color, clots, mucus, and sediment.	Some hematuria is expected after augmentation surgery; copious, bright red blood and blood clots are not expected and may represent significant hemorrhage; mucus will be copious and may obstruct the catheter.
	Irrigate the augmented bladder as directed (typically q 2 h) during the immediate postoperative period; irrigate, using a 60 ml catheter-tipped syringe.	Irrigation with sterile saline removes mucous secretions from the augmented bladder, ensuring catheter patency; copious mucus is expected during irrigation.
	Do not forcibly evacuate saline after injection; gently withdraw saline and instill another 60 ml if needed for gentle irrigation.	Vigorous irrigation with forcible aspiration may disrupt the healing bowel-to-bladder anastomosis.
	Before discharge, teach the patient how to irrigate the augmented bladder.	Mucus is a persistent problem in the augmented bladder; it is likely to be most significant for the first year after surgery. Although mucus itself is not harmful, it tends to coagulate and may block the catheter, preventing complete emptying.
	Advise the patient to drink at least 8 ounces (and as much as 16 ounces) of cranberry juice a day; encourage him to drink pure juice rather than premixed preparations; if he does not like the taste, advise him to mix the pure juice with ginger ale or other beverages.	Although 8 to 16 ounces of cranberry juice will not significantly alter urinary pH or prevent urinary infection, it has been shown to encourage formation of a mucolytic agent, hippuric acid, that thins the mucus, allowing better bladder evacuation.[90]

NURSING DIAGNOSIS	NURSING INTERVENTIONS	RATIONALE
Pain related to surgical trauma	Identify the location, character, and duration of pain, as well as aggravating and alleviating factors.	Incisional pain produces a chronic, dull, boring pain in the midline; spasms of the augmented bladder produce a sharp, cramping pain in the suprapubic area that is relieved by bladder evacuation; flank pain may indicate an upper urinary tract obstruction.
	Administer analgesic or narcotic agents for incisional pain as directed.	Narcotic or analgesic drugs temporarily relieve postoperative incisional pain.
	Administer antispasmodic agents as directed for bladder spasm pain.	Bladder spasms result from smooth muscle contraction against a closed (catheterized) bladder outlet; antispasmodic drugs relieve pain by inhibiting these contractions.
	Contact the physician promptly if the patient develops flank pain.	Flank pain may indicate upper urinary tract obstruction; postoperative ureteral stents are left in place to minimize the risk of obstruction; relieving the obstruction will relieve flank pain.
	Institute nonpharmacologic measures to relieve pain as appropriate; keep lighting dim, and use pillows and proper positioning to limit discomfort.	Nonpharmacologic interventions also limit pain from the surgical incision or bladder spasms; flank pain will not respond to these interventions.
Fluid volume deficit (potential) related to nasogastric tube	Monitor the nasogastric tube for patency and volume and nature of output.	A nasogastric tube is needed for gastrointestinal decompression after surgical bowel manipulation; blockage of the tube encourages fluid volume deficit and vomiting.
	Maintain suction to the nasogastric tube as directed; irrigate if necessary.	Continuous suction using gentle negative pressure removes gastric secretions until normal peristalsis returns; irrigation removes plugs or thicker material from the tube.
	Administer intravenous fluids as directed.	Fluids and electrolytes lost via the nasogastric tube are replaced by parenteral fluids.
	Auscultate the abdomen daily for return of peristaltic bowel sounds.	The return of peristalsis indicates the end of postoperative ileus.
	Clamp the nasogastric tube after peristalsis returns, and offer the patient sips of liquids as directed; remove the tube as directed when the patient can tolerate liquids.	Even after the return of peristalsis, the bowel must be slowly reintroduced to regular foods; premature discontinuation of the nasogastric tube causes nausea and vomiting, requiring replacement of the tube with prolonged ileus.

NURSING DIAGNOSIS	NURSING INTERVENTIONS	RATIONALE
	Slowly advance the diet to full liquids, then to soft foods, and then to regular foods.	Prematurely rapid introduction increases the risk of prolonged ileus and reintroduction of the nasogastric tube.
Impaired physical mobility (imposed) related to needs of wound healing	Instruct the patient not to lift any heavy objects for the first month after surgery.	Lifting heavy objects increases the risk of disrupting the healing anastomosis between bowel and bladder.
	Advise the patient that strenuous exercise, contact sports, or impact aerobics are strictly contraindicated for the first month after surgery.	These activities increase the risk of disrupting the healing anastomosis between bowel and bladder.
	Advise the wheelchair-bound patient that weight shifts and transfers must be done without exertion for the first month after surgery; help the patient obtain a Hoyer lift as indicated.	The physical exertion required for normal weight shifts and transfers increases the risk of disrupting the healing bowel-to-bladder anastomosis.

PATIENT TEACHING

1. Before surgical reconstruction, teach the patient to perform intermittent catheterization.
2. After the surgery, teach the patient to irrigate the augmented bladder. Reinforce this instruction as indicated.
3. Teach the patient to avoid strenuous activities and exercise until the delicate bowel-to-bladder anastomosis has healed.
4. Teach the patient to catheterize the bladder regularly to avoid rupture of the augmentation enterocystoplasty.

Urinary Retention

Urinary retention is the failure of the bladder to empty itself by means of urination. Dribbling, overflow incontinence with frequent urination, compromised force of stream, and nocturia are the presenting symptoms of urinary retention.

For videourodynamic image of urinary retention, see Color Plate 5, page xi.

PATHOPHYSIOLOGY

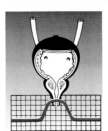

Acute urinary retention is a complete inability to void; as bladder volume increases, bladder pain and discomfort intensify. Acute retention is a medical emergency requiring catheter drainage. Chronic urinary retention is the inability to evacuate the bladder completely. Micturition occurs, but some urine remains in the bladder, resulting in more frequent attempts to empty the bladder and predisposing the individual to urinary in-

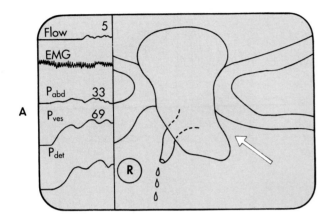

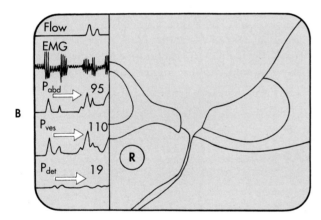

FIGURE 5-8
A, Diagram of urinary retention caused by bladder outlet obstruction in a female. A large cystocele causes much of the bladder to lie below the outlet, producing mild mechanical obstruction. Arrow on the top left indicates poor flow, and arrow near the bottom indicates high voiding pressure (69 cm H$_2$O). Arrow on the right indicates large cystocele. **B,** Diagram of urinary retention caused by deficient detrusor contractility in a male patient. Arrow on the upper left indicates straining pattern noted in intravesical and abdominal pressure channels, and arrow on the bottom left shows flat detrusor pressure tracing with absent contraction.

URINARY RETENTION: DEFICIENT CONTRACTILITY

Transient causes

Medications
  Antispasmodic drugs
  Antidepressant drugs
  Narcotics
  Psychotropic drugs
  Antiparkinsonian drugs
  Recreational drugs (hallucinogens, cannabis)
  Calcium channel blockers
Constipation/fecal impaction
Hysterical retention
Immobility/acute illness
Herpes zoster of sacral nerve roots
Acute overdistention injury

Chronic causes

Spinal injury of sacral nerve roots
Peripheral neuropathies (diabetes mellitus, chronic ethanol abuse)
Lifelong habit of infrequent voiding
Cauda equina syndrome
Tabes dorsalis
Postpolio deficit

fection. Two pathophysiologic conditions cause urinary retention—obstruction and deficient detrusor contractility.

Bladder outlet obstruction principally affects men, although obstruction occasionally is seen in women (Figure 5-8, *A*). Prostatic outlet obstruction in men manifests as prostatitis, benign glandular hypertrophy, or prostate cancer. Functional bladder outlet obstruction is caused by dyssynergia of the striated or smooth muscle components of the sphincter mechanism. Detrusor-sphincter dyssynergia or vesicosphincter dyssynergia typically accompanies spinal disease or injury, resulting in instability (reflex) incontinence. Dyssynergia of the smooth muscle of the urethrovesical outlet is called *bladder neck dyssynergia*. Congenital urethral valves or polyps, congenital or acquired strictures, and stenosis of the urethral meatus also cause bladder outlet obstruction in men.

Bladder outlet obstruction is relatively uncommon in women. Women may experience obstruction because of urethral distortion from pelvic descent or specific trauma. Bladder outlet obstruction is an uncommon complication of urethropexy or periurethral injection, and women with spinal disease or injury may have bladder neck or vesicosphincter dyssynergia. Idiopathic bladder neck dyssynergia is particularly rare among women.[70]

Bladder outlet obstruction predisposes the urinary system to the adverse effects of increased voiding pressure and urinary stasis. The pathophysiology of obstructive uropathy is discussed in Chapter 6.

In contrast to obstruction, deficient detrusor contractility affects both women and men. Transient detrusor deficiency can be traced to a reversible cause, whereas chronic deficiency is traced to a chronic condition that may or may not be reversible. The box on page 144 outlines common causes of transient and chronic deficient detrusor contractility (Figure 5-8, *B*).

Urinary retention caused by deficient detrusor con-

tractility adversely affects the urinary system. Incomplete bladder evacuation causes urinary stasis and contributes to bladder ischemia, increasing the risk of urinary tract infection. Fortunately, because deficient contractility is associated with low or no voiding pressure, obstructive uropathy is avoided unless the condition is complicated by bladder wall hypocompliance.

COMPLICATIONS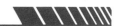

Urinary tract infection
Febrile urinary tract infection
Vesicoureteral reflux
Compromised or insufficient renal function

DIAGNOSTIC STUDIES AND FINDINGS

Diagnostic Test	Findings
Urodynamics/ videourodynamics	Pressure flow analysis demonstrates high-pressure contraction with poor or intermittent flow pattern, indicating obstruction or low pressure, or poorly sustained or no contraction with intermittent or poor flow, indicating deficient detrusor contractility. Bladder wall hypocompliance and detrusor instability may be noted. Fluoroscopy may show trabeculation, diverticula of obstruction, or smooth-walled bladder of deficient contractility. Urethral obstruction may be visualized during micturition.
Cystogram/voiding cystogram	Trabeculation and diverticula indicate obstruction; the level of obstruction is detectable during micturition urethrogram. Deficient contractility is noted as smooth-walled bladder with large capacity.
Intravenous pyelogram/ urogram (**IVP/IVU**)	Normal upper urinary tract or hydronephrosis and compromised renal function, indicating obstructive uropathy.

MEDICAL MANAGEMENT

GENERAL MANAGEMENT AND DRUG THERAPY

Double voiding or timed voiding program

Administration of cholinergic drug to improve deficient contractility

Administration of alpha adrenergic blocking drug to diminish bladder outlet resistance

Intermittent catheterization (rather than indwelling catheter) for urinary drainage

SURGICAL MANAGEMENT

Surgical resection of obstructive lesion

Dilation of stricture or surgical repair of pelvic descent

1 ASSESS

ASSESSMENT	OBSERVATIONS
Urinary retention	Postvoid residual greater than 25% of total bladder capacity (sum of voided volume and residual volume)
Obstructive symptoms	Poor force of stream; hesitancy to initiate stream; sensations of incomplete bladder evacuation
Irritative symptoms	Urgency to urinate; diurnal urinary frequency (more often than q 2 h) and nocturia (more than one episode per night)
Urinary tract infection	Foul-smelling urine with bacteriuria, pyuria (fever may be present)

2 DIAGNOSE

NURSING DIAGNOSIS	SUBJECTIVE FINDINGS	OBJECTIVE FINDINGS
Urinary retention related to deficient detrusor contractility or bladder outlet obstruction	Reports poor or intermittent urinary stream, hesitancy to urinate or combination of urgency to void with hesitancy to initiate stream and sensations of incomplete bladder evacuation	Postvoid urinary residual volume exceeds 25% of total bladder capacity (sum of voided volume and residual urinary volume)
Potential for infection (urinary) related to urinary retention	Reports signs and symptoms of urinary tract infection	Urine culture reveals more than 100,000 CFU/ml of urine

3 PLAN

Patient goals

1. Urinary retention will resolve, and spontaneous voiding will result in complete bladder evacuation.
2. Urinary retention will resolve, and bladder evacuation will be achieved by catheterization.
3. Symptoms of instability (urge) incontinence will resolve or be controlled.
4. The patient will have no urinary tract infection.

4 IMPLEMENT

NURSING DIAGNOSIS	NURSING INTERVENTIONS	RATIONALE
Urinary retention related to deficient detrusor contractility or bladder outlet obstruction	Teach the patient the technique of double voiding; instruct the patient to void and then to wait on the toilet for 3 to 5 min before voiding again.	Double voiding is designed to improve the voided volume by allowing the detrusor to contract, relax and rest, and then contract again; this technique may significantly reduce urinary retention in mild to moderate cases of obstruction or deficient contractility.

NURSING DIAGNOSIS	NURSING INTERVENTIONS	RATIONALE
	Instruct the patient with deficient detrusor contractility and diminished sensations of filling to void on a timed schedule of q 3-4 h.	Timed voiding prevents the overdistention of the bladder that contributes to deficient detrusor contractility among individuals with peripheral neuropathies, such as those produced by diabetes mellitus.
	Institute a fluid control program (see Fluid Intake: What, When, and How Much, page 303).	Spacing fluids throughout the day while ensuring adequate fluid intake avoids bladder overdistention that may exacerbate symptoms of retention and reduces the risk of urinary infection.
	Administer or teach the patient to self-administer a cholinergic medication as directed.	Bethanechol chloride is a cholinergic analog that increases sensory urgency and has the potential to improve contractility during micturition. Bethanechol may improve bladder evacuation among patients with deficient contractility, although it is contraindicated when retention is caused by obstruction.
	Administer or teach the patient to self-administer an alpha adrenergic blocking agent as directed (see box on page 130).	Alpha adrenergic blocking drugs relax smooth muscle of the bladder neck, prostatic urethra, and rhabdosphincter. These drugs may be used to relieve urinary retention caused by prostatic outlet obstruction, vesicosphincter dyssynergia, and bladder neck dyssynergia, or as an adjunct with bethanechol chloride for patients with deficient contractility.
	Institute an intermittent catheterization program, or teach the patient to perform self-catheterization in consultation with the physician and patient.	Intermittent catheterization provides regular, complete evacuation of the bladder with less risk for symptomatic bacteriuria than an indwelling catheter.
	Help the patient choose an appropriate intermittent catheter.	The ideal intermittent catheter should be relatively small to minimize discomfort with insertion (approximately 12 to 14 French for adults) and should be constructed of a material that allows washing and several uses; the catheter should be relatively short to allow easy storage.
	Insert an indwelling catheter, or help the physician insert an indwelling catheter as directed.	An indwelling catheter may be the only alternative for urinary retention; its use is reserved for patients who are unable or unwilling to manage retention by other means.

→ > >

NURSING DIAGNOSIS	NURSING INTERVENTIONS	RATIONALE
	Select a catheter according to French size and material of construction.	A smaller catheter may offer greater comfort; catheters made of hydrogel materials offer potential advantages of greater biocompatibility, reduced friction and irritation of urethral mucosa, and reduced bacterial adherence compared to Silastic, Teflon-coated, or silicone catheters.[89]
	Select a catheter with optimum drainage capacity.	The ratio of external diameter to diameter of the catheter lumen influences the likelihood of effective drainage; a catheter with a relatively thin external wall is preferred over a catheter with a thicker wall, since it provides greater internal drainage capacity.
	Help the patient choose and put on a leg bag for urinary collection.	The ideal leg bag contains a relatively large volume of urine, is backed by a breathable surface that is comfortable when worn on the skin, and has a drainage port that is easily opened and readily closed. The straps should be made of elastic cloth or Velcro so that skin irritation is minimized. The bag should be designed to spread urine through the device, minimizing bulging that creates an obvious defect when worn under clothing. The tubing from catheter to leg bag should be long enough to avoid placing traction on the catheter.
	Help the patient choose a bedside collection bag.	The bedside bag should have an adequate volume (approximately 2,000 ml or more) to prevent excessive filling through sleep; the drain valve should be easily opened and readily closed; the tubing from catheter to drainage bag should be long enough to allow movement in bed.
	Advise the patient that irritative voiding symptoms (frequency of urination, nocturia, urgency to urinate, and urge incontinence) may be caused by instability incontinence.	Detrusor instability may coexist with bladder outlet obstruction; a causal relationship has been postulated.[66,69]
	Institute a timed voiding schedule with a fluid management program in consultation with the physician.	Timed voiding may reduce instability incontinence by ensuring bladder evacuation before the onset of unstable detrusor contractions; a fluid management program is designed to ensure adequate daily intake and to avoid consumption of boluses of fluids that exacerbate both retention and instability.

NURSING DIAGNOSIS	NURSING INTERVENTIONS	RATIONALE
	Administer or teach the patient to self-administer antispasmodic medications as directed to pharmacologically "paralyze" the detrusor; institute an intermittent catheterization program as directed.	Antispasmodic medications are likely to produce complete urinary retention in the obstructed patient with detrusor instability; intermittent catheterization is instituted to ensure regular, complete bladder evacuation.
Potential for infection (urinary) related to urinary retention	Teach the patient to recognize the signs and symptoms of urinary tract infection (i.e., foul-smelling urine with suprapubic or lower back pain, hematuria, fever, or chills) and to seek prompt treatment if these symptoms occur (see Cystitis/Urinary Tract Infection, page 52).	A urinary tract infection may worsen existing retention, causing acute urinary retention and leading to systemic disease unless appropriately managed.
	Consult the physician about using prophylactic antiinfective therapy for bacteriuria.	Suppressive or prophylactic antiinfective drug therapy is used selectively among individuals with urinary retention, weighing potential untoward effects of treatment, such as the emergence of antibiotic-resistant bacterial strains.
	Instruct the patient to drink adequate fluids (at least 1,500 ml, or about six 8-ounce glasses, for adults each day).	The antegrade movement of urine through the kidneys and ureters into the bladder is an important defense mechanism against bacterial infection.
Knowledge deficit	See Patient Teaching.	

5 EVALUATE

PATIENT OUTCOME	DATA INDICATING THAT OUTCOME IS REACHED
Urinary retention has resolved; spontaneous voiding results in complete bladder evacuation.	Spontaneous voiding continues after obstructive lesion has been treated by surgical or pharmacologic measures. Postvoid urinary residual volume is less than 25% of total bladder capacity.
Urinary retention has resolved; bladder evacuation has been attained by catheterization.	Patient is able to perform self intermittent catheterization.
Symptoms of instability (urge) incontinence have resolved or are adequately managed.	Diurnal voiding frequency is more often than q 2 h, episodes of nocturia are one or none per night; *or,* urinary leakage and sensations of marked urgency to void are absent between catheterizations.
Patient has no urinary tract infection.	Urine culture shows no bacteriuria.

PATIENT TEACHING

1. Teach the patient the names, dosages, administration, action, and potential side effects of medications used to manage urinary retention.
2. Teach the patient with bladder outlet obstruction to avoid stimuli likely to increase the risk of acute urinary retention (e.g., bladder overdistention, chilling, excessive alcohol intake).
3. Teach the patient with bladder outlet obstruction to avoid medications that predispose to acute urinary retention, including antidepressant medications, psychotropic drugs, antispasmodic drugs, over-the-counter decongestants (alpha adrenergic agonists), and antiparkinsonian medications.
4. Teach the patient using intermittent catheterization or an indwelling catheter how to distinguish the symptoms of significant urinary infection (cloudy, odorous urine with symptoms of fever, hematuria, and chills) from the asymptomatic bacteriuria inevitable with bladder management by intermittent or indwelling catheters.

Extraurethral Incontinence

Extraurethral incontinence is the uncontrolled leakage of urine by some communication that bypasses the urethral sphincter mechanism. Urinary leakage is continuous and relatively unaffected by physical exertion or sensations of urgency to void. In some cases extraurethral leakage manifests as a continuous dribble coexisting with a relatively normal voiding pattern; in other instances leakage is severe, replacing normal voiding.

PATHOPHYSIOLOGY

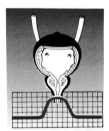

Extraurethral leakage arises from one of three sources: reconstructive surgical procedures, urinary ectopia, or urinary fistula. **Reconstructive surgical procedures,** such as the Bricker ileal conduit or sigmoid conduit, deliberately bypass the bladder and urethra because of a tumor or particularly severe hostile neuropathic function. **Urinary ectopia** is the result of a congenital defect of the bladder. An *ectopic ureter* may open into the urethra below the level of the urethral sphincter or vagina. With ectopia of the bladder (exstrophy/epispadias defects), part of the bladder is externalized and there is no urethral sphincter mechanism (Figure 5-9).

A **urinary fistula** is a tract that provides abnormal communication between pelvic organs or between a pelvic organ and the skin. Fistulae are acquired defects; the tract is named by describing its origin and terminal points. For example, a *vesicovaginal fistula* is a communication between the bladder and the vaginal vault, and

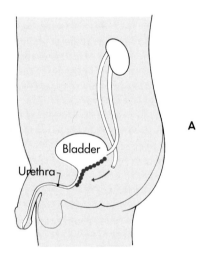

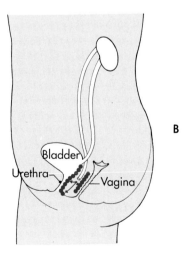

FIGURE 5-9
Common sites for ureteral ectopia. **A,** Male. **B,** Female.

a *urethrovaginal fistula* is a tract between the urethra and the vagina. Fistulae also may connect the bladder or urethra with the skin. A *urethrocutaneous fistula* produces leakage when it bypasses the sphincter mechanism, and a *vesicocutaneous fistula* allows leakage directly from the bladder.

On a worldwide basis, the most common cause of fistulae is complications of labor and delivery. In the United States, however, fistulae most commonly occur as a complication of hysterectomy or other pelvic surgical procedures. Other causes of urinary fistulae are penetrating trauma, perineal wounds, and invasive tumors (Figure 5-10).[92,93]

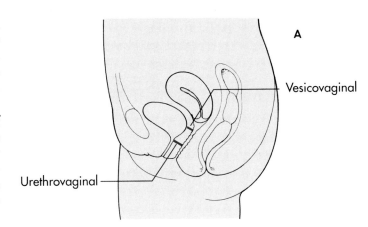

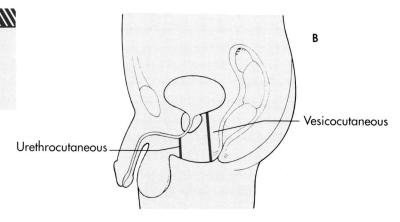

COMPLICATIONS

Urinary tract infection
Febrile urinary tract infection
Altered skin integrity
Shame, humiliation, social isolation

FIGURE 5-10
Common fistulae. **A,** Female. **B,** Male.

DIAGNOSTIC STUDIES AND FINDINGS

Diagnostic test	Findings
Cystogram/voiding cystogram	Urinary fistula with extravasation of contrast materials
Intravenous pyelogram/ urogram (IVP/IVU)	Ectopic ureter or extravasation of contrast material with fistula
Endoscopy	Fistula noted on cystourethroscopy; methylene blue test (instillation of methylene blue into bladder) may be used to detect small vesicovaginal or urethrovaginal fistulae; ectopic ureter with orifice in urethra can be detected with urethroscopy; ectopic ureteral orifice opening into vagina may be detected by colposcopy or IVP/IVU

MEDICAL MANAGEMENT

GENERAL MANAGEMENT AND DRUG THERAPY

Urinary containment with or without Foley catheter
Topical application of tetracyline to fistulous tract
Prophylaxis with antiinfective drugs in some cases

SURGICAL THERAPY

Closure of repair of urinary ectopia
Closure of urinary fistula

1 ASSESS

ASSESSMENT	OBSERVATIONS
Extraurethral incontinence	Continuous urinary leakage not correlated with urgency to void or physical exertion
Altered skin integrity	Moist, odorous, perineal skin with lesions or rashes
Social isolation	Patient reports avoiding activities that require social interaction, or fears that others will discover the urinary leakage problem

2 DIAGNOSE

NURSING DIAGNOSIS	SUBJECTIVE FINDINGS	OBJECTIVE FINDINGS
Extraurethral (total) incontinence related to urinary ectopia, urinary fistula	Reports constant urinary leakage that may range in severity from dribble to failure of bladder storage; leakage is not associated with urgency or physical exertion	Voiding diary demonstrates conditions ranging from continuous dribbling leakage superimposed on normal pattern of diurnal frequency to absence of spontaneous voiding with continuous leakage, requiring diaper containment
Impaired skin integrity related to extraurethral incontinence	Reports rashes or lesions of perineal skin	Examination of perineal skin reveals moist, odorous skin with lesions or specific rashes
Social isolation related to urinary leakage, odor, and fear of embarrassment and discovery	Reports avoiding activities requiring social interaction and fears that others will detect urinary leakage	May have unkempt appearance and poor hygiene; may report feelings of depression and loneliness.

3 PLAN

Patient goals

1. Extraurethral incontinence will be resolved, *or* urinary leakage will be adequately contained by a Foley catheter with or without a containment system.

2. Skin integrity will be restored and maintained.
3. Social isolation will be resolved.

4 IMPLEMENT

NURSING DIAGNOSIS	NURSING INTERVENTIONS	RATIONALE
Extraurethral (total) incontinence related to urinary ectopia, urinary fistula	Help the patient choose and obtain a urinary containment device; typically, individuals with very mild extraurethral leakage use a small pad; those with more significant leakage require a diaper-type device.	Extraurethral leakage is continuous, so that even relatively small ectopic orifices or fistulae produce a significant volume of urine over a 24-hour period.

NURSING DIAGNOSIS	NURSING INTERVENTIONS	RATIONALE
	Insert an indwelling urethral catheter, or help the physician place a suprapubic tube as directed.	An indwelling catheter sometimes is inserted to divert urine from a fistula; depending on its anatomic relation to the fistula, the catheter may ablate, alleviate, or fail to affect incontinence.
	Teach the patient to care for the suprapubic or urethral catheter.	An indwelling catheter is left in place until surgical repair is completed or as a permanent management program.
	Administer or help the physician administer tetracycline mixed in saline to sclerose the fistulous tract.	Tetracycline is a caustic substance administered topically; controlled application to a fistula may produce sufficient scarring to prevent incontinence.
Impaired skin integrity related to extraurethral incontinence	Help the patient choose and obtain an appropriate urinary collection device.	The ideal urinary collection device protects the skin by completely absorbing leakage, minimizing the time urine is in contact with the skin.
	Teach the patient the principles of a skin care program (i.e., regular washing, complete drying, applying a moisture barrier or skin sealant, and using a collection device).	Maintaining healthy skin depends on regular cleansing and complete drying; moisture barriers or skin sealants offer some protection from exposure to urinary leakage, and collection devices protect the skin by minimizing exposure to urine.
	Administer or teach the patient to self-administer a cream or powder for monilial rash as prescribed.	Monilial rashes are managed by routine skin care and local application of an antifungal cream or powder.
	Teach the patient with ammonia contact dermatitis to clean the skin with soap and water; thoroughly dry the skin; and direct warm, dry air to the area for 15 minutes each day; advise the patient to use a hand-held hair dryer set at the lowest warm setting; between treatments, teach the patient to apply a skin sealant or a moisture barrier and to use an appropriate containment device.	Ammonia contact dermatitis occurs as a result of prolonged exposure of the skin to urine; regular, complete drying and using a moisture barrier or skin sealant and collection device minimize exposure.
Social isolation related to urinary leakage, odor, and fear of embarrassment and discovery	Encourage the patient to seek a definitive management program for instability incontinence.	Many patients are advised by families, friends, or even health care professionals to "live with" their condition; treatment and resolution are realistic goals that prevent complications such as social isolation.
	Reassure the patient with extraurethral incontinence that the condition is not incurable, even though the leakage may be quite severe.	Extraurethral incontinence may be particularly frustrating, since it arises from a source other than the detrusor muscle or sphincter and is not affected by traditional management strategies for other forms of incontinence.

→ > >

NURSING DIAGNOSIS	NURSING INTERVENTIONS	RATIONALE
	Help the patient contact an advocacy or support group such as Help for Incontinent People (HIP), the Simon Foundation, or Continence Restored, Inc. (see the box on page 93).	Patient advocacy groups provide support and help participants obtain health care for urinary leakage; advocacy groups also help the patient identify strategies for coping with leakage until a definitive management program has been completed.

5 EVALUATE

PATIENT OUTCOME	DATA INDICATING THAT OUTCOME IS REACHED
Extraurethral incontinence has resolved, *or* **urinary leakage is adequately contained by a Foley catheter with or without a containment system.**	Extraurethral incontinence is absent, or leakage is completely contained by collection device; no odor of urine is detectable; the collection device is not readily detectable under the patient's clothing.
Skin integrity has been restored and is maintained.	Perineal examination reveals no lesions or rashes; patient can accurately describe principles of skin care for an incontinent individual.
Social isolation has resolved.	Patient reports less fear of engaging in social activities.

PATIENT TEACHING

1. Teach the patient that extraurethral incontinence is the result of anatomic defects that bypass the sphincter mechanism and that it will not respond to traditional management strategies for incontinence.
2. Teach the patient how tetracycline is administered, potential side effects, and the goals of therapy.

Functional Incontinence

Functional incontinence is urinary leakage caused by impaired physical mobility, dexterity, or cognition rather than by organic dysfunction of the urinary system. Functional incontinence is particularly important because it affects the character and management options of all individuals who experience a voiding dysfunction.

PATHOPHYSIOLOGY

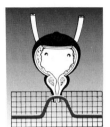

Functional incontinence can be divided into one of four broad categories. **Impaired mobility** affects the individual's ability to reach the bathroom and to maneuver onto the toilet in response to the need to urinate. An elderly individual's mobility may be limited by poor sight, limited physical endurance, neurologic deficits, or joint pain and arthritis. Individuals with neuropathic bladder dysfunction may be confined to a wheelchair or may walk with assistive devices such as a cane or walker.

Impaired mobility is profoundly influenced by issues related to **access.** For example, even the most skilled paraplegic patient may be unable to successfully empty the bladder if available bathrooms have inaccessible, narrow doorways or stalls. Similarly, elderly individuals may be unable to use the toilet simply because there are no hand rails to lower themselves onto the toilet or because the toilet is placed too low for reasonable access. Other barriers to toilet access include stairs, poor lighting, and environmental hazards such as slick-soled shoes or loose throw rugs.

Impaired dexterity also affects an individual's predisposition to incontinence. Once the toilet has been reached, the individual must manipulate the clothing to be able to urinate. Manipulating zippers, buttons, hooks, undergarments, and other aspects of clothing requires time and varying degrees of dexterity and visual acuity. Impaired dexterity also influences the range of bladder management programs available for the person with coexisting chronic incontinence. For example, from a purely urologic perspective, a quadriplegic individual is best managed by intermittent catheterization; however, this program is unrealistic for many quadriplegics because they cannot manipulate clothing and perform catheterization independently. Using a condom with a reflex voiding program, although less urologically ideal, is a more appropriate bladder management program for many quadriplegics because of the functional limitations imposed by the demands of catheterization.

Altered cognition also affects urinary continence. The mentally challenged patient may fail to grasp the significance of signals of urgency or the social significance of continence. In addition, the person experiencing significant short-term memory loss from Alzheimer's disease or other diseases may gain continence by routine prompting to urinate.

Like all incontinent individuals, the person with functional incontinence faces issues of skin integrity, prevention of urinary tract infection, and the potential for urinary system distress. In the context of this discussion, however, the discussion of the nursing management of functional incontinence is limited to interventions designed specifically to enhance the individual's access to toilet facilities, ability to manipulate clothing to prepare for toileting, and ability to perceive and act on the knowledge that continence is a desirable and attainable goal.

COMPLICATIONS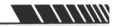

Social isolation
Urinary tract infection
Altered skin integrity
Upper urinary tract distress

DIAGNOSTIC STUDIES AND FINDINGS

Diagnostic test	Findings
Urodynamics/ videourodynamics	Normal bladder function or urinary incontinence coexisting with functional deficit
Voiding diary	Normal or small functional capacity with reasonably predictable episodes of urinary leakage; enuresis is not uncommon

MEDICAL MANAGEMENT

Referral for physical therapy to maximize mobility

Referral for mental health care for cognitive or motivational defects

Referral to occupational therapy to maximize manual dexterity

Referral to nursing to institute bladder management program designed to reverse or minimize functional incontinence

1 ASSESS

ASSESSMENT	OBSERVATIONS
Impaired physical mobility	Observe gait and use of assistive devices
Access to toilet	Distance to toilet in patient's home and work place; need for particular assistive devices or structural alterations; environmental barriers to bathroom access
Impaired manual dexterity	Observe manipulation of clothing, specifically ability to manipulate buttons, hooks, snaps, Velcro, and laces
Altered cognition	Observe ability to respond to request to toilet or to complete toileting when prompted by assisted placement on a toilet; observe behaviors related to incontinent episodes (does patient ask for assistance with toileting or acknowledge urge to urinate?)

2 DIAGNOSE

NURSING DIAGNOSIS	SUBJECTIVE FINDINGS	OBJECTIVE FINDINGS
Functional incontinence related to impaired mobility/access	Reports difficulty walking or inability to walk; needs more time to gain access to toilet or is unable to gain access to toilet	Abnormal gait; difficulty initiating or stopping ambulation; needs assistive device or is unable to walk, requiring wheelchair; visual impairment also may affect efficiency of ambulation; environmental barriers limit or preclude independent access to the toilet
Functional incontinence related to impaired dexterity	Reports difficulty manipulating clothing	Difficulty manipulating zipper, button, hook, snap device, Velcro
Functional incontinence related to impaired cognition	Unaware or unconcerned about incontinence	Disorientation to person, place, time; significant short-term memory loss or is unable to process signals of urinary urgency and translate them into toileting behavior

3 PLAN

Patient goals

1. Impaired mobility will be alleviated or overcome.
2. Barriers to toilet access will be removed, or other devices are used.
3. Clothing will be manipulated in a reasonable time frame for toileting.
4. Toileting will be completed with prompting and assistance as needed.

4 IMPLEMENT

NURSING DIAGNOSIS	NURSING INTERVENTIONS	RATIONALE
Functional incontinence related to impaired mobility/access	Encourage the physically impaired patient to obtain the services of physical therapy as indicated.	Physical therapy helps the patient maximize muscle strength, mobility, and balance.
	Help the physically handicapped patient to obtain and use assistive devices as indicated.	Wheelchairs, canes, walkers, or other assistive devices allow the otherwise immobile patient to maneuver and control the environment, including access to the toilet.
	Encourage the patient with mildly compromised ambulation to obtain and wear supportive, nonskid walking or running shoes.	Slick-soled shoes or house slippers limit mobility by impairing balance and increase the risk of a serious fall.
	Encourage the removal of environmental barriers to the toilet, including loose rugs and poor lighting.	Environmental barriers exacerbate functional incontinence by limiting access to the toilet.
	Instruct the family to install hand rails for the toilet at home, or provide hand rails in the institutional toilet.	Hand rails enhance access and mobility by helping individuals raise and lower themselves onto the toilet.
	Install a raised toilet seat as indicated.	A raised toilet seat minimizes the need to raise or lower the trunk during transfers.
	Provide the patient with a bedside toilet seat as indicated; help the patient select an appropriate seat with sturdy anchored or wheeled legs, a padded seat, and adequate receptacle for urine.	The bedside commode is placed at the patient's bedside or near the living area, bypassing the need to reach a distant toilet. The commode also provides greater access to a receptacle for urine for the patient with severely limited mobility. The patient is likely to require assistance emptying and cleaning the bedside toilet.
	Provide the patient with a hand-held urinal as indicated.	The hand-held urinal gives the patient immediate access to a receptacle for urination; the patient may require assistance emptying and cleaning the hand-held urinal.
	Help the patient obtain eyeglasses and hearing aids (which increase sensory input) based on appropriate health evaluation.	Sensory deficits limit mobility and increase the risk of falls.

→ > >

NURSING DIAGNOSIS	NURSING INTERVENTIONS	RATIONALE
Functional incontinence related to impaired dexterity	Encourage the patient with limited dexterity to consult a physical or occupational therapist as indicated.	Dexterity is maximized by therapy, exercise, and use of assistive devices; care may be coordinated by a physical or occupational therapist.
	Help the patient obtain clothing that maximizes dexterity; eliminate excessive layers of clothing, and substitute elastic waistbands and Velcro for buttons, zippers, snap devices, hooks, or laces whenever feasible.	Easily managed clothing improves access to the toilet by reducing the time required to remove clothing for urination.
	Help the patient obtain eyeglasses and hearing aids (which increase sensory input) based on appropriate health evaluation.	Sensory deprivation limits the ability to manipulate clothing for effective toileting.
Functional incontinence related to impaired cognition	Institute a patterned-urge toileting program. Evaluate a voiding pattern for the patient using an electronic data logger or intensive observation for a specified period of time. Design an individualized pattern of prompted toileting based on this observed pattern. Help caregivers implement this pattern by prompting the patient to void and helping him reach the toilet. Provide verbal or other rewards to encourage establishment of a regular toileting pattern and elimination of incontinent episodes.	A patterned-urge toileting program assumes that incontinence among elderly or demented individuals represents the effects of cognitive impairment and institutional care patterns, as well as changing bladder function. Observation of the individual's incontinent toileting pattern allows evaluation of bladder capacity and the individual's potential for regular toileting. Prompting the patient provides a visual and audible stimulus for toileting with assistance to the toilet as needed. Providing rewards reinforces the significance of toileting behaviors that promote continence.[68]
	Institute a behavioral modification program to encourage toileting behaviors in mentally impaired individuals. Begin the program by helping the patient toilet on a regular schedule based on evaluation of incontinence patterns. As the patient begins to exhibit greater competence in these toileting behaviors, assistance is slowly withdrawn until a pattern of independent toileting has been established.	A toileting program for mentally impaired individuals requires that there be no serious underlying voiding dysfunction and that the patient have adequate mental facilities to integrate social and sensory input into effective toileting behaviors.[72]
Knowledge deficit	See Patient Teaching.	

5   EVALUATE

PATIENT OUTCOME	DATA INDICATING THAT OUTCOME IS REACHED
Impaired mobility has been alleviated or overcome.	Patient demonstrates the ability to maneuver into the bathroom and onto the toilet seat in a reasonable period for effective urination.

PATIENT OUTCOME	DATA INDICATING THAT OUTCOME IS REACHED
Barriers to toilet access have been removed, or other devices are used.	Patient's toilet is equipped with hand rails, an elevated seat, and adequate lighting, *or* the patient uses an alternative to the toilet (e.g., bedside commode or hand-held urinal).
Clothing is manipulated in a reasonable time frame for toileting.	Patient can remove clothing without assistance; there are no excessive layers, and zippers, buttons, hooks, and laces have been replaced by Velcro and elastic waistbands that the patient can manipulate.
Toileting is successfully completed with prompting and assistance as needed.	Patient can toilet on a regular schedule with little or no assistance or prompting.

PATIENT TEACHING

1. Teach the patient and family the causes and pathophysiology of functional incontinence. Tailor comments to an appropriate level for the patient's cognitive abilities.
2. Teach the patient with impaired mobility to use assistive devices as indicated.
3. Teach the patient and caregivers how to use and clean bedside commodes or hand-held urinals.
4. Teach caregivers the goals and process of a prompted-urge response toileting program or a bladder retraining program. Emphasize the need for consistency in executing these programs and the importance of strictly avoiding punitive actions.
5. Explain the goals of the prompted-urge response toileting program or bladder retraining program to the patient, using appropriate language. Emphasize the goals of the program throughout its execution.

CHAPTER 6

Obstructive Uropathies

Obstruction is a dynamic process that results when the inflow or outflow in a physical or biologic system is blocked. In the urinary system, obstruction may occur at any point from the calyx to the distal urethra. Obstruction causes stasis (slowing or arrest) of the urinary flow above the obstructive lesion that affects the entire urinary tract. The deleterious effects of obstruction are described by the concept **obstructive uropathy** (Figure 6-1).

An obstructive lesion may be described by its location and by its nature as intrinsic, extrinsic, or functional. Intrarenal obstructive lesions may be congenital or acquired. **Hydrocalycosis** is the dilation of one or more calyces as a result of obstruction. Congenital infundibular stenosis or infundibulopelvic stenosis may obstruct an individual calyx. Acquired hydrocalycosis may be caused by inflammation, urinary calculus (stone), renal tumor, or trauma. Extrinsic factors such as an aberrant blood vessel or extrinsic tumor also may compress a single calyx, causing hydrocalycosis. **Megacalycosis** is a generalized enlargement of the calyces of one or both kidneys. The condition typically is congenital, causing abnormal development of the kidney and parenchymal thinning.[114]

The **ureteropelvic junction** (UPJ) is the most common site of upper urinary tract obstruction in infants and children and a common site of obstruction in adults.[110] Intrinsic obstruction affects the muscle bundles at the junction of the renal pelvis and proximal ureter. During embryogenesis, the ureteropelvic junction is a solid structure that undergoes canalization to allow urine to pass from the upper to the lower urinary tract. When canalization does not occur (because of unclear embryonic conditions), congenital ureteropelvic junction obstruction results.[118] Because the ureteropelvic junction is relatively narrow, urinary calculi may obstruct it as they attempt to exit the relatively capacious pelvis and enter the narrow ureter. Extrinsic sources of obstruction include kinks, bands, and adhesions that distort the anatomy of the ureteropelvic junction. Aberrant blood vessels also contribute to obstruction, presumably because they distort the renal pelvic and ureteral anatomy.[111]

Ureteral obstruction also arises from intrinsic or extrinsic sources. Urinary calculi may obstruct the ureter as they pass through the narrow ureteropelvic junction, the area where the ureters cross the iliac arteries and the ureterovesical junction. Ureteral obstruction may occur as the result of strictures from intrinsic abnormalities or from extrinsic sources, including retroperitoneal fibrosis and tumors. **Distal ureteral atresia** is the termination of the ureter in a blind cul-de-sac. **Megaureter** is a congenital condition in which the ureter is massively enlarged and tortuous; its distal segment typically is stenotic and aperistaltic. Intrinsic ureteral obstruction is also caused by relatively uncommon conditions such as **ureteral valves** or **ureteral diverticula**. Aberrant blood vessels may obstruct the ureters if they distort the normal ureteral course. For example, a **retrocaval ureter** courses behind the inferior vena cava, obstructing the passage of urine from the kidney to the bladder. The underlying defect is in the embryogenic development of the vena cava rather than the ureter.[121]

The bladder outlet also is prone to obstruction from intrinsic or extrinsic lesions or functional causes. **Bladder neck hypertrophy** and **bladder neck contracture**

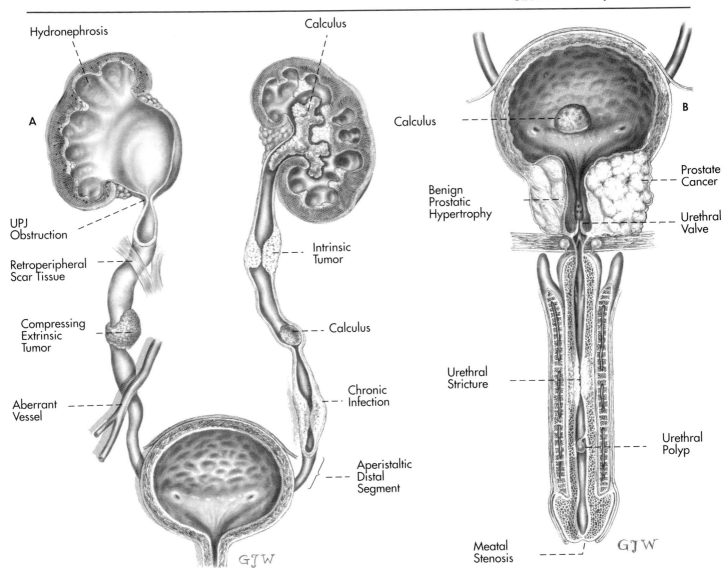

FIGURE 6-1
A, Obstruction of kidneys and ureters. **B,** Obstruction of bladder and urethra.

are intrinsic lesions that narrow the urethrovesical opening, with subsequent obstruction. These lesions may be congenital or acquired. In contrast, **bladder neck dyssynergia** is a functional obstruction of the outlet that results when the smooth muscle bundles at the bladder outlet fail to relax during micturition. Bladder neck dyssynergia is an acquired disorder caused by a spinal lesion or psychogenic distress. **Prostatic outlet obstruction** occurs as a result of inflammation, a tumor, or benign hypertrophy. Obstruction affects the bladder neck and proximal (prostatic) urethra. Extrinsic obstruction of the bladder outlet may occur as the result of extrinsic tumors or prolapse of a ureterocele into the proximal urethra.

Urethral obstruction may be intrinsic, extrinsic, or functional. **Urethral stricture** is a congenital or acquired intrinsic lesion that obstructs the outflow of urine from the bladder. The membranous urethra is the

most amenable to obstruction, although any portion of the urethra may be affected by stricture from trauma and infection. **Meatal stenosis** is the narrowing of the urethral meatus. Typically congenital, stenosis distorts the urinary stream and may cause clinically significant obstruction. **Urethral valves** are an intrinsic, congenital anomaly that causes significant obstruction. Valves occur exclusively in males and may be located in the posterior (sphincteric) or anterior (conduit) urethral segments. Intrinsic urethral polyps or cysts are rare intrinsic sources of obstruction; their clinical presentation resembles that of urethral valves. **Vesicosphincter dyssynergia** is a functional obstruction of the urethra affecting the striated muscular components of the sphincter mechanism. Vesicosphincter dyssynergia occurs as the result of spinal lesions or as a behavioral phenomenon coexisting with unstable bladder dysfunction in children.

Regardless of its location, the significance of an obstructive lesion depends on the severity of the urinary stasis, infection, and dilation it causes. The deleterious effects of obstruction affect the urinary system above the level of the lesion. For example, the dilation caused by calyceal obstruction is limited to the affected calyx, whereas ureteropelvic junction obstruction affects the entire kidney; bladder outlet obstruction may dilate both upper urinary tracts, including the ureters and kidneys. The term **hydronephrosis** is used to describe the anatomic result of obstruction affecting the kidney. The cascade of events that produces hydronephrosis represents the urinary system's initial attempts to overcome or compensate for obstruction. When these compensatory mechanisms fail, parenchymal atrophy and compromised renal function ensue.

The deleterious effects of hydronephrosis are affected by time, the severity of obstruction (percentage of urinary outflow blocked), and whether infection occurs. In a completely obstructed kidney, tissue damage following hydronephrosis is seen within 7 days of obstruction. If the kidney remains obstructed for only about 2 weeks, renal function retains the potential for nearly complete recovery after the obstruction is removed. After 3 weeks, however, the affected kidney will recover only 50% or less of its previous filtration ability. The histologic changes caused by hydronephrosis initially are noted in the distal nephron and eventually reach the glomerulus. Arterial blood flow is markedly reduced and venous drainage is impaired, further intensifying ischemia and subsequent parenchymal compromise. The severity and rapidity of these effects are intensified by infection of the urinary system.[105]

Urine exits the affected kidney across the obstructive lesion or by extravasation or pelvolymphatic or pelvovenous backflow. If obstruction is unilateral, the contralateral kidney partly compensates for compromised renal function through hyperplasia and hypertrophy. The kidney that undergoes **compensatory renal hypertrophy** becomes significantly larger than the affected (obstructed) kidney without evidence of hydronephrosis. As expected, this hypertrophy is reversed when the obstruction is relieved.

Obstruction of the ureter also causes it to increase in length and width, called tortuosity. As the obstructed ureter fills with urine, its baseline pressure increases and peristaltic waves decrease in strength and frequency. The pacemaker system of the ureter is also affected, rendering it dependent on hydrostatic pressure in the renal pelvis for antegrade movement of urine. Thus ureteral dilation and obstruction create increased baseline pressure that aggravates hydronephrosis and its deleterious effects.[126]

Obstruction of the bladder outlet or urethra adversely affects the detrusor muscle. With obstruction, the detrusor muscle undergoes hypertrophy in an attempt to sustain more powerful contractions. Initially the smooth muscle bundles undergo hypertrophy, and collagen is deposited. Over time, however, there is a general disruption of the neuromuscular junctions of the bladder wall, and trabeculation is noted. Neurologic and histologic changes in the detrusor may increase the baseline pressure in the bladder vesicle during its filling/storage phase. This condition, known as **compromised compliance,** creates pressure opposing normal ureteral peristalsis. As a result, the kidneys are predisposed to stasis, hydronephrosis, infection, and reflux.

Benign Prostatic Hypertrophy (Hyperplasia)

Benign prostatic hypertrophy (BPH) is the enlargement of the prostate gland during the later decades of life. It becomes clinically significant when the extrinsic obstruction caused by the gland obstructs the bladder outlet, including the bladder neck and prostatic portion of the proximal urethra.

PATHOPHYSIOLOGY

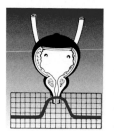

The cause and natural history of benign prostatic hypertrophy are not clearly understood. The prostate grows relatively slowly between birth and puberty. During pubescence, rapid growth and maturation continue to a steady state attained at age 20.[78] This steady state lasts to age 45 to 50, when another gradual increase in prostatic size and weight occurs.[107]

Contrary to popular belief, no persuasive evidence exists concerning risk factors for the condition. Sexual activity (or celibacy), tobacco or alcohol use, diabetes, or social factors are not connected with an increased incidence. Obstructive symptoms of benign prostatic hypertrophy tend to be seen earlier in black men than among white men, and Japanese men have a lower incidence than white men, but the reason for these racial variances is unknown. The two factors necessary for the development of the condition are aging and functioning testes.[78,107]

The critical role of testicular androgens in benign prostatic hypertrophy is demonstrated by the absence of the condition in males who have undergone castration before puberty and the marked reduction in incidence among men castrated before 40 years of age. However, castration of men with existing benign prostatic hypertrophy has not produced significant relief of obstructive symptoms in many studies.[78]

Testosterone is the principal hormonal product of the testes. In the prostate it serves as a precursor for dihydrotestosterone, which is the prominent interstitial androgen that influences prostatic growth. Dihydrotestosterone is known to play a crucial role in normal prostatic growth throughout maturation; however, its role in the development of benign prostatic hypertrophy remains unclear.[78]

Endogenous estrogens have also been implicated in the development of benign prostatic hypertrophy.[78] In human males it is important to note that although plasma testosterone levels are falling off, estradiol and androstenediol levels remain relatively unchanged. Thus, alteration of the synergy between testosterone and its derivatives and the endogenous estrogens in the male is responsible for the proliferation of benign prostatic hypertrophy, although their role in the generation of prostatism is not established.[78,107]

Although the development of benign prostatic hypertrophy itself is not harmful, the sequelae produced by this condition cause significant morbidity and may prove fatal. The signs and symptoms of benign prostatic hypertrophy are a result of bladder outlet obstruction resulting from gradual encroachment of the prostatic capsule into the proximal urethra. Early changes include hesitancy initiating micturition, decreased force in urinary stream, diurnal frequency, and nocturia. Compensatory hypertrophy of the detrusor muscle results in trabeculation, diverticula, and hypertrophy of the trigone. Paradoxically, this may produce a reduction in symptoms but does not indicate any objective improvement in bladder outlet obstruction.[78,107]

Later changes produced by bladder outlet obstruction stemming from benign prostatic hypertrophy include myogenic decompensation when compensatory hypertrophy is no longer effective. The bladder wall then becomes increasingly noncompliant and hypotonic, resulting in increasing postvoid residuals and greater chance of infection. Increased resistance at the ureterovesical junction results in ureteral dilation and progressive hydronephrosis. Unless infection is present in the upper urinary tract, few symptoms are perceived by the individual, although renal function is impaired. In certain cases incompetence of the ureterovesical junction combined with increased voiding pressure may result in vesicoureteral reflux that compromises the hydrodynamic function of the renal pelvis and ureters and promotes the likelihood of pyelonephritis.[78]

The two primary complications of benign prostatic hypertrophy are urinary tract infection and acute urinary retention. Urinary tract infection results from the presence of postvoid residuals that cause hypoxemia of the bladder wall and decreased resistance to bacterial invasion.[78] Acute urinary retention is a surprisingly common complication.

COMPLICATIONS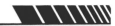

Acute urinary retention
Urinary tract infection
Obstructive uropathy with ureteral dilation, hydronephrosis
Compromised renal function
Detrusor decompensation

DIAGNOSTIC STUDIES AND FINDINGS

Diagnostic test	Findings
Voiding diary	Urinary frequency more often than q 2 h while awake; two or more episodes of nocturia per night; urgency and urge incontinence may coexist
Intravenous pyelogram/ urogram (IVP/IVU)	(Reserved for cases in which obstructive uropathy is suspected) dilation of the ureters with hydronephrosis; delayed excretion of contrast medium; parenchymal thinning in advanced cases
Urinary flow study	Poor flow pattern with low maximum and average flow rates; prolonged voiding time and postvoid residual volume greater than 100 ml or 25% of total bladder capacity

Continued.

DIAGNOSTIC STUDIES AND FINDINGS—cont'd

Diagnostic test	Findings
Urodynamics/ videourodynamics	(Reserved for patients with known coexisting voiding dysfunction or neuropathic conditions that raise suspicion of dysfunction) large cystometric capacity with sensory urgency and/or detrusor instability; bladder wall compliance may be compromised; voiding pressure study demonstrates high-pressure contraction with poor flow pattern, indicating outlet obstruction, *or* decompensation of the detrusor with low-pressure, poorly sustained contractions; videourodynamics demonstrates narrowed prostatic urethra characteristic of BPH, trabeculation of the bladder in advanced cases; vesicoureteral reflux occasionally is present
Endoscopy	Narrowing of the prostatic urethra; trabeculation of the bladder may be noted
Prostatic ultrasound	Bilateral enlargement of the gland with no hypoechogenic areas suspicious for malignant tumor; bright prostatic calculi may be noted
Urinalysis and urine culture	Infection noted in certain cases
Serum creatinine and blood urea nitrogen (BUN)	Elevated in unusually severe cases with markedly compromised renal function

MEDICAL MANAGEMENT

GENERAL MANAGEMENT AND DRUG THERAPY

"Watchful waiting" routine evaluation of the patient with minimal to moderate obstruction that is not associated with significant obstructive uropathy or complications of acute urinary retention or infection

Pharmacologic endocrine therapy, including estrogens, androgen antagonists, luteinizing hormone–releasing hormone antagonists, and a 5-alpha-reductase inhibitor

Alpha-adrenergic blocking drugs (antagonists)

Indwelling catheterization for episodes of acute urinary retention; intermittent or indwelling catheterization may be used for temporary management when urinary retention is severe

SURGICAL INTERVENTIONS/SPECIAL PROCEDURES

Open prostatectomy

Transurethral prostatectomy or transurethral incision of the prostate

Balloon dilation of the prostate

Transurethral microwave therapy

Implantation of intraurethral prostatic stent

Table 6-1

HORMONAL AGENTS USED FOR BPH

Antiandrogen agents: Flutamide, Anandron, Kasadex

Pharmacologic actions: Selectively block androgenic receptors

Potential side effects: Impaired libido, erectile dysfunction, gynecomastia, diarrhea

Aromatase inhibitors: Testolactone

Pharmacologic actions: Blocks conversion of testosterone to estrogen

Side effects: Headache, rare loss of libido, erectile dysfunction

Gonadotropin releasing hormone analogs: leuprolide

Pharmacologic actions: Inhibits secretion of leutinizing hormone from pituitary, diminishes serum levels of testosterone and dihydrotestosterone

Side effects: Impaired libido, erectile dysfunction, estrogen-type effects including hot flashes and gynecomastia

5-Alpha-reductase inhibitors: Finesteride, Proscar,* MK906*

Pharmacologic actions: Blocks 5-alpha-reductase enzyme that converts testosterone to dihydrotestosterone

Side effects: Headache, occasional loss of libido

From Finkbiner and Bissada[103a]; Grayhack and Kozlowski.[107]
*These drugs are under evaluation in FDA approved clinical trials.

Table 6-2

ALPHA-ADRENERGIC BLOCKERS

Agents

Phenoxybenzamine
    Dosage: 5-10 mg po bid
Prazosin
    Dosage: 1-5 mg bid
Terazosin
    Dosage: 1-10 mg at hs
Doxazosin
    Dosage: 1-16 mg at hs

Pharmacologic action

Phenoxybenzamine produces alpha 1 and alpha 2 adrenergic blockade; all other agents provide selective alpha 1 adrenergic blockade

Side effects

General: Postural hypotension, tachycardia, drowsiness, significant fatigue, rhinitis

Specific: Postural hypotension associated with prazosin administration may be intensified by hyponatremia; serum sodium is evaluated prior to start of therapy

From Lepor.[113a]

Table 6-3

ALTERNATIVE TREATMENTS FOR BENIGN PROSTATIC HYPERTROPHY

Transurethral prostate incision

Description: Limited transurethral incisions of the prostatic capsule from bladder neck to lateral or upper border of verumontanum; typically limited to patients with mild enlargement
Complications: Significant bleeding is a rare complication
Potential advantages: Less extensive resection reduces morbidity associated with classic transurethral resection technique; bleeding typically is minimal

Microwave therapy

Description: Transurethral application of heat using microwave technology; single or multiple applications are described
Complications: Transient but severe local inflammation with intensification of irritative voiding symptoms; acute urinary retention requiring catheter drainage
Potential advantages: Beneficial for patients who are poor candidates for surgical resection

Balloon dilation

Description: Transurethral passage of a balloon that is inflated in the prostatic urethra, thus dilating the obstructing lesion
Complications: Recurrence of symptoms may necessitate repeated treatments
Potential advantages: Surgical incision and related complications of bleeding and retention are avoided

Continued.

Table 6-3—cont'd

ALTERNATIVE TREATMENTS FOR BENIGN PROSTATIC HYPERTROPHY—cont'd

Intraurethral stent

Description: Transurethral placement of a titanium wire mesh (stent) that remains securely fixed in the prostatic urethra; in time the urethra epithelializes the device

Complications: Migration, dislodgment of device, infection or calculus formation, local inflammation with irritative voiding symptoms

Potential advantages: Surgical resection and associated complications of hemorrhage and acute retention are avoided; device may be removed if local inflammation or infection occurs*

From Grayhack and Kozlowski[107]; Lepor.[113a]
*Not approved for this use by the FDA.

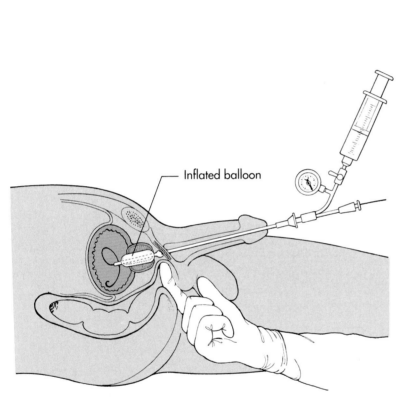

FIGURE 6-2
Transurethral balloon dilation. Inflated balloon in prostatic urethra.

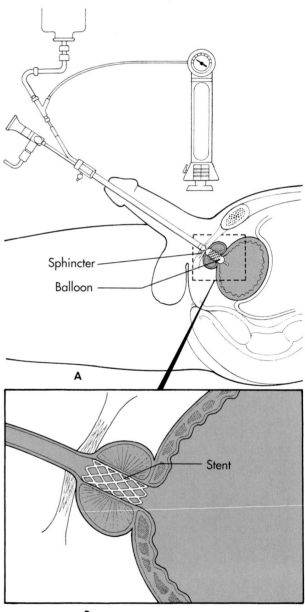

FIGURE 6-3
Prostatic stent. **A,** Placement of stent. **B,** Stent in place increases prostatic urethral lumen.

1 ASSESS

ASSESSMENT	OBSERVATIONS
Prostate gland enlargement	Digital rectal examination demonstrates symmetric glandular enlargement with no nodules or induration
Poor urinary stream	Voided urinary stream reveals diminished caliber (less than a pencil lead); patient shows intermittence with straining to enhance evacuation, hesitancy to initiate stream, and prolonged voiding time
Altered patterns of urinary elimination	Obstructive symptoms (diurnal frequency, nocturia, poor force of stream, hesitancy) with or without irritative symptoms (urgency, urge incontinence)
Chronic urinary retention	Obstructive voiding symptoms with documented urinary residual greater than 100 ml or 25% of total bladder capacity
Acute urinary retention	Total inability to urinate with acute onset
Urinary tract infection	Irritative symptoms with dysuria and bacteriuria noted on urine culture

2 DIAGNOSE

NURSING DIAGNOSIS	SUBJECTIVE FINDINGS	OBJECTIVE FINDINGS
Altered patterns of urinary elimination related to BPH	Complains of obstructive symptoms (diurnal frequency, nocturia, diminished force of stream, and hesitancy) with or without irritative symptoms (urgency to void, urge incontinence)	Diurnal frequency greater than q 2 h; nocturia two episodes or more per night; urinary flow reveals poor stream with hesitancy and prolonged voiding time
Urinary retention (chronic) related to BPH	Reports sensations of incomplete bladder emptying	Documented urinary residual greater than 100 ml or 25% of total bladder capacity
Urinary retention (potential for acute) related to BPH	Reports a sudden inability to urinate and suprapubic discomfort that intensifies with bladder filling	Catheterization reveals large urinary volume despite inability to urinate
Potential for infection (urinary tract) related to BPH and urinary stasis	Complains of irritative voiding symptoms with dysuria; hematuria and fever occasionally occur	Urine culture reveals bacteriuria with more than 100,000 CFU*/ml; bacteriuria and pyuria noted on urinalysis

*Colony-forming units.

3 PLAN

Patient goals

1. Patterns of urinary elimination will return to normal.
2. Chronic urinary retention will resolve.
3. Acute urinary retention will be avoided or promptly reversed.
4. Urinary tract infection will be avoided or promptly managed.

→ › ›

4   IMPLEMENT

NURSING DIAGNOSIS	NURSING INTERVENTIONS	RATIONALE
Altered patterns of urinary elimination related to BPH	Instruct the patient with mild or moderate obstructive symptoms to void on a timed schedule q 2-3 h.	Regular bladder emptying prevents over-distention, which places the bladder at risk of acute retention and infection.
	Institute a fluid management program. Advise the patient to obtain adequate daily fluid intake (at least 1,500 ml, or about six 8-oz glasses, per day). Instruct him to limit beverages with meals to 8 ounces and to restrict fluids 2 hours before sleep to sips. Encourage him to sip beverages throughout the day.	A fluid management program ensures an adequate daily fluid intake while avoiding bolus intake of fluids with meals, which increases the risk of acute urinary retention, detrusor instability, and infection.
	Teach the patient with mild to moderate retention to double void: instruct him to void as usual, wait on the toilet for 3 to 5 minutes of rest, and then urinate again.	Double voiding may produce more complete bladder evacuation in a patient with mild to moderate obstructive symptoms.
	Administer or teach the patient to self-administer anticholinergic medications for unstable detrusor contractions.	Anticholinergic medications diminish the occurrence of unstable detrusor contractions and associated irritative bladder symptoms.
	Advise the patient that antispasmodic medications may intensify urinary retention, creating the need for intermittent catheterization to ensure regular, complete bladder evacuation.	Antispasmodic medications reduce bladder contractility; this may produce total urinary retention in a patient with preexisting retention.
Urinary retention (chronic) related to BPH	Teach the patient with severe obstructive symptoms and significant urinary retention to perform self intermittent catheterization as directed.	Intermittent catheterization provides regular, complete bladder evacuation.
	Administer or teach the patient to self-administer hormonal agents as directed (see Table 6-1).	Hormonal agents reduce prostatic enlargement by antagonizing testosterones and related androgens at the level of the hypothalamus, testis, or prostatic tissue receptors.
	Administer or teach the patient to self-administer alpha-adrenergic blocking drugs as directed (see Table 6-2).	Alpha-adrenergic blocking drugs diminish the obstruction caused by BPH by acting on the smooth muscle bundles in the bladder neck and prostatic capsule; relaxation of these muscle bundles diminishes the resistance to outflow during urination.
	Prepare the patient for transurethral or open resection prostatectomy (see Open Prostatectomy, page 176, and Transurethral Prostatectomy, page 171).	Resection of excessive prostatic tissue diminishes retention and obstruction by increasing the caliber of the bladder outlet and disrupting smooth muscle bundles at the bladder neck and prostatic capsule.

NURSING DIAGNOSIS	NURSING INTERVENTIONS	RATIONALE
	Prepare the patient for transurethral microwave therapy of prostatic hypertrophy as directed.	Microwave therapy uses hyperthermia to perform a prostatectomy (Table 6-3).
	Prepare the patient for transurethral balloon dilation of the prostate as directed.	Transurethral balloon dilation of the prostate reduces obstruction and retention by enlarging the lumen of the proximal urethra (see Table 6-3 and Figure 6-2).
	Prepare the patient for placement of a urethral stent as directed.	The prostatic stent is a wire mesh implanted directly into the proximal (prostatic) urethra; it diminishes retention and obstruction by mechanically increasing the prostatic urethral lumen (see Table 6-3 and Figure 6-3). (The prostatic stent has not been approved by the FDA for this use.)
Urinary retention (potential for acute) related to BPH	Advise the patient to avoid over-the-counter decongestants or combination decongestant/antihistamine medications.	Decongestant medications are alpha sympathomimetics; besides relieving congestion in the upper airways, they increase tone at the bladder neck and prostatic urethra, increasing the patient's predisposition to acute urinary retention.
	Advise the patient to avoid over-the-counter diet pills.	Like decongestants, diet pills rely on alpha sympathomimetics for their appetite-suppressant actions.
	Advise the patient to avoid excessive intake of alcohol.	Alcohol predisposes the patient to acute urinary retention by its diuretic effect, causing bladder overdistention.
	Advise the patient to avoid trying to urinate after prolonged exposure to cold temperatures; teach him to warm his body before trying to urinate.	Exposure to cold predisposes the patient to urinary retention, possibly as a result of increased urethral tone indirectly related to shivering or possibly because of blood being shunted away from the detrusor to prevent hypothermia; rewarming the body before urination reverses these effects.
	Advise the patient with acute urinary retention to promote voiding by trying to urinate in a warm, private bathroom. The patient should assume a sitting position, place both feet firmly on the floor, and relax as much as possible. Drinking warm tea further stimulates micturition.	Privacy and a warm bathroom promote relaxation of the pelvic floor muscles and micturition. A sitting position is necessary, since the process may require some time. Warm tea serves as a mild bladder stimulant, increasing the desire to void.
	If the patient still cannot void, advise him to stand in a warm shower or sit in a tub filled with warm water to promote urination. Reassure him that it is best to proceed with urination without trying to move to the toilet.	Warm water encourages micturition, possibly by relaxing the pelvic floor muscles and promoting local blood flow; moving to the toilet is avoided, since the bladder contraction may be suppressed by postponing urination while moving.

→ > >

NURSING DIAGNOSIS	NURSING INTERVENTIONS	RATIONALE
	Advise the patient to seek urgent medical care if acute urinary retention persists for 6 hours or if suprapubic pain and urgency become unmanageable.	Acute urinary retention is a medical emergency; catheterization is required to prevent bladder rupture and subsequent infection if attempts to spontaneously urinate are unsuccessful.
Potential for infection (urinary tract) related to BPH and urinary stasis	Advise the patient to avoid chronically reducing fluid intake as a strategy to reduce urinary frequency.	Patients may reduce fluid intake in an attempt to reduce urinary frequency and nocturia; ironically, this strategy only concentrates the urine, increasing bladder irritability and urinary frequency while predisposing the urinary system to infection.
	Teach patient the signs and symptoms of urinary infection and pyelonephritis; advise patient to obtain a urine specimen for urinalysis and culture and seek prompt care should symptoms of infection occur.	Urinary infection is intensified by an obstruction; prompt care minimizes these risks (see Cystitis/Urinary Tract Infection, page 52).
Knowledge deficit	See Patient Teaching.	

5   EVALUATE

PATIENT OUTCOME	DATA INDICATING THAT OUTCOME IS REACHED
Patterns of urinary elimination have returned to normal.	Diurnal frequency returns to q 2 h or less often; nocturia returns to one or no episodes per night.
Chronic urinary retention has resolved.	Postvoiding residual volumes are less than 100 ml or 25% of total bladder capacity.
Acute urinary retention has been avoided or promptly reversed.	Episodes of acute urinary retention are avoided; patient accurately describes a strategy for managing acute urinary retention should it occur.
Urinary tract infection has been avoided or promptly managed.	Urine culture demonstrates no bacteriuria.

PATIENT TEACHING

1. Teach the patient the natural history of benign prostatic hypertrophy, including the significance of obstruction of the urinary system.
2. Teach patient specific strategies to reduce risk of acute urinary retention, such as avoiding overdistention of the bladder, excessive chilling or alcohol intake, and medications that can cause retention.
3. Teach the patient specific strategies for managing the complications of benign prostatic hypertrophy, including urinary tract infection and acute urinary retention.
4. Teach the patient the names, dosages, administration, and potential side effects of any medications used to treat his condition.

TRANSURETHRAL PROSTATECTOMY

Transurethral prostatectomy is the surgical resection of the prostate gland under endoscopic control. A rigid cystoscope is inserted into the urethra and bladder, and the prostatic urethra is localized. Obstructive prostatic tissue is removed by a resectoscope (Figure 6-4). A glycine or sorbitol solution is irrigated through the resectoscope during the procedure, removing blood and tissue from the operative field. The solution also allows electrocauterization of the prostatic vascular bed, which prevents excessive hemorrhage without burning adjacent tissue. The area of resection varies with each patient but typically includes the bladder neck and prostatic fossa. The trigone, ureteral orifices, and verumontanum are carefully avoided to prevent potential complications of vesicoureteral reflux and stress incontinence.[107]

INDICATIONS

Obstructive uropathy related to benign prostatic hypertrophy (BPH)

Acute urinary retention related to prostatic hypertrophy

Recurrent urinary infections or febrile urinary infection related to benign prostatic hypertrophy

CONTRAINDICATIONS

Prostatic enlargement without obstructive uropathy

Inability to tolerate anesthesia or surgical resection

COMPLICATIONS

Hemorrhage	Stress urinary incontinence
Transurethral resection (TUR) syndrome	Erectile dysfunction
Acute urinary retention	

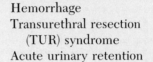

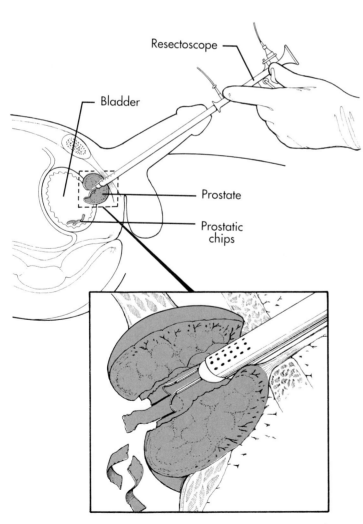

FIGURE 6-4
Transurethral resection of the prostate (TURP).

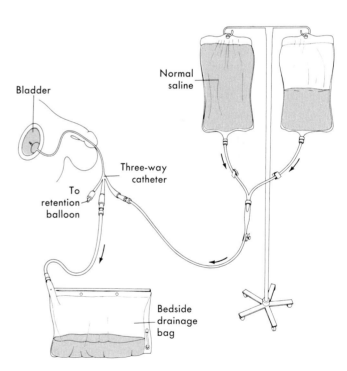

FIGURE 6-5
Continuous irrigation of the bladder requires a three-way Foley catheter that allows simultaneous infusion and drainage of an irrigating solution (normal saline) through the bladder. The solution is infused rapidly into the bladder, and the bedside drainage bag is assessed for evidence of excessive bleeding and then drained every 1 to 2 hours (From Beare P and Myers J: *Principles and practice of adult health nursing,* St Louis, 1990, Mosby–Year Book.)

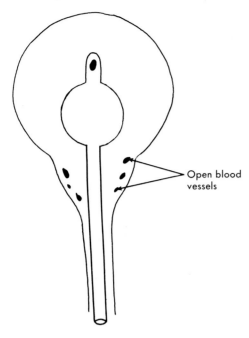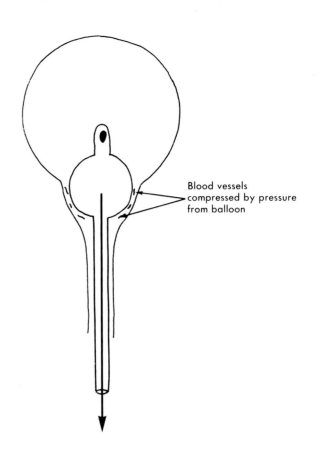

Open blood vessels

Blood vessels compressed by pressure from balloon

FIGURE 6-6
Gentle traction is maintained against the prostatic vascular bed to prevent excessive bleeding following transurethral resection. (From Lerner J and Kan Z: *Mosby's Manual of urologic nursing,* St Louis, 1982, Mosby–Year Book, Inc.)

PREPROCEDURAL NURSING CARE

NURSING DIAGNOSIS	NURSING INTERVENTIONS	RATIONALE
Knowledge deficit related to procedure, goals, anesthesia, and potential untoward effects	Reinforce preoperative teaching, including the procedure, its goals, anesthesia to be used, potential untoward effects, and expected nursing care.	Anxiety before surgical resection reduces the patient's ability to learn and retain information; repeating it decreases anxiety and improves retention.
	Advise the patient that general and spinal anesthesia has been used for transurethral resection of a prostatic adenoma; consult the physician and anesthetist about which type is likely to be used for this patient, and prepare the patient according to hospital protocols.	Because incision is avoided, either general or spinal anesthesia is suitable for transurethral prostate resection; the choice is affected by the patient's preference and medical history and the size of the adenoma.
	Advise the patient that transurethral resection is expected to change ejaculatory function; reassure him that retrograde ejaculation will not render him unable to attain or sustain an erection, although it is expected to alter his fertility potential.	Resection of the prostatic fossa produces retrograde ejaculation (semen is expelled into the bladder rather than propelled out of the urethra with orgasm); this condition alters fertility potential, although it should not produce erectile dysfunction.
	Advise the patient that stress incontinence may occur after transurethral resection of the prostate; this incontinence is expected to improve with time.	Mild stress incontinence may occur after prostatic resection; often the leakage is transient.

NURSING DIAGNOSIS	NURSING INTERVENTIONS	RATIONALE
	Advise the patient that a three-way Foley catheter will be left in the urethra after the surgery; irrigation is discontinued and the catheter is removed after expected post-operative bleeding ceases.	A three-way catheter allows irrigation of the bladder, which prevents acute urinary retention caused by clots in the catheter and provides hemostasis against the prostatic vascular bed.
	Reassure the patient that even a relatively small amount of bleeding will discolor a large volume of urine and irrigating fluid; advise him that his nurses will routinely monitor his urinary output to ensure that excessive bleeding does not occur.	Hemorrhage of the prostatic vascular bed discolors a large volume of irrigant and urine, which may frighten the patient, leading him to believe that he is bleeding significantly; reassurance *before* surgical resection alleviates this anxiety.

POSTPROCEDURAL NURSING CARE

NURSING DIAGNOSIS	NURSING INTERVENTIONS	RATIONALE
Altered tissue perfusion (peripheral, prostatic vascular bed) related to surgical incision	Maintain three-way Foley catheter with gentle traction as directed (Figure 6-5).	The catheter and traction produce hemostasis against the newly resected prostatic fossa.
	Monitor urine output q 1-2 h for evidence of excessive bleeding (large volume of bright red blood with clots).	Excessive bleeding may occur after surgical resection of the prostatic vascular bed; although some bleeding is expected, significant blood loss is noted as a large volume of blood mixed with urine output.
	Obtain a serum hemoglobin and hematocrit as directed; compare postprocedural values with presurgical levels.	Significant prostatic bleeding causes a decline in serum hematocrit and hemoglobin.
	Monitor vital signs for evidence of significant bleeding with hypovolemic shock.	Rapid pulse with increased blood pressure is followed by declining blood pressure when bleeding is severe.
	Maintain traction on indwelling catheter as directed (Figure 6-6).	Gentle traction prevents bleeding by compressing vessels of the prostatic urethra.
	Following removal of the catheter (approximately 36 to 72 hours after surgery), provide the patient with several bottles to monitor hematuria; instruct him to save some urine from each voiding episode to evaluate resolution of hematuria.	Flecks of blood and pink-tinged urine are common after catheter removal. As hematuria clears, the urine regains its clear, yellow color. Successive bottles of urine demonstrate this sequence of events and provide evidence of persistent hematuria if healing is incomplete before the catheter is removed.
	Reinsert an indwelling catheter as directed if marked hematuria persists for more than 24 hours after removal or if significant hematuria occurs.	The catheter is reinserted to provide sustained hemostasis when wound healing is delayed.

NURSING DIAGNOSIS	NURSING INTERVENTIONS	RATIONALE
	Reassure the patient that flecks of dark blood and lightly tinged urine may recur for about 10 to 14 days after catheter is removed.	Dark flecks of blood and minimal hematuria may occur after the scabs from the surgical resection spontaneously fall off.
Altered tissue perfusion (deep leg veins) related to surgical position for transurethral resection of prostate	Have the patient wear antiembolic stockings (obtained and fitted before surgery) after prostate resection.	Because transurethral resection of the prostate requires keeping the legs in stirrups for a prolonged period, deep vein thrombosis may occur; antiembolic stockings reduce the risk of thrombosis by promoting venous return.
	Raise the foot of the bed 20 to 30 degrees during the first postoperative day.	Mild elevation of the bed encourages venous return from the deep veins of the leg, using a favorable pressure gradient created by gravity.
	Teach the patient to perform passive leg exercises until the catheter has been removed and he is ambulatory.	Contracting the leg muscles encourages the return of blood from the deep veins of the leg.
	Maintain adequate fluid intake (at least 1,500 ml per day); administer intravenous fluids as directed to prevent dehydration.	Dehydration intensifies the risk of deep vein thrombosis by increasing the viscosity of the blood.
Urinary retention (potential) related to surgical resection of prostate adenoma	Maintain continuous irrigation with three-way catheter for 24 h after transurethral resection as directed.	Continuous irrigation mechanically removes clots from the bladder, preventing clogging of the catheter and urinary retention.
	Irrigate the catheter with saline, or help the physician irrigate the catheter as directed.	Irrigation evacuates large blood clots and prevents urinary retention.
	Empty drainage bag q 1-2 h when continuous irrigation occurs and every shift while catheter is in place; use large drainage bag (2 L or more) after prostatectomy.	Continuous irrigation causes rapid filling of the drainage bag and urinary retention unless it is emptied regularly.
	Advise the patient that his urologist may gently dilate the urethra during an outpatient follow-up visit; reassure him that the procedure will be performed with adequate pain control.	Bladder neck contracture may complicate transurethral prostatectomy; gentle dilation with a metal sound is used to prevent this potential complication.
Potential for TUR syndrome related to surgical resection of benign prostatic adenoma	Monitor patient for signs of TUR syndrome (bradycardia, tachypnea, vomiting, agitation, and altered alertness) during first postoperative day.	TUR syndrome is caused by fluid volume excess and electrolyte imbalance following prostate resection.
	Maintain adequate fluid intake (at least 1,500 ml) using oral or intravenous administration routes as directed.	Maintaining adequate hydration minimizes the risk of electrolyte imbalance and TUR syndrome.
	Promptly inform the physician if signs of TUR syndrome occur.	Left untreated, TUR syndrome can be fatal.

NURSING DIAGNOSIS	NURSING INTERVENTIONS	RATIONALE
Pain related to prostatic resection	Administer anticholinergic medications as directed to prevent painful bladder spasms and leakage around the catheter.	Unstable bladder contractions may occur after prostatic resection; anticholinergic medications reduce discomfort and prevent unstable contractions.
	Advise the patient that mild dysuria (burning with urination) may occur after catheter removal; advise the patient to drink at least 1,500 ml of clear liquids (about six 8-ounce glasses) to reduce dysuria.	Irritation of the urethra may cause mild discomfort after removal of the catheter; clear liquids and urination reduce this discomfort.
	Administer urinary analgesics as directed following removal of the catheter.	Urinary analgesics diminish dysuria through pharmacologic actions that are unclear.
Altered patterns of urinary elimination related to surgical resection of prostate	Advise the patient that he will have urinary frequency and urgency for a short period after catheter removal.	Irritation from surgical resection and the Foley catheter causes transient urinary urgency and frequency following removal of the catheter.
	Teach the patient with dribbling and stress incontinence how to do pelvic exercises (see page 304).	Pelvic exercises strengthen the periurethral muscles, reducing or ablating stress incontinence.
	Advise the patient with stress incontinence that leakage should regress and disappear within the first year after surgery.	Sphincter damage is a rare complication of transurethral resection of the prostate; persistent stress incontinence is the outcome of this rare complication.
	Advise the patient to consult his urologist or a continence nurse specialist for definitive management of urinary incontinence.	Stress incontinence is a treatable condition that may be managed by physiotherapy, medications, or other means under the care of a qualified specialist.
	Advise the patient with symptoms of instability (urge) incontinence that this symptom may disappear or persist after prostate resection.	Detrusor instability may be reversed by relieving the obstruction in some cases; in other cases, instability related to neuropathy may persist despite relief of obstruction.[96]
	Advise the patient with persistent instability (urge) incontinence to seek definitive management from a urologist or continence nurse specialist.	Persistent instability incontinence is a treatable condition manageable by behavioral therapy, medications, or other means under the care of a qualified specialist.

PATIENT TEACHING

1. Teach the patient the potential complications of transurethral prostatectomy, including bladder neck contracture, incontinence, and altered fertility potential. Help the patient formulate strategies for managing any complications.
2. Teach the patient the significance of follow-up evaluations after transurethral resection of a prostatic adenoma.
3. Inform the patient of the potential for regrowth of a benign prostatic adenoma (usually 10 years or more after surgery). Emphasize the importance of routine prostate evaluation, even after surgical resection.

OPEN PROSTATECTOMY

Open prostatectomy is the surgical resection of the prostate gland without the capsule, using a suprapubic, retropubic, or perineal approach. Once the incision has been made, the bladder is opened and the prostate enucleated with blunt or sharp instruments, leaving the prostatic capsule intact. Urethral and suprapubic tubes are left in the bladder to provide hemostasis and urinary drainage (a retroprostatic Penrose drain is left in when a perineal enucleation is done). Open surgical enucleation of the prostate is reserved for cases of benign prostatic hypertrophy (BPH) when the prostate virtually closes the urethral outlet. Open surgery is also useful when the gland is exceptionally large or when benign prostatic hypertrophy is associated with a pathologic bladder condition such as bladder calculi or diverticula. The suprapubic and retropubic approaches are most commonly used for benign adenomas; retropubic prostatectomy is typically reserved for radical surgery when adenocarcinoma is present.[107]

INDICATIONS

Hyperplastic prostate too large for transurethral resection

Benign prostatic hypertrophy with bladder complications such as calculi or bladder neck diverticula

CONTRAINDICATIONS

Prostatic adenomas amenable to transurethral resection or incision

COMPLICATIONS

Stress incontinence
Epididymitis
Erectile dysfunction
Hemorrhage
Fistula

Bladder neck contracture (stricture)
Osteitis pubis (painful infection or inflammation of the symphysis pubis bone)

PREPROCEDURAL NURSING CARE

NURSING DIAGNOSIS	NURSING INTERVENTIONS	RATIONALE
Knowledge deficit related to procedure, goals, anesthesia, and potential untoward effects	Reinforce preoperative teaching, including the procedure, its goals, anesthesia to be used, potential untoward effects, and expected nursing care.	Anxiety before surgical resection reduces the patient's ability to learn and retain instruction; repeating it decreases anxiety and improves retention.
	Advise the patient that general anesthesia will be used unless otherwise directed.	Open prostatectomy requires open surgical incision and extensive resection, so general anesthesia typically is required.
	Advise the patient that he will have suprapubic and urethral catheters when he returns from surgery.	The urethral catheter is used primarily for hemostasis of the enucleated prostatic capsule and the suprapubic catheter for urinary drainage.
	Advise the patient undergoing perineal prostatectomy that a retroprostatic drain (collapsible rubber drain) will be placed in the perineal area behind the scrotum.	A Penrose drain is used to drain the retroprostatic space when a perineal approach is elected, since there is a risk of hemorrhage and drainage into this space.
	Advise the patient that continuous or intermittent irrigation of the bladder may be necessary for the first 24 h after surgery.	Continuous drainage is not always required for open resection of the prostate, since an additional suprapubic tube is used to drain the bladder; continuous or intermittent irrigation evacuates blood clots and prevents urinary retention.

NURSING DIAGNOSIS	NURSING INTERVENTIONS	RATIONALE
	Advise the patient that the catheters typically are removed 36 to 72 h after surgery.	The catheter is removed after active bleeding of the prostatic capsule has stopped.
	Advise the patient that antiinfective medications may be administered after surgery to prevent infection.	Antiinfective medications help prevent urinary tract infections and osteitis pubis.

POSTPROCEDURAL NURSING CARE

NURSING DIAGNOSIS	NURSING INTERVENTIONS	RATIONALE
Altered tissue perfusion (peripheral, prostatic capsular, vascular bed) related to surgical enucleation of benign adenoma	Maintain traction on urethral catheter as directed (see Figure 6-6).	The Foley catheter and balloon provide gentle hemostasis for the vascular bed until active bleeding stops.
	Administer anticholinergic medications, and ensure adequate bladder drainage after surgery.	Bladder spasms (unstable detrusor contractions) increase the risk of bleeding and disruption of the surgical site; overdistention of the bladder is avoided because it promotes unstable contractions, and anticholinergic medications are used to inhibit bladder spasms.
	Monitor the urine from the urethral and suprapubic tubes for evidence of excessive bleeding (bright red output with clots); pink-tinged urine is expected.	Although blood-tinged urine is expected after prostatectomy, passage of excessive, bright red blood and clots may indicate significant, uncontrolled hemorrhage.
	Monitor serum hematocrit and hemoglobin values, and compare to preoperative data.	Hematocrit and hemoglobin decline if significant postoperative bleeding occurs.
	Monitor vital signs for evidence of significant bleeding with hypovolemic shock (hypertension with rapid pulse followed by declining blood pressure with weakened pulse); contact the physician immediately if any signs of significant bleeding occur.	Severe, uncontrolled bleeding alters vital signs and will cause hypovolemic shock unless treated quickly.
	After the catheter has been removed, reassure the patient that pink-tinged urine is expected; give him several bottles for collecting urine from consecutive voids.	Small amounts of blood will color the urine pink after the catheter has been removed; monitoring a string of bottles provides documentation of gradual cessation of this bleeding as the urine changes from pink to its usual clear, yellow tint.
	Consult the physician if bleeding persists for longer than 24 to 48 hours or if a large amount of bright red urine with clots is noted.	Bright red urine with clots indicates persistent significant bleeding, justifying reinsertion of the urethral catheter for more vigorous hemostasis.

NURSING DIAGNOSIS	NURSING INTERVENTIONS	RATIONALE
Urinary retention (potential) related to surgical enucleation of prostatic adenoma	Maintain continuous irrigation or perform intermittent irrigation of the urethral and suprapubic catheters as directed.	Irrigating the catheters mechanically removes clots and prevents clogging of the tubes, with subsequent urinary retention.
	Maintain separate drainage systems for the suprapubic and urethral catheters.	Separate systems allow discrimination of output from each catheter so that occlusion can be isolated and corrected by irrigation.
	Help the patient maintain an adequate fluid intake (at least 1,500 ml/day); administer intravenous fluids for hydration as directed.	Adequate hydration flushes the urinary system, reducing the risk of the catheter becoming clogged by clots.
	After the catheter has been removed, monitor intake and urinary output.	Poor urinary output is an indication of urinary retention, possibly as a result of urethral obstruction from clots or debris.
	Advise the patient that his urologist may gently dilate the urethra with a metal sound to ensure that there is no bladder neck contracture; reassure the patient that the procedure will be performed with adequate pain control.	Bladder neck contracture may complicate open prostatectomy; gentle dilation prevents this complication.
Pain related to surgical incision and prostate gland enucleation	Assess the location, character, and duration of pain.	Pain from open prostatectomy may arise from the surgical incision or from bladder spasms; incisional pain typically is a dull, boring pain in the midline, whereas bladder spasms cause cramping pains of sudden onset and short duration in the suprapubic area.
	Administer analgesic/narcotic medications as directed for incisional pain and antispasmodic medications for bladder spasms.	Analgesic medications diminish incisional pain, and antispasmodic medications prevent bladder spasms.
	Implement nonpharmacologic strategies to minimize pain (e.g., proper positioning, minimizing environmental distractions, and preventing bladder overdistention).	Nonpharmacologic interventions are no less important than drugs in promoting the patient's comfort.
	Advise the patient that he may have moderate dysuria (discomfort with urination) for several days after the catheter is removed.	Irritation from the surgical enucleation and Foley drainage may occur after the catheter is removed.
	Advise the patient to drink an adequate volume of clear liquids (at least 1,500 ml/day, or about six 8-ounce glasses).	Adequate hydration dilutes the urine, minimizing dysuria.

NURSING DIAGNOSIS	NURSING INTERVENTIONS	RATIONALE
	Administer urinary analgesics (see Chapter 11) for a brief period after catheter removal as directed.	Urinary analgesics minimize dysuria through pharmacologic actions that are unclear.
Altered patterns of urinary elimination related to surgical enucleation of obstructive prostatic adenoma	Advise the patient that in rare cases dribbling and stress incontinence occur after open prostatectomy.	Surgical enucleation of an obstructive prostate may cause transient or chronic sphincter incompetence with stress incontinence.
	Teach pelvic floor muscle exercises to the patient with dribbling or stress incontinence.	Pelvic floor muscle exercises minimize or stop stress incontinence by strengthening periurethral striated muscles.
	Advise the patient with chronic stress incontinence (persisting for longer than 1 year after surgery) to consult a urologist or continence nurse specialist for definitive management of stress incontinence.	Stress incontinence is a treatable condition that may be managed by physiotherapy, medications, or surgery under the direction of a qualified specialist.
	Advise the patient with symptoms of instability (urge) incontinence that this symptom may disappear or may persist after prostate resection.	Detrusor instability may be reversed by relieving the obstruction in some cases; in other cases, instability related to neuropathy may persist despite relief of obstruction.
	Advise the patient with persistent instability (urge) incontinence to seek definitive management from a urologist or continence nurse specialist.	Persistent instability incontinence is a treatable condition that may be managed by behavioral therapy, medications, or other means under the care of a qualified specialist.

PATIENT TEACHING

1. In consultation with the urologic surgeon, inform the patient of the possible postoperative complications, including urinary incontinence, altered fertility potential, and osteitis pubis. Help the patient identify appropriate strategies for managing any complications.
2. Inform the patient of the possibility of bladder neck contracture following open prostatectomy. Encourage strict adherence to follow-up visits to minimize the potential for contracture formation.
3. Teach the patient the signs and symptoms of urinary infection and strategies to manage an infection should it occur.

Urinary Calculi

Calculi are stones that form from precipitate materials in the urine. Urinary calculi that pass spontaneously without causing discomfort or infection present no serious threat to health. In contrast, calculi that obstruct the urinary system, cause significant pain, transiently or permanently compromise renal function, and predispose the system to infection represent a significant threat to health, demanding prompt diagnosis and management.

PATHOPHYSIOLOGY

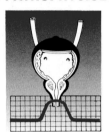

The cause of calculi formation is complex and incompletely understood. Urinary calculi are approximately 97.5% crystalline and 2.5% mucoprotein or glycoprotein matrix and are described by their predominant salt content. To understand the pathophysiologic process of stone formation in the urinary tract, it is necessary to understand basic principles of biologic crystallization. Calculi formation requires the following conditions in the urinary tract. A solution has a given solubility product that is constant. Once this product has been reached, adding further solute (such as calcium oxalate or other stone salt) will not raise its concentration within the solution. Supersaturation occurs when further solute is added to the solute (urine). At a formation concentration the supersaturated solute spontaneously precipitates from the solution, forming the beginning of a potential calculus. Unlike the solubility product, the formation concentration varies with circumstances. Calculus formation requires the initiation of a crystal from precipitation of a stone salt from the urine, followed by crystal growth and aggregation. This process requires energy that is obtained from urine in a supersaturation.[104]

Two predisposing epidemiologic factors have been identified in association with an increased likelihood of stone formation: predisposing anatomic or biochemical factors, such as the inherited predisposition for cystinuria or medullary sponge kidney, and environmental factors, such as diet, climate, fluid intake patterns, and occupation.[97]

Several theories have attempted to explain calculus formation in the urinary tract. The *precipitation-crystallization theory* is based on the general principles of biologic crystallization; it delineates four necessary steps for stone formation. The first step is the nucleation phase, in which the smallest unit of a crystal is formed in the urine. This nucleus may be of homogeneous or heterogeneous form relative to the remaining portion of the calculus. In the second phase the crystal form grows and aggregates into a larger form. For this growth to occur, supersaturation of the urine persists and circumstances allowing a formation concentration to be attained continue. The greater the degree of supersaturation, the greater the rate of stone formation. The third stage of stone formation occurs when the crystal becomes entrapped in the upper urinary tract. Otherwise, the crystal is passed into the urine, and no clinically apparent disease occurs. The final stage of the precipitation-crystallization process involves continued growth of the trapped particle, resulting in clinically significant disease.[104,119]

The *inhibitor lack theory* attempts to explain why some persons form stones and others do not, even though both groups excrete urine that is supersaturated with certain substances that inhibit crystallization and subsequent calculi. These substances have been identified as magnesium, pyrophosphate, citrate, mucoproteins, and various peptides.[104]

The *matrix initiation theory* observes the finding that the matrices of calculi in certain persons are mucoproteins that typically act as crystal inhibitors. In this case mucoproteins are hypothesized to contain a qualitative defect that renders them dysfunctional; thus they predispose the person to calculi formation rather than serve as a crystal inhibitor as they do in normal individuals.[78,104]

The *epitaxy theory* attempts to account for the presence of mixed urinary calculi and the process by which a crystal is formed with layers of different substances. The crystalline lattice of a specific substance is organized in a predictable manner that may closely resemble other crystalline lattices. Certain calculi may have an inner core of uric acid and an outer covering of calcium oxalate. Thus one crystal forms upon the latticework of a similar substance, resulting in a mixed urinary stone.[104]

Which of these factors relevant to urinary stone formation will prove predominant and which will prove secondary remains to be elucidated. A *final theory* of stone formation will be based on elucidation of the process of biologic crystallization and the role of the kidneys and urinary transport organs for maintaining a crystal- and stasis-free system.[78]

A urinary calculus typically is discovered when the stone becomes entrapped, resulting in the abrupt onset of acute renal or bladder colic. The most common sites of entrapment are a calyx or calyceal diverticulum, the ureteropelvic junction, the segment of ureter at or near the pelvic brim adjacent to the point where the ureter crosses the iliac vessels, the posterior pelvic portion of the ureter in women, and the ureterovesical junction. Of all the areas of anatomic narrowing, the ureterovesical junction is the most difficult for a calculus to pass.[78]

The renal colic typically occurs at night or during the early morning hours when the patient is sedentary. The pain begins in the flank and radiates to the groin and testes in men or the labia majora and broad ligament in women. As the stone moves to the midureter, the pain radiates to the lateral portion of the flank and lower abdomen. As the calculus moves toward the ureterovesical junction, the pain associated with the initial renal colic may recur, associated with irritable voiding symptoms of urinary urgency or urge incontinence. Colic is perceived most intensely as the calculus moves or if it implants at a certain site. Movement of the stone also causes localized pain resulting from obstruction.

Bladder colic is characterized by bladder pain that crescendoes immediately after micturition. A stabbing pain may be felt when changing position, and urinary urgency and urge incontinence are commonly associated.[78]

Because visceral pain such as renal colic is mediated by the autonomic nervous system via the celiac ganglia, nausea and vomiting, intestinal stasis, and ileus may occur. Patients typically are restless as they change position to reduce discomfort. Grunting respirations signaling distress may be present. The pulse and blood pressure may be elevated in response to pain. Fever is rare unless a urinary tract infection is present.

A stone more than 4 mm in diameter is unlikely to pass through the ureter. Even smaller stones that are securely implanted in the wall of a calyx or ureter are less likely to pass and more likely to be obstructive or cause infection.

Aggressive removal of urinary calculi is considered for any patient who has a single kidney or significant renal insufficiency. Age and general health status, however, may make a patient a poor candidate for the anesthesia necessary for calculus manipulation.[78]

COMPLICATIONS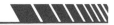

Infection (bacteriuria, pyelonephritis, systemic sepsis)
Hematuria
Obstructive uropathy
Compromised renal function

Although the cause of calculus formation remains unclear, the following specific risk factors increase the likelihood that an individual will form urinary stones.[108]

Renal tubular acidosis (RTA) is a condition that occurs when the kidneys cannot excrete an acidic urine. As a result, systemic hyperchloremic acidosis ensues. Individuals with untreated renal tubular acidosis develop hypercalciuria and often form calcium stones.

Cystinuria is another risk factor for urinary calculi. Excessive cystine in the urine probably represents a metabolic abnormality that predisposes these individuals to the formation of cystine calculi.

Hypercalcemia, or excess calcium in the blood, predisposes an individual to hypercalciuria. The most common cause of hypercalcemia is *hyperparathyroidism,* or excessive secretion of the hormone parathormone, causing mobilization of calcium from body storage into the blood.

Xanthinuria, excessive excretion of xanthine in the urine, predisposes a person to urinary calculi. The condition may be an untoward effect of allopurinol administration or of a genetic deficiency.

Hyperoxaluria predisposes the affected individual to oxalate calculi. The condition may occur as the result of excessive dietary intake or a metabolic disorder.

Urinary infection may predispose a person to calculi, particularly when the pathogen can split urea molecules.

Immobility, neuropathic bladder dysfunction, and urinary retention also predispose an individual to urinary stones. All of these conditions cause urinary stasis, which enhances the precipitation of stone-forming salts from the urine while slowing urinary transport, thus giving the potential stone nidus a greater chance of forming an obstructive latticework.

DIAGNOSTIC STUDIES AND FINDINGS

Diagnostic test	Findings
Kidney-ureter-bladder (KUB) x-ray	Radiopaque urinary calculi
Intravenous pyelogram/ urogram (IVP/IVU)	Used to determine whether calculi are present in the urinary system; also provides detailed evaluation of extent of obstructive uropathy and some indication of renal (excretory) function
Voiding cystourethrogram/ cystogram	Filling defect in bladder may be noted on preliminary (scout) film and early filling films
Retrograde pyelogram (RPG)	Localization of calculi not detected by routine means (KUB, IVP/IVU)
Ultrasonography	Calculi produce a nonechogenic bright spot with a shadow below the calculus
Radionuclide studies	Renal scan demonstrates compromised focal scars of parenchyma or abnormal vascular perfusion related to recurrent stone disease with infection
Stone analysis	Chemical analysis of urinary calculi is useful for determining the principal elements in the stone and thus helps guide therapy
Urinalysis	Elevated calcium in patients with renal tubular acidosis and stones; elevated oxalate in patients with calcium oxalate stones; urinary pH may show abnormal acidosis or alkalosis
Urine culture	>100,000 CFU*/ml with urinary system infection
24-Hour urine chemistries	Used to determine abnormal metabolism of calcium, phosphorus, uric acid, oxalate, cystine, citrate, sodium, and magnesium
Serum electrolytes	Used to determine abnormal metabolism of calcium, phosphorus, uric acid, alkaline phosphates, and parathormone
Blood urea nitrogen (BUN), creatinine	Used to determine effects of urolithiasis on renal function

*Colony-forming units.

MEDICAL MANAGEMENT

GENERAL MANAGEMENT

Adequate fluid intake to prevent calculi formation and to encourage passage of urinary calculi

Dietary changes to minimize calculus formation (Table 6-4)

Medications to minimize calculus formation (Table 6-5)

Chemolysis to dissolve calculi

Extracorporeal shock wave lithotripsy or direct lithotripsy under endoscopic control for upper ureteral, pelvic, and renal stones

Endoscopic basket retrieval for stones in lower third of ureter

Endoscopic retrieval or electrohydraulic lithotripsy of bladder stones

SURGERY

Nephrolithotomy, ureterolithotomy for renal or ureteral stones

Vesicolithotomy for bladder calculi

Table 6-4

DIETARY MANIPULATION AND URINARY CALCULI

Calculi	Common dietary sources
Calcium stones (reduction of dietary calcium among patients with specific disorders of calcium absorption or metabolism) (moderate restriction, 400-600 mg/day recommended)	Milk, ice cream, cheeses, other dairy products Sardines Canned salmon Dark green, leafy vegetables
Oxalate stones (reduction of dietary oxalates, emphasizing specific foods high in oxalates)	Asparagus, beets, spinach, rhubarb Raspberries, cranberries, plums Cranberry juice, grape juice, grapefruit juice Almonds, cashews Worcestershire sauce
Uric acid stones (reduction of foods rich in uric acid)	Organ meats (e.g., liver, kidney), lean meats Whole grains

From Jenkins.[108]

Table 6-5

PHARMACOLOGIC MANAGEMENT OF URINARY CALCULI

Calculi	Agent
Cystine stones	D-Penicillamine (binds with cystine to render it in a more soluble form) α-Mercaptopropinoglycide (similar to D-penicillamine) Captopril (similar to D-penicillamine and may be even more effective, although postural hypotension limits therapeutic dosage range)
Uric acid stones	Allopurinol (a xanthine oxidase inhibitor, it reduces urinary excretion of uric acid) Sodium bicarbonate or citrate (raises urinary pH; if pH remains at 6.5 with output of 3 L, existing uric acid calculi will dissolve)
Oxalate stones	Pyridoxine (reduces urinary oxalate excretion in patients with primary hyperoxaluria) Cholestyramine (binds oxalate in the gut for patients with enteric hyperoxaluria)
Calcium and calcium/oxalate stones	Sodium bicarbonate or citrate (inhibits calcium excretion and increases urinary citrate levels in patients with renal tubular acidosis) Hydrochlorothiazide, trichlormethiazide (reduces urinary calcium excretion among persons with idiopathic hypercalciuria; may offer some benefit to individuals with normal calcium urine levels and recurrent calcium stones) Orthophosphate (decreases urinary calcium excretion and increases inhibitor activity among persons with hypercalciuria and normocalciuria) Cellulose phosphate (diminishes calcium absorption by binding calcium in the gut) Potassium citrate (reduces calcium stone formation in individuals with hypocitriuria)

From Jenkins.[108]

1   ASSESS

ASSESSMENT	OBSERVATIONS
Pain	Dull, aching pain in flank, lower back, suprapubic area, or groin; pain is not relieved by position, movement, or urination
Infection	Dysuria with cloudy, odorous urine; systemic infection with fever, flank pain, nausea, and vomiting may be present

2 DIAGNOSE

NURSING DIAGNOSIS	SUBJECTIVE FINDINGS	OBJECTIVE FINDINGS
Pain related to urinary calculi causing obstruction	Complains of intense pain in flank, lower back, suprapubic area, or groin	Pain is described as dull and boring and is not relieved by position changes or urination; patient typically is restless and in apparent distress
Potential for infection (urinary system) related to obstruction, urinary stasis	Complains of irritative voiding symptoms (frequency, urgency, dysuria) with or without fever, nausea, vomiting, and flank pain	Urine culture demonstrates >100,000 CFU/ml of bacteria and systemic temperature over 37.7° C (100° F)
Altered patterns of urinary elimination related to urinary calculi	Reports irritative symptoms with or without urge incontinence	Voiding diary demonstrates diurnal urinary frequency more often than q 2 h with or without urge incontinence
Altered peripheral tissue perfusion (renal) related to obstruction	Relates history of urinary calculi	Serum creatinine and BUN are abnormal, or radionuclide studies demonstrate compromised renal function

3 PLAN

Patient goals

1. Urinary calculi will be passed spontaneously or removed through extracorporeal lithotripsy, endoscopic retrieval, or open surgery, thus relieving the obstruction.
2. Recurrent urinary calculi will be prevented.
3. Recurrent urinary calculi that occur despite preventive program will be promptly detected and treated.
4. Urinary system infection will be avoided or promptly managed.
5. Renal perfusion and parenchymal function will be preserved.

4 IMPLEMENT

NURSING DIAGNOSIS	NURSING INTERVENTIONS	RATIONALE
Pain related to urinary calculi causing obstruction	Assess the character, location, and duration of pain; evaluate alleviating and aggravating factors.	Renal colic caused by an obstructing urinary calculus is centered in the flank when the stone is located in the kidney or upper ureter. As the stone nears the lower ureter and ureterovesical junction, the pain shifts to the groin and irritative voiding symptoms appear. Renal colic often occurs in bouts of severe pain; these episodes may occur in the early morning, interrupting sleep, and are not relieved by position changes, urination, or movement. Distinguishing renal colic from other forms of flank or groin pain is important for effective treatment.

NURSING DIAGNOSIS	NURSING INTERVENTIONS	RATIONALE
	Advise the patient that "anticipatory watching" is done before invasive or extracorporeal interventions to give the body time to pass obstructing calculi spontaneously. Reassure the patient that aggressive pain management is maintained during anticipatory watching and that stones will be manipulated without delay should they become embedded or should other symptoms occur, prompting other management.	As many as half of all urinary calculi pass spontaneously, and patients are given the opportunity to pass a calculus spontaneously before other procedures are implemented. Nonetheless, when the stone embeds or threatens urinary system function, prompt intervention is undertaken.
	Administer or teach the patient to self-administer analgesic or narcotic medications as directed.	The pain caused by an obstructing urinary calculi is intense and not easily relieved by nonpharmacologic means; narcotic analgesia typically is required.
	Minimize environmental distractions, including noise, sound, and too many visitors.	Controlling noise and environmental distractions facilitates rest and minimizes nausea associated with renal colic, promoting the pain relief action of analgesic medications.
	Observe the patient for changes in the intensity of pain.	Intensification of pain may indicate embedding of the stone, with increased obstruction; acute relief from pain may indicate passage of the calculus through an anatomically narrow area.
	Apply warm compresses to the patient's flank.	Local application of heat may provide relief from renal colic.
	Help the patient to ambulate and to obtain adequate fluids (as much as 3,000 ml/day in certain circumstances).	Adequate fluid intake and controlled ambulation may assist in the passage of obstructing calculi, relieving associated pain.
Potential for infection (urinary system) related to obstruction, urinary stasis	Obtain urinalysis and urine culture and sensitivity as directed (see Cystitis, page 52).	Urinary tract infection often coexists with obstructing urinary calculi; a positive urine culture will identify the bacteria causing the infection.
	Evaluate the patient for signs of febrile urinary tract infection (i.e., irritative voiding symptoms with fever and flank pain).	Febrile urinary tract infection is a serious complication of obstructing urinary calculus that requires prompt treatment *before* any invasive intervention to remove calculus.
	Administer prophylactic antiinfective medications as directed before invasive interventions to manipulate urinary stones.	Manipulation of a urinary calculus by endoscopic, surgical, or extracorporeal means can cause tissue trauma and bleeding. Bacteria-laden urine can rapidly move into the bloodstream, causing septicemia and shock. Prophylactic antiinfective therapy eliminates or greatly reduces this risk.

→ › ›

NURSING DIAGNOSIS	NURSING INTERVENTIONS	RATIONALE
	Encourage adequate fluid intake (at least 1,500 ml/day); provide intravenous fluids as directed if the patient cannot tolerate oral fluids.	Adequate fluid intake promotes antegrade urinary movement (even in a partly obstructed system), promoting the passage of an obstructing stone and the passage of bacteria from the urinary system.
Altered patterns of urinary elimination related to urinary calculi	Reassure the patient that irritative voiding symptoms associated with urinary calculus are temporary.	Irritative voiding symptoms are caused by inflammation from the calculus and intensified when bacteriuria occurs; relief from the calculus reverses these symptoms.
	Advise the patient that urinary frequency will persist for several days after an acutely obstructing stone is removed, crushed, or passed spontaneously.	A brief period of diuresis follows relief of acute obstruction.
	Advise the patient with urge incontinence that leakage is transient and will be relieved when the stone is removed or passes spontaneously.	A urinary calculus in the bladder vesicle or at the ureterovesical junction causes sufficient detrusor irritation to trigger unstable contractions; passage or removal of the stone reverses these symptoms.
Altered peripheral tissue perfusion (renal) related to obstruction	Advise the patient of the possibility that urinary calculi may recur, and emphasize the need for prevention and prompt management.	Urinary calculi that cause obstruction and infection can compromise renal function; preventing stones and prompt treatment if they do occur minimize this risk.
	Teach the patient to strain all urine when engaged in anticipatory watching for spontaneous passage of a urinary calculus.	Straining of the urine allows retrieval and subsequent analysis of stones that are spontaneously passed with urination; analysis of these calculi helps guide medical management designed to prevent recurrence of stone disease.
	Teach the patient to drink an adequate amount of clear liquids daily—at least 1,500 ml/day (45 ounces).	Clear liquids dilute the urine, decreasing the likelihood that stone-forming elements will precipitate in the urine and promoting the early passage of stones before they become large enough to obstruct.
	Consult with the physician about dietary changes to reduce the recurrence of urinary stones.	Restricting dietary calcium, oxalates, or uric acid may reduce the risk of recurrent stones in some patients (see Table 6-4).
	Administer or teach the patient to self-administer pharmacologic agents designed to reduce the likelihood of recurrent urinary calculi (see Table 6-5).	Pharmacologic agents are used to manipulate the urinary constituents to reduce the likelihood of calculus formation.
	Instruct the patient that pharmacologic treatment for urinary calculi will be ongoing, possibly for many years or a lifetime.	Metabolic disorders that predispose toward urinary calculi are chronic, lifelong conditions requiring ongoing prophylaxis to reduce existing stones and prevent future ones.

NURSING DIAGNOSIS	NURSING INTERVENTIONS	RATIONALE
	Help the patient reduce reversible risk factors for urinary calculi.	Immobility, restricted fluid intake, and an indwelling catheter in the bladder are potentially alterable risk factors; modifying these risk factors affects the likelihood of recurrent calculi.
	Prepare the patient for extracorporeal shock wave lithotripsy, percutaneous or endoscopic stone retrieval, or lithotripsy or surgical lithotomy as directed (see special sections on each procedure).	Obstructive or embedded calculi that are unlikely to pass spontaneously with the urine are managed aggressively to prevent complications from urinary obstruction and infection.
Knowledge deficit	See Patient Teaching.	

5   EVALUATE

PATIENT OUTCOME	DATA INDICATING THAT OUTCOME IS REACHED
Urinary calculi have been passed spontaneously or removed using extracorporeal lithotripsy, endoscopic retrieval, or open surgery, thus relieving the obstruction.	Renal colic and obstruction have resolved; x-ray or ultrasonic imaging studies show no obstructive calculi.
Recurrent urinary calculi are prevented.	Serial imaging studies show no recurrent urinary calculi; patient accurately describes a management program (dietary, pharmacologic, or other means) for preventing stone recurrence.
Urinary calculi that have recurred despite the preventive management program are promptly detected and treated.	Patient describes a reasonable strategy for seeking prompt health care, both near her home and when traveling, if symptoms of renal colic occur.
Urinary system infection has been avoided or promptly managed.	Urine culture demonstrates no bacterial growth; there are no signs of febrile urinary infection.
Renal perfusion and parenchymal function have been preserved.	Radionuclide imaging studies show good bilateral renal perfusion and parenchymal function; serum creatinine and BUN levels are within normal limits.

→ > >

PATIENT TEACHING ▪▪

1. After the medical evaluation and stone analysis have been completed, teach the patient about the type of stone she had and reinforce any prescription for ongoing medical therapy to prevent recurrence.
2. Teach every patient about the chance of recurrence of urinary calculi and the need for an adequate daily fluid intake to prevent stone recurrence.
3. Teach every patient to avoid excessive alcohol intake, which causes dehydration and increases the risk of stone formation.
4. Teach the patient to include an adequate volume of *clear* liquids in her diet and to refrain from drinking too many beverages with sugar or other additives.
5. Teach the patient the names, dosages, administration, and potential side effects of any medications used to prevent the recurrence of urinary calculi.
6. Teach the patient the signs and symptoms of urinary tract infection and the association between urinary calculi and infection.
7. Help the patient become more knowledgeable about seeking prompt health care when the symptoms of urinary stone disease occur. Teach him how to seek urgent care both at home and when traveling in another city or country.

EXTRACORPOREAL SHOCK WAVE LITHOTRIPSY

Extracorporeal shock wave lithotripsy (ESWL) uses shock waves to reduce calculi to small particles that can pass into the bladder and out with the urine. Shock waves differ from ultrasonic waves in several significant aspects. Ultrasonic sound waves create a sinusoidal wave pattern with gentle peaks and valleys, whereas shock waves constitute a single positive pressure front with several frequencies with a sharp onset and more gradual decline. When transmitted through relatively degassed water or water-containing body tissue, shock waves lose only a small amount of their original energy and do not cause significant tissue damage. Shock waves cause mechanical stress in brittle elements (such as most urinary calculi) that pulverize the stone with repeated application. As a single shock wave reaches the stone, the stone's front and rear surfaces are disrupted. This disintegration of the outer aspects of the stone exposes new surfaces that are disrupted in turn, causing fragmentation of a larger, obstructive stone into smaller particles that can pass through the urinary system[106] (Figure 6-7).

Extracorporeal shock wave lithotripsy is performed in a specially designed stationary or mobile suite (the latter is contained in the cab of a large truck) containing a large reservoir of degassed water, a spark gap generator that can produce shock waves, and fluoroscopic or ultrasonic imaging equipment capable of locating the stone within a three-dimensional perspective (Figure 6-8). The patient is given appropriate anesthesia (the procedure is painful and requires control of movement to prevent misdirection of shock waves to body areas

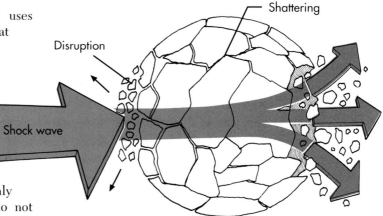

FIGURE 6-7
Shock waves cause disruption of front and rear surfaces while shattering the center of the calculus.

other than the calculus) and placed in the degassed water "bath" with a mobile chair (Figure 6-9). The urinary calculus is localized through fluoroscopy or ultrasonography, and carefully controlled doses of shock waves are used to reduce the stone to small fragments that can pass with the urine. Often a nephrostomy tube, "double J," or pigtail catheter extending from the renal pelvis to the bladder is passed before lithotripsy to prevent obstruction as the steinstrasse (column of sandlike fragments) is passed. In other cases ureteroscopy and ureterolithotripsy, endoscopic extraction, or ureteral meatotomy is used to resolve obstructive steinstrasse.

The first lithotriptors were used on patients in Germany as early as 1980. In the United States, several regional universities were recipients of dedicated lithotriptors several years later. As urologists gained experience in using lithotripsy to treat patients with urinary calculi, mobile units and second-generation units were developed (Table 6-6). For example, the traditional bath of degassed water has been modified so that "minibath" and "membrane" lithotriptors deliver shock waves without submersion. The spark gap generator also has been modified so that shock waves can be generated from a piezoceramic element (piezoelectric), a 10 mg lead azide pellet, or an electromagnetic shock wave generator.[106,109]

INDICATIONS

Obstructing renal or pelvic stones
Ureteral stones (ureteroscopic manipulation may be required)
Staghorn calculi (often in combination with other approaches)

CONTRAINDICATIONS*

Bleeding disorders
Lower ureteral stones amenable to basket extraction
Obstruction below the calculi
Marked anatomic abnormalities that make correct positioning impossible

*Many traditional contraindications to extracorporeal shock wave lithotripsy, such as pacemakers, metal clips near the kidneys, obesity, small children, stones in a pelvic kidney, and calculi near the sacrum, have been overcome with greater experience using this relatively new technology.[106]

COMPLICATIONS

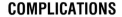

Transient hematuria
Incomplete excretion of stone (residual stone fragments)
Renal colic pain with obstructing steinstrasse

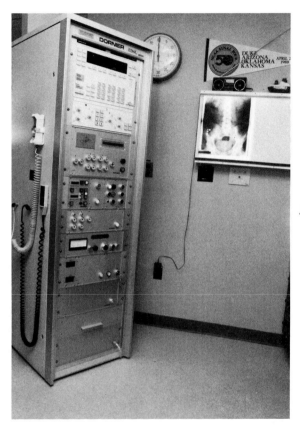

A

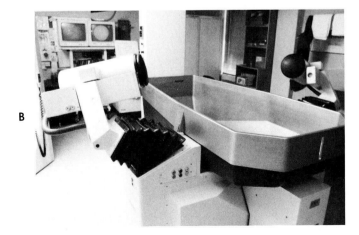

B

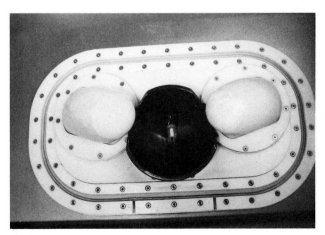

C

FIGURE 6-8

A, ESWL control panel and x-ray (see stones in left kidney and marker on right). **B,** Tub for extracorporeal shock-wave lithotripsy. **C,** Source of impulse located in bottom of tub. (From Brundage D: *Renal disorders,* St Louis, 1992, Mosby–Year Book.)

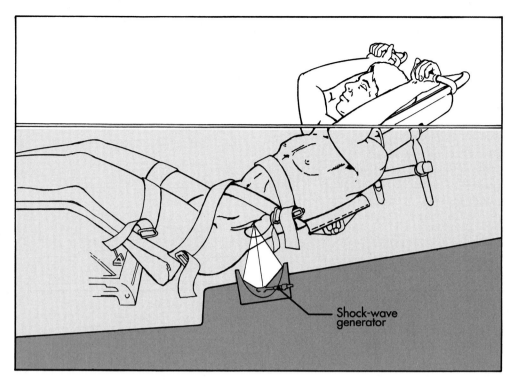

FIGURE 6-9
Patient positioned for shock-wave lithotripsy using spark gap generator. Area of flank is exposed for effi-cient shock-wave conduction. (From Brundage D: *Renal disorders,* St Louis, 1992, Mosby–Year Book.)

Table 6-6

COMMON LITHOTRIPTORS

Device	Shock wave source	Imaging device	Anesthetic required
"Bath" lithotriptors			
Dornier HM3*	Spark gap	Fluoroscopy	Yes
Yash-Yoda	Chemical explosion	Fluoroscopy	Yes
Dornier New Generator and Ellipsoid	Spark gap	Fluoroscopy	Intravenous sedation only
"Minibath" lithotriptors			
Wolf Piezolith 2200	Piezoelectric	Ultrasound	No†
Technomed Sonolith 3000	Spark gap	Ultrasound and fluoroscopy	Yes
"Membrane" lithotriptors			
Dornier MPL 5000	Spark gap	Ultrasound and fluoroscopy	Possibly intravenous sedation
Dornier HM4	Spark gap	Fluoroscopy	Yes
Siemens Lithostar	Electromagnetic	Fluoroscopy	No†
EDAP-LT01	Piezoelectric	Ultrasound	No†
Northgate SD-3	Spark gap	Ultrasound	Intravenous sedation or general
Direx Tripter X-1	Spark gap	Fluoroscopy	(Undergoing FDA trials)
Diasonics Therasonic	Piezoelectric	Ultrasound and fluoroscopy	(Undergoing FDA trials)
Storz Modulith	Electromagnetic	Ultrasound and fluoroscopy	No†
Breakthrough Medical Corp.	Spark gap	Ultrasound or fluoroscopy	General or epidural

From Gillenwater[106] and Jenkins.[109]
†The use of analgesic or sedative medications is based on the clinical judgment of the attending physician rather than the manufacturer's recommendations.

PREPROCEDURAL NURSING CARE

NURSING DIAGNOSIS	NURSING INTERVENTIONS	RATIONALE
Knowledge deficit related to procedure, goals, anesthesia, and potential untoward effects	Reinforce prepreprocedural teaching, including the procedure, its goals, potential untoward effects, and expected nursing care.	Anxiety before the procedure reduces the patient's ability to learn and retain information; repeating it decreases anxiety and improves retention.
	Reassure the patient that ESWL does not require an incision, although endoscopic or percutaneous procedures may be done along with ESWL.	Endoscopic or percutaneous placement of catheters may be used to ensure adequate drainage following ESWL.
	Reassure the patient that anesthesia or needed sedation will be given before or during the procedure.	Lithotriptors use different technologies to disrupt urinary stones; general anesthesia, intravenous sedation, or other measures may be used to reduce anxiety and control pain.
	Advise the patient that some hematuria (pink to light red urine) is expected after the procedure.	ESWL causes some trauma to the kidney, producing transient hematuria.
	Advise the patient that he is expected to pass small fragments of urinary calculi over the first week after ESWL; teach him to strain the urine for fragments as directed.	ESWL produces shock waves that pulverize larger stones into small fragments that can be excreted from the urinary system; the patient may strain the urine for stone analysis when indicated.
	Advise the patient that renal colic (pain) may occur after ESWL, particularly when a large stone burden is pulverized.	Obstructing steinstrasse may occur after ESWL, producing renal colic; the urologist may elect to place a ureteral catheter or nephrostomy tube when obstructive steinstrasse is likely.
Altered peripheral tissue perfusion (renal) related to inherent bleeding disorder aggravated by ESWL	Question the patient about use of anticoagulant drugs (including aspirin) and history of bleeding or clotting disorders before ESWL; promptly inform the physician if any disorders are discovered or if previously unknown anticoagulant drugs are being used.	ESWL produces trauma to renal tissue and transient hematuria; anticoagulant medications or uncontrolled bleeding disorders may lead to serious hemorrhage.[106]
	Obtain prothrombin time (PT) and partial thromboplastin time (PTT) before the procedure.	Tests of prothrombin time and partial thromboplastin time are used to detect unsuspected bleeding disorders before ESWL.[106]
	Obtain imaging studies of the urinary system as directed.	Imaging studies of the urinary system assist in localization of urinary calculi before the procedure, minimizing the number of shock waves required and associated hematuria.

➜ ❯ ❯

NURSING DIAGNOSIS	NURSING INTERVENTIONS	RATIONALE
	Administer bowel preparation as directed.	A bowel preparation is required for individuals with neuropathic bowel or for those with normal gastrointestinal function who have sufficient fecal contents to obscure fluoroscopic visualization of the kidneys.
Potential for infection (urinary system or systemic) related to obstructive urinary calculi and ESWL	Obtain a urine culture as directed.	Bacteriuria is eradicated before ESWL or endoscopic manipulation of the urinary tract.
	Obtain vital signs and a complete blood count before ESWL as directed.	Systemic infection or febrile urinary infection is controlled before the procedure.
	Prepare the patient for percutaneous nephrostomy before the procedure.	Percutaneous nephrostomy may be used to control bacteriuria when obstruction is sufficiently severe that systemic antiinfective therapy is unlikely to control urinary infection.[106]

POSTPROCEDURAL NURSING CARE

NURSING DIAGNOSIS	NURSING INTERVENTIONS	RATIONALE
Altered peripheral tissue perfusion (renal) related to ESWL	Monitor the patient for hematuria after ESWL.	Some hematuria is expected; however, bright red, bloody urine with clots indicates significant bleeding.
	Teach the patient to monitor the urine at home for resolution (or persistence) of hematuria; instruct the patient to call the physician should bleeding persist.	Most patients are discharged from an ESWL facility (e.g., hospital) the day of the procedure; teaching the patient to monitor his urine helps him know when to seek care for persistent hematuria if necessary.
	Emphasize the necessity of follow-up evaluation for bleeding after ESWL.	Perirenal hematoma is a very rare complication following ESWL that may require surgical drainage or other medical management.
Pain (potential) related to ESWL, passage of stone fragments	Assess pain after ESWL for location, character, duration, intensity, and alleviating and aggravating factors.	Obstructing fragments produce a renal colic–type pain, whereas bladder spasms or urinary infection causes discomfort in the suprapubic area with dysuria; the management of each type of pain is different.
	Prepare the patient for additional endoscopic, ESWL, or percutaneous procedures as directed.	Renal colic from embedded urinary calculi fragments may require manipulation to relieve obstruction.
	Administer or teach the patient to self-administer analgesics as directed.	Analgesics are used before stone fragments are passed to prevent pain from their passage.

NURSING DIAGNOSIS	NURSING INTERVENTIONS	RATIONALE
	Help the patient maintain adequate intake of clear liquids (at least 1,500 ml/day).	Fluid intake assists in the passage of stone fragments after ESWL.
Altered patterns of urinary elimination related to passage of urinary calculi and ESWL	Encourage the patient to drink an adequate volume of clear liquids after ESWL.	Fluids flush the urinary system of fragments or other debris that can cause irritative voiding symptoms.
	Administer or teach the patient to self-administer antispasmodic medications or urinary analgesics as directed.	Antispasmodics or analgesics reduce irritative voiding symptoms and unstable contractions while stone fragments are being passed after ESWL.
	Reassure the patient that irritative voiding symptoms, including urge incontinence (if present), are transient.	The passage of stone fragments into the bladder may cause sufficient irritation to trigger unstable contractions of the detrusor and urinary urgency and frequency; these symptoms are expected to diminish after the fragments have been passed.

PATIENT TEACHING

Refer to page 188.

PERCUTANEOUS OR ENDOSCOPIC STONE RETRIEVAL/LITHOTRIPSY

In addition to extracorporeal shock wave lithotripsy (ESWL), a variety of other methods can be used to remove urinary calculi. The lower third of the ureter and bladder may be approached by cystoscopy, and higher segments of the ureter may be treated through ureteroscopy. The renal pelvis and upper ureter may be approached through a percutaneous nephrostomy tract established through a flank approach. Smaller stones may be retrieved by means of a *stone basket*. Larger stones and embedded calculi may be pulverized using ultrasonic or laser lithotripsy probes placed directly against the calculus (Figure 6-10). The fragments are irrigated from the urinary tract via the endoscope or left to be excreted during urination.

The indications for percutaneous nephroscopic stone lithotripsy have changed dramatically with the development and successful clinical use of extracorporeal lithotripsy.[106,113] Percutaneous nephrolithotomy typically is used for calculi larger than 2.5 cm and for staghorn stones in the renal pelvis. These relatively large stones are broken into fragments by direct contact with an ultrasonic lithotriptor or electrohydraulic probe. Ureteral and bladder stones are retrieved when

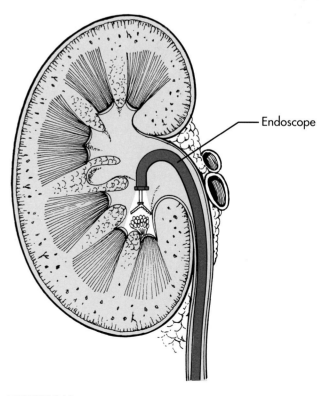

— Endoscope

FIGURE 6-10
Endoscopic stone retrieval.

possible or pulverized using electrohydraulic, laser, or ultrasonic lithotripsy. Bladder calculi are debulked with an electrohydraulic lithotriptor.

INDICATIONS

Cystoscopic lithotripsy or basket retrieval: Stones in the lower third of the ureter not easily reached by ESWL; bladder calculi

Ureteroscopic lithotripsy or basket retrieval: Stones embedded in the ureter that are not readily amenable to ESWL; obstructing steinstrasse (adjunctive therapy for ESWL)

Percutaneous nephroscopic lithotripsy or retrieval:

Adjunctive therapy to ESWL for large staghorn calculi

CONTRAINDICATIONS

Urinary system infection
Upper urinary tract calculi readily amenable to ESWL

COMPLICATIONS
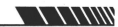

Systemic or febrile urinary tract infection
Hematuria
Incomplete excretion of stone fragments (residual calculi)

PREPROCEDURAL NURSING CARE*

NURSING DIAGNOSIS	NURSING INTERVENTIONS	RATIONALE
Knowledge deficit related to procedure, goals, anesthesia, and potential untoward effects	Reinforce preoperative teaching, including the procedure, its goals, anesthesia to be used, potential untoward effects, and expected nursing care.	Anxiety before the procedure reduces the patient's ability to learn and retain information; repeating it decreases anxiety and improves retention.
	Advise the patient that a surgical incision is not required for cystoscopic or ureteroscopic procedures.	Endoscopic technology allows visualization and manipulation of the bladder and ureter without surgical incision.
	Advise the patient that a percutaneous tract for nephroscopic manipulation does not require open surgery.	The percutaneous nephroscope is inserted via a tract from the flank; the kidney is not exposed, as it is for surgical lithotomy.
	Advise the patient that hematuria is expected after basket retrieval or lithotripsy of urinary calculi.	Stone retrieval or direct-contact lithotripsy causes some trauma to adjacent tissues, with resulting hematuria.
	Advise the patient that a catheter may be left in place for a brief period following calculi manipulation or removal.	An indwelling catheter may be used for urinary drainage after endoscopic manipulation.
	Consult with the physician and anesthetist about the choice of anesthesia, and prepare the patient according to hospital protocol.	General or spinal anesthesia may be used for more invasive and extensive procedures, whereas intravenous sedation and local anesthesia may be sufficient for more limited cystoscopic procedures.
Potential for infection (urinary system) related to calculi disease and endoscopic manipulation of stones	Obtain a urine culture as directed.	Bacteriuria is controlled before endoscopic or percutaneous stone manipulation to prevent systemic spread of bacteria during the procedure.

*See also Endoscopy, page 39.

NURSING DIAGNOSIS	NURSING INTERVENTIONS	RATIONALE
	Administer antiinfective medications as directed for urinary tract infection.	Antiinfective medications are given before stone manipulation to control or prevent urinary infection.
	Before stone manipulation, prepare the patient for a percutaneous nephrostomy tube or other form of urinary drainage as directed.	Urinary drainage may be required to control urinary tract infection before manipulation.
Altered peripheral tissue perfusion (renal, urinary system) related to manipulation of urinary calculi	Question the patient for any history of bleeding or clotting disorders or use of anticoagulant drugs.	Calculi manipulation causes local tissue trauma and bleeding that may be complicated by uncontrolled clotting disorders or anticoagulant medications.
	Obtain a prothrombin time (PT) and partial thromboplastin time (PTT) before stone manipulation.	PT and PTT results indicate any unsuspected or uncontrolled bleeding disorders.

POSTPROCEDURAL NURSING CARE

NURSING DIAGNOSIS	NURSING INTERVENTIONS	RATIONALE
Altered peripheral tissue perfusion (renal, urinary system) related to trauma, calculus disease	Observe the urine for evidence of excessive bleeding (bright red blood with clots).	Some hematuria is expected after endoscopic manipulation of urinary calculi; excessive bleeding is unexpected and requires prompt management.
	Observe any drains or tubes for urinary output and signs of bleeding.	Nephrostomy or other drainage tubes may be placed after endoscopic manipulation of urinary calculi; bleeding may be noted from these tubes.
	Obtain hematocrit and hemoglobin as directed, and compare values to preprocedural data.	Bleeding will cause declining serum hematocrit and hemoglobin.
	Monitor vital signs for evidence of severe bleeding (rapid pulse with hypertension followed by decline in the blood pressure).	Severe bleeding alters vital signs.
Potential for infection (urinary system) related to calculi manipulation	Monitor the patient for signs of urinary tract or systemic infection; obtain urine culture as directed.	Urinary infection may occur following manipulation of urinary calculi; systemic infection may occur because the integrity of the urinary system has been compromised by manipulation of calculi.
	Monitor vital signs for signs of systemic infection; obtain blood cultures as directed.	A low-grade fever may occur after stone manipulation; however, a fever exceeding 38° C (101° F) indicates a probable systemic infection, requiring prompt management.

NURSING DIAGNOSIS	NURSING INTERVENTIONS	RATIONALE
	Administer antiinfective medications as directed.	Antiinfective medications are used to control urinary system or systemic infection.
Pain related to urinary calculi and subsequent manipulation	Assess pain for location, duration, character, intensity, and aggravating and alleviating factors.	Cystoscopic manipulation of urinary stones may cause irritative voiding symptoms and bladder spasms; obstructing stone fragments may cause renal colic–type pain. Each form of pain is managed differently.
	Administer or teach the patient to self-administer analgesics as directed.	Analgesics reduce pain as stone fragments pass.
	Provide heat to the flank area for discomfort.	Local heat may relieve the discomfort associated with percutaneous or endoscopic manipulation of the urinary system.
	Help ensure that the patient drinks an adequate amount of clear liquids (at least 1,500 ml/day).	Clear liquids flush the urinary system, reducing irritative voiding symptoms and promoting excretion of stone fragments.
	Administer anticholinergic or urinary analgesic medications as directed.	Anticholinergic medications relieve the discomfort of bladder spasms by inhibiting unstable detrusor contractions; urinary analgesics relieve irritative voiding symptoms through pharmacologic actions that are unclear.

PATIENT TEACHING

Refer to page 188.

OPEN SURGICAL LITHOTOMY

Surgical lithotomy was once the standard of care for removing urinary calculi that failed to pass spontaneously. Because of advances in endoscopic manipulation and extracorporeal lithotripsy, surgery now is reserved for specific indications, such as deeply embedded calculi that are not amenable to other forms of manipulation. *Nephrolithotomy* (Figure 6-11, *A*) is the surgical removal of calculi from the kidney, and *pyelolithotomy* is the removal of a stone from the renal pelvis (Figure 6-11, *B*). The kidney and renal pelvis typically are approached from a flank incision, although a posterior lumbotomy or anterior transperitoneal approach is used for patients who are not physically suited for the flank position. The kidney is entered through its surgical planes, and major vessels are carefully avoided; the pelvis usually is approached from its lateral aspect. The goal of the procedure is maximum preservation of functioning parenchyma. Carefully avoiding major blood vessels and intraoperative cooling of the kidney to 15° to 20° C (59° to 68° F) with an iced slush minimizes the deleterious effects of ischemia on parenchymal function.

Ureterolithotomy is the surgical removal of a urinary calculus from the ureter (Figure 6-11, *C*). The surgical approach is influenced by the level of the obstructive stone. A flank incision is used for stones in the upper segments of the ureter. Alternately, a posterior lumbar incision may be used on severely impacted stones. Stones in the midureter are approached by means of a

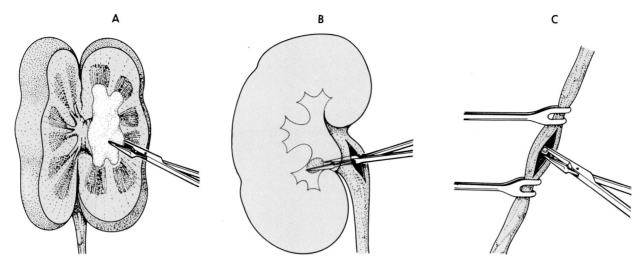

FIGURE 6-11
Location and methods of removing renal calculi from upper urinary tract. **A,** Nephrolithotomy, removal of staghorn calculus from renal parenchyma (kidney split). **B,** Pyelolithotomy, removal of stone through renal pelvis. **C,** Ureterolithotomy, removal of stone from ureter. (From Beare P and Myers J: *Principles and practice of adult health nursing,* St Louis, 1990, Mosby–Year Book.)

subcostal flank incision or an extraperitoneal approach with the incision extending from below the tip of the twelfth rib and extending anteriorly. In contrast, stones in the lower third of the ureter are approached endoscopically unless they are so severely embedded that this approach is unlikely to prove beneficial. The lower ureter is approached from a modified Gibson incision (lower flank approach), a midline paramedian incision, or a transverse incision of the lower abdomen. In rare cases a transvesical approach is required when a stone is embedded in the ureterovesical junction. Regardless of the approach, the ureter is exposed and the stone removed, guarding against unexpected migration of the calculus. Ureteral stents may be placed to prevent obstruction from postoperative edema, and Penrose drains also may be used, depending on the surgical approach.

INDICATIONS

Renal or ureteral calculi not amenable to extracorporeal lithotripsy or endoscopic manipulation

CONTRAINDICATIONS

Calculi likely to pass spontaneously
Calculi amenable to less invasive manipulations

COMPLICATIONS

Renal ischemia and parenchymal damage
Hypertension
Infection
Urinary leakage from the ureter
Ureteral stricture
Paralytic ileus (rare)

PREPROCEDURAL NURSING CARE

NURSING DIAGNOSIS	NURSING INTERVENTIONS	RATIONALE
Potential for infection (urinary system and systemic sepsis) related to obstructive calculus	Obtain urinalysis, urine culture and sensitivity as directed.	Bacteriuria must be treated before invasive manipulation of an obstructing urinary stone to prevent systemic spread and septic shock.
	Evaluate the patient for signs of pyelonephritis (urinary infection with fever and flank pain).	Pyelonephritis must be treated before invasive manipulation of a urinary calculus.

→ › ›

NURSING DIAGNOSIS	NURSING INTERVENTIONS	RATIONALE
	Prepare the patient for preliminary urinary drainage with a percutaneous nephrostomy before stone surgery as directed.	Preliminary drainage may be required to control infection before lithotomy.
Knowledge deficit related to procedure, goals, anesthesia, and potential untoward effects	Reinforce preoperative teaching, including the procedure, its goals, anesthesia to be used, potential untoward effects, and expected nursing care.	Anxiety before the lithotomy reduces the patient's ability to learn and retain information; repetition decreases anxiety and improves retention.
	Advise the patient that ureteral stents or an indwelling catheter may be left in place for a brief period after surgery.	Temporary catheter drainage is used to prevent obstruction from postoperative inflammation and to promote healing of any loss of ureteral integrity.
	Advise the patient that intravenous fluids will be administered for a brief period after surgery; intravenous antibiotics will also be administered.	Intravenous fluids are administered until oral fluids can be tolerated; the venous access site also allows for administration of intravenous antibiotics.
	Assure the patient that postoperative pain will be managed aggressively, but that renal colic will be relieved by surgical removal of the obstructing stones.	Renal colic is ablated by removal of the obstructing calculus.

POSTPROCEDURAL NURSING CARE

NURSING DIAGNOSIS	NURSING INTERVENTIONS	RATIONALE
Pain related to surgical trauma, bladder spasm, or urinary tract obstruction	Evaluate location, character, and duration of pain; identify alleviating and aggravating factors.	Incisional pain is expected after surgical lithotomy. It is localized to the area of the incision, dull, and prolonged. Bladder spasms produce a characteristic cramping pain of short duration. Obstruction pain mimics renal colic; it is more intense than incisional pain and requires prompt intervention to prevent renal compromise.
	Administer narcotic analgesics as directed for incisional pain and anticholinergic medications for bladder spasms.	Narcotic analgesics relieve incisional pain, and anticholinergic medications prevent the unstable detrusor contractions that cause bladder spasms.
	Provide nonpharmacologic pain-relief measures (e.g., minimize environmental distractions); position the patient and provide splints when coughing and doing deep-breathing exercises.	Nonpharmacologic pain-relief measures work with pharmacologic agents to maximize the patient's comfort.

NURSING DIAGNOSIS	NURSING INTERVENTIONS	RATIONALE
	Promptly contact the physician should renal colic–type pain occur after surgical lithotomy.	Renal colic indicates urinary obstruction, which demands prompt treatment to relieve the pain and prevent renal damage.
Altered peripheral tissue perfusion (renal, ureteral) related to surgical trauma	Monitor urine for evidence of excessive bleeding (bright red urine with clots).	Excessive bleeding from a surgical lithotomy site may be noted in the urine.
	Monitor Penrose drains for evidence of bloody discharge.	A significant amount of bloody discharge from a Penrose drain indicates operative site hemorrhage.
	Evaluate hemoglobin and hematocrit values, and compare these with preoperative data.	Diminishing hemoglobin and hematocrit indicate blood loss, probably from surgical site.
	Monitor vital signs for signs of hypovolemic shock (rapid pulse with hypertension followed by decreasing blood pressure).	Changes in vital signs indicate advanced, severe blood loss that warrants immediate intervention.
Potential for infection (urinary system, systemic) related to urinary calculi disease and surgical lithotomy	Regularly monitor patient for signs of systemic or febrile urinary infection (fever, chills, and cloudy, odorous urine).	Systemic or febrile urinary infection is a serious, potentially life-threatening complication unless promptly managed.
	Administer parenteral and oral antiinfective medications as directed.	Antiinfective medications prevent serious urinary system or systemic infections.
	Obtain urine for culture and sensitivity as directed.	Bacteriuria is treated promptly after surgical lithotomy before signs of febrile infection appear.
Ineffective airway clearance related to flank incision	Place particular emphasis on postoperative pulmonary toilet (turning, coughing, and deep-breathing maneuvers).	Pulmonary toilet is routinely emphasized after surgery; these maneuvers are particularly significant after a procedure requiring a flank incision, which may cause discomfort with even normal respiratory excursion.
	Splint the chest whenever deep-breathing and coughing maneuvers are done.	Splinting the chest with a pillow reduces the discomfort associated with these maneuvers.
	Arrange the pulmonary toilet schedule with the narcotic analgesic schedule to provide maximum effect before pulmonary toilet.	Pulmonary toilet is better tolerated near peak action of medications rather than near the time for administration of a subsequent dose.

PATIENT TEACHING

Refer to page 188.

CHAPTER 7

Genitourinary Cancer

Genitourinary tumors affect the urinary system or the male reproductive system. Urinary system tumors affect the kidneys, ureters, bladder, and urethra; reproductive system tumors primarily affect the prostate, testes, and penis. Although the general principles of urologic oncology apply to any tumor of the genitourinary tract, the discussion in this chapter is limited to cancers of the kidney, bladder, prostate, and testis.

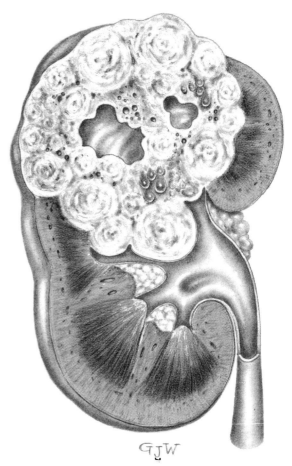

RENAL CELL CARCINOMA

Renal Tumors

Renal tumors arise from primary or metastatic malignancies. Primary tumors of the kidneys are relatively rare, accounting for only 6% of all cancer cases in adults.

Adenocarcinoma (renal cell carcinoma, or hypernephroma) is the most common primary tumor of the kidney. Renal sarcomas are relatively rare, accounting for only 1% to 3% of primary kidney tumors. Metastatic renal tumors are also relatively uncommon. Metastatic tumors may arise from malignancies of the breast, lung, and stomach.[174,176] This discussion is limited to the pathophysiology and care of renal cell carcinomas.

The cause of renal cell carcinoma remains unclear; weak correlations with cigarette smoking and environmental and work-related toxins, including asbestos, have been noted.[149,161] Renal cell carcinomas have been associated with specific syndromes, including von

Hippel-Lindau disease, adult polycystic disease, and horseshoe renal anomalies. Rare instances of familial occurrence have been observed, probably related to an autosomal dominant gene containing a specific karyotypic aberration.[137] Analgesic abuse, particularly excessive consumption of drugs containing phenacetin, has also been linked with renal cell carcinoma.[156] Renal cell carcinoma is most commonly noted in the fifth and sixth decades of life, although it occasionally occurs among younger adults or children. Men are affected approximately twice as often as women.[180]

PATHOPHYSIOLOGY

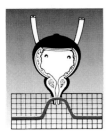

The pathophysiologic significance of a renal cell carcinoma arises from its markedly aggressive propensity for local invasion and metastasis to distant sites. Renal cell carcinoma is such an aggressive neoplasm that many patients have distant metastasis, and even with aggressive treatment, significant morbidity and death occur.[150]

Renal cell carcinomas occur in both kidneys from either the upper or lower pole. The tumor originates from the proximal renal tubular epithelial cells. Grossly, these tumors grow from the inner aspect (cortex) of the kidney toward the periphery, producing the characteristic bulging mass noted on imaging studies. As the tumor grows, it distorts normal pelvocalyceal architecture, causing splaying of the calyces. The tumor often contains cystic structures, areas of necrosis, and fat, and it may obstruct the kidney through compression of individual calyces.

A renal cell carcinoma may invade adjacent structures. These tumors often extend into the renal and perirenal vasculature. As many as 20% of renal cell carcinomas invade the renal vein, and up to 15% invade the inferior vena cava. The thrombi created by these invasive extensions may reach the right atrium. The tumor also may invade the perirenal fat before disrupting the renal capsule, increasing the risk of metastasis to adjacent organs.[141,180]

In addition to its propensity for local invasion, a renal cell carcinoma is likely to spread by metastasis. The lungs and bones are the most common sites of metastasis, but other common sites are the paraaortic and other regional lymph nodes, adrenal gland, brain, and other adjacent organs, including the liver, pancreas, and colon. Metastatic spread occurs via hematogenous or lymphatogenous routes.

Staging of tumors is used to determine care and as a general guideline for prognosis. Although various staging systems have been proposed, all have basic commonalities. Perhaps the most commonly used system,

proposed by Robson and his associates,[167] comprises four stages. Stage I tumors are confined to the renal capsule. Stage II tumors extend into the perirenal fat and/or ipsilateral adrenal gland but are contained by Gerota's fascia. Stage IIIa tumors have metastasized to the renal vein or inferior vena cava, and stage IIIb tumors have spread to regional nodes by a lymphatogenous route. Stage IV tumors have invaded beyond Gerota's fascia to adjacent organs, and stage IVb tumors have produced metastases in the lungs, bones, or other distant organs.

The tumor, node, metastasis (TNM) classification system also has been applied to renal cell carcinomas.[180] Although it is more complex than the Robson system, it also is more descriptive. The letter "T" is used to describe the primary tumor. A T_1 tumor is small enough to be entirely contained within the renal capsule without causing distortion of the pelvocalyceal system. A T_2 tumor is also contained within the capsule but is large enough to distort the inner architecture of the kidney. T_1 and T_2 tumors are comparable to the stage I tumor of the Robson system. A T_{3a} tumor extends into the perirenal fat or ipsilateral adrenal gland, comparable to a Robson stage II tumor. A Robson stage IIIa tumor is described by three TNM tumor grades: a T_{3b} tumor is one that has spread to the renal vein; a T_{3c} tumor involves the renal vein and inferior vena cava below the diaphragm; and a T_{4b} tumor affects the inferior vena cava above the diaphragm.

The descriptor "N" in the TNM system is further subdivided into grades 0 (no nodal involvement), 1 (involvement of a single node on the same side as the primary tumor), 2 (involvement of several regional nodes on the same or opposite side as the primary tumor), 3 (fixed regional nodes), and 4 (nodal involvement beyond the renal region). Robson stage III tumors involve the lymphatic system and are described as "N" 1 through 4 via the TNM classification taxonomy. The letter "M" is used to describe the presence of metastasis. The descriptor "M_0" indicates no metastases, and "M_1" indicates distant metastatic tumors comparable to Robson stage IV tumors.

COMPLICATIONS

Urinary obstruction
Pain
Hypertension
Bleeding
Anemia
Liver dysfunction*
Colon dysfunction*
Central nervous system disorders*
*Related to metastatic disease.

DIAGNOSTIC STUDIES AND FINDINGS

Diagnostic test	Findings
Complete blood count	Anemia related to blood loss, or erythrocytosis related to excessive secretion of erythropoietin
Sedimentation rate	Elevated in many cases (limited assistance in differential diagnosis)
Serum electrolytes	Hypercalcemia may be noted
Urinalysis	Gross or microscopic hematuria
Urine cytologic studies	Nonspecific findings (rarely helpful for diagnosis of renal cell carcinoma)
Intravenous pyelogram/ urogram (IVP/IVU)	Distortion of the internal renal architecture with splaying of the calyces; tumor may have calcified elements; obstructive uropathy may be present
Renal arteriography	Neovascularity of tumor and tumor invasion into renal vein or inferior vena cava
Ultrasound	Solid renal mass
Abdominal computed tomography (CT)	Solid tissue mass (Hounsfield units help differentiate tumor from fluid-filled cyst or stone); also useful for detecting larger nodal metastasis, invasion of the inferior vena cava, and larger distant metastases
Magnetic resonance imaging (MRI)	Tumor and any local invasion

---

BIOLOGIC RESPONSE MODIFIERS AND RENAL CELL CARCINOMA

Agents

Leukocyte-derived interferon alpha
interferon beta
interferon gamma
IL-2/LAK (interleukin-2)

Action

Exploits antigen markers specific to renal cell carcinoma tumor cells to intensify the body's immune response to the malignancy

Side effects

Pyrexia, nausea, vomiting, fatigue

From Dreicer and Williams.[141]

MEDICAL MANAGEMENT

GENERAL MANAGEMENT AND CHEMOTHERAPY

Single-agent or combination-agent chemotherapy

Hormonal agents to impede tumor growth (box)

Immunotherapeutic agents to intensify immune system response to tumor

Radiotherapy for palliation of patients with distant metastasis and tumor debulking before surgery

SURGERY

Radical nephrectomy to remove contained unilateral tumor

Regional lymphadenectomy to stage tumor (therapeutic value remains unclear)

Surgical removal of vena caval thrombi

1 ASSESS

ASSESSMENT	OBSERVATIONS
Abdomen	Palpable mass in upper quadrants of abdomen may be caused by primary tumor
Hematuria	Gross hematuria may be noted, or microscopic hematuria may be diagnosed on urinalysis
Pain	Flank pain may be associated with obstruction (uncommon), and bone pain may indicate metastasis
Fatigue, pallor	Anemia may result in intolerance of physical exertion and pallor
Nutritional status	Weight loss, suppressed appetite with metastasis, advanced disease

2 DIAGNOSE

NURSING DIAGNOSIS	SUBJECTIVE FINDINGS	OBJECTIVE FINDINGS
Altered protection related to renal neoplasm with potential for local invasion and metastasis	Notes symptoms consistent with renal cell carcinoma	Pathologic diagnosis, imaging studies demonstrate renal cell carcinoma
Pain related to primary tumor, metastasis	Reports chronic, aching skeletal pain or flank pain	Bony pain described as chronic; aching of back, lower extremities, or specific joints; evidence of metastatic disease may be present; flank pain described as intense or moderate, or pressure associated with increased fluid intake; pain may be noted during early morning hours; flank pain may arise from primary tumor compression of urinary outflow
Altered tissue perfusion (cardiovascular, renovascular) related to vascular invasion of renal vein, inferior vena cava, erythrocytosis, or anemia	Complains of headache and sensations of pressure in the head or fatigue and intolerance of physical exertion	Elevated blood pressure; jugular distention may be noted; complete blood count (CBC) reveals erythrocytosis (excessive erythrocytes with several immature forms) or anemia (inadequate hematocrit [Hct] and hemoglobin [Hb]); pallor may be noted
Altered nutrition: less than body requirements related to renal cell carcinoma, chemotherapy, radiotherapy	Reports loss of appetite or nausea and vomiting with intolerance of foods	Weight loss; negative nitrogen balance may be noted

→ > >

NURSING DIAGNOSIS	SUBJECTIVE FINDINGS	OBJECTIVE FINDINGS
Potential for trauma related to bony metastasis with risk of pathologic fractures	Reports bone pain	Pain may be specific to one extremity or more generalized; mobility is limited, and guarding of fractured limb is common
Anticipatory grieving related to guarded prognosis of advanced-stage renal cell carcinoma	Reports fear of cancer, its treatment, and prognosis	Patient and family express fear, distress, and anxiety related to potential loss of loved one

3 PLAN

Patient goals

1. Protective defenses will be maintained or enhanced.
2. Flank or bone pain will be relieved or adequately managed.
3. Blood pressure, hematocrit, and hemoglobin will be kept within normal limits.
4. The patient will be able to ingest adequate amounts of essential nutrients daily.
5. Physical injury or pathologic fractures will be avoided.

4 IMPLEMENT

NURSING DIAGNOSIS	NURSING INTERVENTIONS	RATIONALE
Altered protection related to renal neoplasm with potential for local invasion and metastasis	Prepare the patient for diagnostic and staging imaging studies as directed.	Diagnostic and imaging studies help determine the primary tumor's size and malignant potential, nodal involvement, and distant metastasis; these data guide the treatment strategy for eradicating the renal cell carcinoma.
	Prepare the patient for radical nephrectomy with or without lymphadenectomy and resection of renal vein or inferior vena caval thrombi as directed (see Radical Nephrectomy, page 208).	Radical nephrectomy is used to manage local (intrarenal) tumor mass in stage I, stage II, and stage IIIa tumors and may be used as a palliative procedure in more advanced tumors. Renal lymphadenectomy is used primarily as a staging procedure, and embolization of the thrombi is indicated when renal invasion of the vasculature is noted.
	Administer systemic chemotherapeutic agents as directed.	Chemotherapeutic agents are used to eradicate malignant cells by various pharmacologic actions directed at rapidly reproducing malignant (and normal) cells.

NURSING DIAGNOSIS	NURSING INTERVENTIONS	RATIONALE
	Prepare the patient for radiotherapy as directed.	Preoperative radiotherapy may be used to debulk the tumor and devitalize growing cells at the tumor periphery, thus reducing the risk of local spread and reducing or eradicating metastases. Radiotherapy is also used for palliation of bone, brain, and lung tumor metastases.
	Administer hormonal agents as directed.	Progesterone, antiestrogens, and androgens have been used to impede tumor growth and spread because estrogens enhanced tumor growth in laboratory animals.[141]
	Administer biologic response modifiers as directed.	Biologic response modifiers are used to intensify the body's immunologic responses to tumor cells (see box on page 202).
Pain related to primary tumor, metastasis	Assess pain for location, duration, character, and aggravating and alleviating conditions.	Obstruction caused by the primary tumor results in moderate to intense flank pain, which can be aggravated by a large fluid intake. Bony pain related to metastasis has a gradual onset and prolonged duration; it typically is located in the spine or long bones of the extremities and may be aggravated by movement.
	Prepare the patient for radical nephrectomy as directed.	Radical nephrectomy relieves flank pain by removing the source of obstruction.
	Administer chemotherapy, radiotherapy, hormonal therapy, or biologic response modifiers as directed.	Nonsurgical pharmacologic agents may relieve flank pain by reducing the tumor's size and thus relieving obstruction.
	Administer or teach the patient to self-administer analgesic, narcotic, or antiinflammatory agents as directed.	Analgesic or narcotic agents relieve flank pain caused by obstruction; bone pain may be relieved by analgesic or antiinflammatory agents.
	Apply heat to the flank or joints for pain.	Gentle heat relieves local discomfort.
	Provide the patient experiencing bone pain with a warm bath as indicated.	A warm sitz bath relieves pain through local application of heat.
	Administer or teach the patient to self-administer sleeping aids as indicated.	Chronic pain, such as that caused by bony metastasis, is aggravated by fatigue; sleeping aids alleviate this effect.

→ > >

NURSING DIAGNOSIS	NURSING INTERVENTIONS	RATIONALE
Altered tissue perfusion (cardiovascular, renovascular) related to vascular invasion of renal vein or inferior vena cava, erythrocytosis, or anemia	Prepare the patient for radical nephrectomy with resection of thrombus as directed.	Surgical removal of the affected kidney reverses renovascular hypertension caused by the renal tumor.
	Administer or teach the patient to self-administer antihypertensive agents as directed.	Antihypertensive agents use different pharmacologic actions to reduce systemic blood pressure; they are useful for controlling blood pressure until the affected kidney is removed or for significant hypertension when nephrectomy is not planned.
	Raise the head of the bed; provide extra pillows during sleep as indicated.	Elevating the head of the bed reduces blood pressure by stimulating the carotid baroreceptors and by relieving pulmonary congestion in cases involving congestive heart failure.
	Monitor the Hct, Hb, and CBC.	Anemia or erythrocytosis will affect these values.
	Prepare the patient for radical nephrectomy, or administer antineoplastic agents as directed.	Radical nephrectomy reduces the anemia or erythrocytosis caused by a bleeding tumor (noted as hematuria) or abnormal erythropoietin secretions; antineoplastic agents reduce blood dyscrasias by eradicating tumor cells.
	Help the patient maintain a diet with adequate iron and nutrients needed to produce viable erythrocytes.	A diet with adequate essential nutrients is crucial for reversing anemia.
Altered nutrition: less than body requirements related to renal cell carcinoma, chemotherapy, radiotherapy	Monitor the patient's weight, dietary intake, and laboratory tests (e.g., total protein, albumin/globulin ratio) to evaluate nutritional status.	Nutritional status is assessed by body weight, dietary intake, and laboratory tests.
	Help the patient choose foods with adequate essential nutrients.	Nausea, vomiting, and loss of appetite are common side effects of chemotherapy and radiotherapy; a diet containing adequate nutrients is crucial for wound healing, immune response, and normal metabolic requirements.
	Provide the patient with frequent small meals.	Small meals are more easily tolerated than large meals by patients receiving antineoplastic therapy.
	Help the patient complete oral hygiene before meals.	Oral hygiene helps the patient tolerate foods by enhancing their taste.
	Provide the patient with food preferences whenever feasible.	Providing food preferences may help stimulate the appetite.

NURSING DIAGNOSIS	NURSING INTERVENTIONS	RATIONALE
	Avoid hot, spicy, and excessively fatty foods.	Spicy, fat-laden foods are more likely to cause nausea and vomiting in patients receiving antineoplastic therapy.
	Administer parenteral, enteral, or oral dietary supplements as directed.	Dietary supplements may be required when appetite suppression and nausea and vomiting are severe.
Potential for trauma related to bony metastasis with risk of pathologic fractures	Advise the patient with bony metastasis that the bones are potentially weak and strenuous exercise should be avoided.	Bony metastasis impedes normal bone architecture, causing weakness and increasing the risk of pathologic fracture.
	Provide a bedside urinal, secure hand rails, overhead trapeze, or other assistive devices as necessary.	Assistive devices reduce the risk of trauma for the patient with limited mobility and increased risk of pathologic fracture.
Anticipatory grieving related to guarded prognosis of advanced-stage renal cell carcinoma	Encourage the patient and family to talk about their feelings and concerns.	Open discussion of feelings of distress and fears is necessary before the patient and family can prepare for their potential loss.
	Provide the patient and family with ongoing information about the patient's plan of care and prognosis in consultation with the physician.	Accurate information helps the patient and family undergo constructive grieving.
	Help the patient and family identify and obtain assistance in completing plans or arrangements for their potential loss.	Making a will and arranging for financial, spiritual, or other concerns help the patient and family cope as they prepare for a potential loss; these arrangements are also helpful following a death.
	Provide support for the patient's family, and encourage them to meet their own physical needs for nutrition, rest, and grieving during the patient's periods of crisis or intensive care.	Family members may neglect their own health in a misdirected attempt to care for the cancer victim; this strategy only impedes the family members as they prepare for the potential loss of a loved one.
	Identify a strategy for contacting the family should death be likely or imminent.	Clearly identifying a means of contacting the family should the patient face a crisis helps alleviate anxiety or guilt associated with leaving the patient to attend to personal needs.

5 EVALUATE

PATIENT OUTCOME	DATA INDICATING THAT OUTCOME IS REACHED
Protective defenses have been maintained or enhanced.	Imaging studies and pathologic studies show regression or eradication of the tumor.

→ > >

PATIENT OUTCOME	DATA INDICATING THAT OUTCOME IS REACHED
Flank or bone pain has been eliminated or is adequately managed.	The patient notes pain relief.
Blood pressure remains within acceptable limits, and hematocrit and hemoglobin remain within normal limits.	Diastolic blood pressure remains below 90 mm Hg; Hct and Hb remain within normal limits for patient's gender and age.
The patient can ingest adequate amounts of essential nutrients daily.	Weight loss is absent or reversed; total protein and albumin/globulin ratio remain within normal limits.
Physical injury and pathologic fractures have been avoided.	Imaging studies show no fractures.

PATIENT TEACHING

1. Teach the patient the pathophysiology and significance of cancer, and reinforce the physician's explanation of the planned treatment program.
2. Teach the patient and family the names, action, schedule of administration, and common side effects of antineoplastic treatments (chemotherapy, hormonal therapy, radiotherapy, and biologic response modifiers) used to treat renal cell carcinoma.
3. Teach the patient ways to maintain adequate nutrition while undergoing antineoplastic therapy.
4. Teach the patient the significance of bony metastasis, as well as strategies for minimizing pain and avoiding pathologic fracture.

RADICAL NEPHRECTOMY

Radical nephrectomy is the surgical removal of the kidney, its surrounding fascia (including Gerota's fascia), the ipsilateral adrenal gland, the proximal half of the ureter, and regional lymph nodes to the level of transection of the renal vessels. An anterior subcostal incision, a flank incision, or a midline incision may be used for radical nephrectomy, depending on the patient's condition and the surgeon's preference.

In some cases renal artery embolization is done before surgery to minimize blood loss during the procedure. A variety of agents, including Gelfoam, detachable balloons, and absolute ethanol, have been used. Absolute ethanol is preferred, because it reduces the risk of postinfarction syndrome.

Lymphadenectomy may be performed at the same time as radical nephrectomy. It is used to stage the tumor, although its therapeutic value remains controversial. Surgical removal of a vena caval thrombus is also undertaken at the time of nephrectomy. Often the thrombus is removed with the aid of a Fogarty catheter.[141,180]

INDICATIONS

Stage I, II, or IIIa renal cell carcinoma
Palliation for advanced tumors (relief of flank pain, significant hematuria, and debilitating paraneoplastic syndromes)

CONTRAINDICATIONS

Solitary kidney
Bilateral tumors

COMPLICATIONS

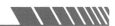

Intraoperative bleeding
Infection
Postinfarction syndrome

PREPROCEDURAL NURSING CARE

NURSING DIAGNOSIS	NURSING INTERVENTIONS	RATIONALE
Knowledge deficit related to surgical procedure, goals, and potential untoward effects	Reinforce preoperative instruction, including a brief explanation of the procedure, its goals, potential untoward effects, and expected nursing care.	Preoperative anxiety diminishes the patient's ability to learn; repeating the information enhances learning and retention and reduces anxiety related to the procedure.
	Prepare the patient for general anesthesia according to hospital protocol.	Radical nephrectomy requires extensive resection, necessitating general anesthesia.
	Advise the patient that intravenous fluids will be administered until oral fluids can be tolerated.	Intravenous fluids and dextrose are used to maintain hydration until oral fluids are tolerated.
	Advise the patient that surgical drains may be placed in the incision to promote wound healing.	Surgical drains are sometimes used to drain fluids from the surgical site, promoting wound healing and minimizing the risk of infection.
	Advise the patient that a urethral catheter will be in place for several days after surgery.	A Foley catheter is used to ensure urinary drainage and to evaluate hematuria after radical nephrectomy.
Altered tissue perfusion (renal) related to renal adenocarcinoma	Prepare patient for preoperative renal artery embolization as directed.	Preoperative renal embolization may be use to reduce bleeding during surgery.
Potential for infection (urinary system) related to renal cell carcinoma causing stasis and obstruction	Obtain urine culture as directed.	Bacteriuria is treated before surgery to prevent systemic infection.
	Administer antiinfective medications as directed.	Antiinfective medications are used to eradicate infection before nephrectomy.

→ > >

POSTPROCEDURAL NURSING CARE

NURSING DIAGNOSIS	NURSING INTERVENTIONS	RATIONALE
Altered tissue perfusion (renal) related to radical nephrectomy with or without renal artery embolization and vena caval thrombectomy	Monitor urinary output for evidence of excessive hematuria.	Hematuria is expected after radical nephrectomy; however, the urine should be only pink tinged; bright red bleeding and clots indicate excessive bleeding, requiring prompt management.
	Monitor hematocrit (Hct) and hemoglobin (Hb) for evidence of postoperative bleeding; compare findings with preoperative values.	Hct and Hb values decrease when bleeding is present; since a renal cell carcinoma may predispose the individual to anemia, postoperative values are compared against a preoperative baseline.
	Monitor vital signs for signs of excessive bleeding (rapid pulse with increased and then declining blood pressure).	Severe postoperative bleeding alters the vital signs, indicating the need for rapid management.
	Monitor patient who has undergone preoperative renal artery embolization for postinfarction syndrome (flank pain, fever, leukocytosis, with/without hypertension).	Postinfarction syndrome may occur after renal artery embolization and may persist for up to 72 hours.
Pain related to radical nephrectomy	Assess pain for location, character, duration, and aggravating and alleviating factors.	Postoperative incisional pain is common after radical nephrectomy, especially since anterior subcostal or flank incisions may be required. This pain is a chronic, dull discomfort that is intense and aggravated by deep inspiration or coughing. Flank pain related on the opposite (contralateral) side is unexpected and warrants prompt investigation.
	Administer analgesic or narcotic agents as directed.	Analgesic or narcotic medications temporarily relieve incisional pain.
	Use nonpharmacologic measures (e.g., limiting environmental distractors and proper positioning) to reduce discomfort.	Nonpharmacologic means are an important adjunct to analgesia in managing acute postoperative pain.
Ineffective airway clearance related to anterior subcostal or flank incision	Maintain scrupulous pulmonary toilet (including turning, coughing, and deep-breathing exercises) after radical nephrectomy.	Pulmonary toilet is instituted after any surgical procedure to prevent potential complications related to ineffective mobilization of pulmonary secretions; surgery requiring a flank or anterior subcostal incision increases the risk of respiratory complications, since coughing or deep breathing aggravates incisional pain.
	Splint the patient with a pillow before pulmonary toilet exercises.	Splinting reduces excessive movement, relieving some discomfort.
	Schedule pulmonary toilet approximately ½ h after administering analgesic medications.	Pulmonary toilet is more effective when pain medications are at their peak effectiveness.

PATIENT TEACHING

1. Reinforce instruction on the role of radical nephrectomy in the overall management of renal cell carcinoma.
2. Teach the patient that symptoms of renovascular hypertension, anemia, hematuria, and certain paraneoplastic syndromes are expected to be relieved or eradicated by radical nephrectomy.
3. Teach the patient how to do pulmonary toilet exercises before surgery, and emphasize the importance of performing these maneuvers despite postoperative discomfort.

Bladder Tumors

Bladder cancers are the second most common malignant tumor of the genitourinary system. They are more common among men than women (3.5:1) and affect whites more often than blacks. Bladder cancers may occur at any age but are particularly common in the sixth decade of life.[134,135]

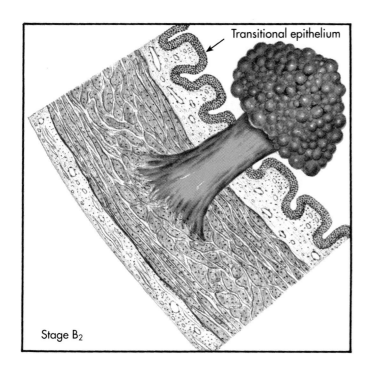

Stage B₂

TRANSITIONAL CELL CARCINOMA OF THE BLADDER (WITH STALK)

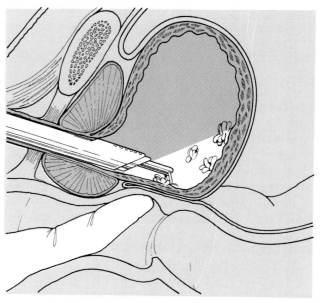

FIGURE 7-1
Resection of bladder tumor.

Transitional cell carcinomas account for approximately 95% of all malignant bladder cancers. Squamous cell carcinomas are relatively uncommon, accounting for only 3% of all vesicle malignancies. Other bladder tumors include adenocarcinomas, urachal adenocarcinomas, small cell carcinomas, and carcinosarcomas. Nonepithelial bladder tumors are particularly rare; leiomyosarcomas or pheochromocytomas affect the muscular tunic of the bladder wall, and primary lymphomas may arise from submucosal lymphoid follicles. This discussion is limited to papillary transitional cell carcinomas and carcinoma in situ.

The cause of bladder cancers remains unclear, although a variety of contributing factors have been identified. Exposure to occupational toxins is linked to as many as one fourth to one third of all tumors in the United States.[138] Aromatic amines found in certain dyes, leather tanning, and exposure to organic chemicals may increase the risk of bladder cancer.[158]

Other risk factors include cigarette smoking, coffee consumption, phenacetin misuse, artificial sweeteners, pelvic irradiation, chronic cystitis, and specific inflammatory bladder lesions. Administration of cyclophosphamides and endogenous tryptophan metabolites also has been correlated with increased risk of bladder malignancies. In addition, familial instances of bladder cancer have been noted.[135]

PATHOPHYSIOLOGY

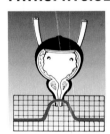

The pathophysiologic significance of transitional cell carcinoma arises from its propensity to grow uncontrolledly, to invade adjacent structures, and to produce distant metastases. The events that lead to the formation of a transitional cell tumor are unclear; however, evidence points to an interaction between oncogene activation and inhibition or loss of cancer suppressor factors in the bladder epithelium. A transitional cell tumor typically grows as a papillary tumor that extends into the bladder vesicle and is anchored to the wall by a slender stalk. This basic papillary structure has many variations, including sessile infiltrating tumors, nodular tumors, and flat, intraepithelial (in situ) tumors. Approximately 70% of all transitional cell carcinomas are papillary, 10% are nodular, and 20% are mixed forms. The malignant potential of transitional cell tumors also varies significantly, ranging from virtually benign papillomas to markedly aggressive carcinomas.[135]

Transitional cell tumors are invasive into the bladder wall. Low-grade tumors are contained entirely within the urothelium, whereas higher stage tumors invade the lamina propria and detrusor muscle before invading the perivesical fat and adjacent organs. Lymphatogenous or hematogenous spread leads to metastatic tumors of the regional (pelvic) lymph nodes, lungs, bones, and liver.

Staging of bladder tumors is important, because the tumor's stage helps to define its malignant potential and size and to determine the best treatment program. Several classification systems may be used for transitional cell carcinoma. The Jewett-Strong-Marshall system classifies tumors using stages 0 and A through D. Stage 0 tumors are entirely contained within the bladder urothelium, and stage A tumors invade the lamina propria. Stage B tumors invade the detrusor muscle; stage B1 tumors are superficially invasive, and stage B2 tumors are deeply invasive. Stage C tumors have invaded the perivesical fat surrounding the bladder, and stage D tumors are associated with distant metastasis. Stage D1 tumors have metastasized to regional lymph nodes, and stage D2 tumors have invaded distant organs.[179]

The TNM (tumor, node, metastasis) system also is widely used to classify transitional cell carcinomas. It was proposed by the International Union Against Cancer and the American Joint Commission on Cancer Staging. The letter "T" is used to denote tumor, the letter "N" denotes nodes, and the letter "M" indicates metastasis. A classification of T_{is} indicates a tumor entirely confined in the bladder urothelium; it is comparable to the stage 0 tumor of the Jewett-Strong-Marshall system. A T_1 tumor has invaded the lamina propria of the bladder, and a T_2 tumor has invaded the superficial detrusor muscle. A T_{3a} tumor has deeply invaded the detrusor muscle, and a T_{3b} tumor has spread to the perivesical fat. A T_4 tumor has spread to adjacent organs. Addition of the letter "N" to the system indicates metastasis to regional nodes, and addition of the letter "M" indicates metastasis to distant organs such as the lungs or bones.[135]

The malignancy of a bladder tumor is further classified by pathologic grading systems.[165] These systems determine the degree of anaplasia in an attempt to predict the malignant potential of an individual tumor. Several grading systems are used. According to one system, 75% of all grade I tumor cells are relatively well differentiated. Grade II tumors show less differentiation (50% of tumor cells are less well differentiated), and in grade III tumors, fewer than 25% of the cells are well differentiated. Grade IV tumors are the most malignant, containing only poorly differentiated cells. As expected, grade III and grade IV tumors are more likely to be invasive and are less responsive to conservative treatment measures than are lower grade tumors.

COMPLICATIONS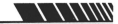

Hematuria	Bone pain*
Obstructive uropathy	Pathologic bone fractures*
Lung dysfunction*	Death
Liver dysfunction*	*Related to metastatic disease.

DIAGNOSTIC STUDIES AND FINDINGS

Diagnostic test	Findings
Urinalysis	Gross or microscopic hematuria; pyuria may be noted
Urine cytologic studies	Malignant cells (voided specimen is acceptable, but specimen obtained after gentle irrigation with saline is preferred)
Flow cytometry	Used to examine DNA content of exfoliated cells obtained from urine cytologic studies; quantitative analysis measures presence of DNA using binding dyes; increased DNA content indicates malignancy (the test is particularly sensitive for high-grade tumors)
Cell surface antigens	Impaired ABH antigen uptake or increased uptake of monoclonal antibodies separates tumor cells from normal surrounding tissue
Intravenous pyelogram/ urogram (IVP/IVU)	Filling defect may be noted on bladder x-rays; periureteral tumors may produce obstructive uropathy; tumors near the bladder base may be associated with trabeculation and bladder outlet obstruction
Voiding cystourethrogram (VCUG)	Filling defect noted on early filling x-rays; this defect typically is obscured as the bladder fill progresses
Endoscopy and biopsy	Visual inspection reveals papillary, nodular tumors; mixed tumors; or flattened lesions of carcinoma in situ; cold-cut biopsy is obtained from obvious tumor, adjacent epithelium, and distant, normal-appearing urothelium; these specimens are used for staging and grading; endoscopy under anesthesia is used to visualize tumors, for biopsy, and for bladder irrigation for urine cytologic studies; bimanual examination for bladder wall thickening and invasive tumor mass is completed during this procedure

MEDICAL MANAGEMENT

GENERAL AND SURGICAL MANAGEMENT: NONINVASIVE TUMORS

Transurethral resection of bladder tumors

Laser fulguration of bladder tumors

Intravesical chemotherapy (see box, page 214)

Routine follow-up endoscopic evaluation with resection of superficial tumors

GENERAL AND SURGICAL MANAGEMENT: INVASIVE TUMORS

Partial cystectomy or radical cystectomy or cystoprostatectomy

Urinary diversion following total (radical) cystectomy consisting of incontinent (ileal or colonic) conduit or continent diversion (Kock pouch, Indiana pouch, Mainz pouch, UCLA pouch)

Adjunct or palliative systemic chemotherapy

Adjunct or palliative external beam radiotherapy

INTRAVESICAL CHEMOTHERAPY FOR BLADDER CANCER

Agent: Thiotepa

Actions: Alkylating chemotherapeutic agent that suppresses tumor growth and recurrence

Side Effects: Transient irritative voiding symptoms (dysuria, urgency, frequency after administration); myelosuppression may be significant, necessitating temporary discontinuation of therapy

Agent: Mitomycin-C

Actions: Antitumor, antibiotic, and alkylating agent that inhibits DNA synthesis of rapidly proliferating tumor cells

Side Effects: Transient irritative voiding symptoms, rash of hands and genitalia may occur if patient does not thoroughly wash after urination of agent; myelosuppression mild and relatively uncommon

Agent: Doxorubicin

Actions: Intercalating agent with antitumor activity

Side Effects: Transient irritative voiding symptoms, rare systemic myelosuppression

Agent: Bacillus Calmette-Guerin (BCG)

Actions: Attenuated strain of *Mycobacterium bovis;* thought to intensify immunologic response to tumor

Side Effects: Transient irritative voiding symptoms and hemorrhagic cystitis; systemic symptoms may require discontinuance of therapy and treatment with isoniazid (INH), rifampin, and/or cycloserine

From Carroll.[134]

1 ASSESS

ASSESSMENT	OBSERVATIONS
Hematuria	Grossly visible blood without pain or dysuria
Altered patterns of urinary elimination	Urinary frequency (greater than q 2 h) and urgency with or without urge incontinence
Pain	Flank pain may be related to ureteral obstruction or retroperitoneal metastasis; chronic bone pain may be caused by skeletal metastasis
Lymphadenopathy	Enlarged pelvic lymph nodes with lymphatic metastasis
Abdominal mass	Hepatomegaly related to hepatic metastasis

2 DIAGNOSE

NURSING DIAGNOSIS	SUBJECTIVE FINDINGS	OBJECTIVE FINDINGS
Altered protection related to malignant bladder tumor with potential for recurrence, local invasion, and distant metastasis	Reports gross, painless hematuria with or without irritative voiding symptoms	Gross or microscopic hematuria without cystitis
Altered patterns of urinary elimination related to bladder tumor and intravesical resection of tumors or chemotherapy	Reports irritative voiding symptoms	Diurnal frequency greater than q 2 h with nocturia greater than one episode per night; urge incontinence may occur
Pain related to urinary obstruction and retroperitoneal or bony metastasis	Complains of flank pain or of aching bone pain	Flank pain is centered in one or both flanks (typically one side only is affected); it is aggravated by drinking large volumes of fluid and relieved by local application of heat. Bone pain is centered in the long bones, pelvis, or spine and aggravated by movement or exercise
Altered tissue perfusion (peripheral, bladder) related to bladder cancer or radiotherapy-induced cystitis	Reports grossly visible blood in the urine	Gross or microscopic hematuria; hematocrit (Hct) and hemoglobin (Hb) values may be affected
Anticipatory grieving related to guarded prognosis in advanced-stage bladder tumors	Reports need to prepare for possible death	Patient's physical condition and the advanced stage of the tumor make guarded prognosis a reality; patient and family demonstrate behavior of preparing for loss of family member

3 PLAN

Patient goals

1. Bladder cancer will be eradicated, and there will be no metastases.
2. Patterns of urinary elimination will return to premorbid parameters, *or* patient will establish new pattern of regular, complete bladder evacuation following creation of ileal conduit or continent urinary diversion.
3. Flank pain will resolve.
4. Bone pain will resolve.
5. Hematuria will resolve.
6. Anticipatory grieving is expressed, and steps to prepare for death are taken in accordance with the patient's and family's wishes.

→ > >

4 IMPLEMENT

NURSING DIAGNOSIS	NURSING INTERVENTIONS	RATIONALE
Altered protection related to malignant bladder tumor with potential for recurrence, local invasion, and distant metastasis	Help the patient who notes grossly visible blood in the urine to obtain prompt medical evaluation.	The presenting sign of bladder cancer typically is gross, painless hematuria; this symptom may also be a sign of renal tumor, ureteral tumor, urinary calculi, or another serious urinary system disorder, indicating prompt medical intervention.
	Advise the patient with irritative voiding symptoms and microscopic hematuria on a routine urinalysis to seek medical evaluation.	Irritative voiding symptoms that coexist with microscopic hematuria may indicate bladder cancer, as well as other urinary tract diseases; medical evaluation allows correct identification and treatment of the underlying disorder, including bladder cancer.
	Obtain voided urine cytologic studies as directed.	Urine cytologic studies help in the identification of malignant cells that have exfoliated into the urine; the test assists in identification of bladder cancer and may provide clues to the tumor grade.
	Prepare the patient for cystoscopy with biopsy, cytologic studies from bladder "washing," and bimanual examination as directed; inform the patient that this procedure requires general anesthesia. (see Endoscopy, page 39).	Endoscopic examination of the vesicle allows evaluation of the tumor's type and growth patterns (size and papillary, nodular, or mixed form), location (bladder base, periureteral, or lateral walls or dome). Biopsy is used to determine the type and grade of tumor and helps in determining stage. Urine cytologic studies from bladder washing assist in grading the tumor, and bimanual examination helps stage the tumor. Because of the invasive nature of the procedure and associated discomfort, general anesthesia may be required.
	Prepare the patient for other diagnostic tests, including IVP/IVU, as directed.	Accurate tumor staging is crucial to determine the proper treatment of a bladder tumor and to identify complications of the disease, including metastasis and obstructive uropathy.
	Prepare the patient for transurethral bladder tumor resection, fulguration, or laser therapy as directed (see Figure 7-1).	Endoscopic resection of bladder tumors is done to debulk or remove noninvasive or superficially invasive malignancies; the tumor can be resected, fulgurated, or treated with a laser.
	Prepare the patient for intravesical chemotherapy as directed (see Table 7-1).	Intravesical chemotherapy is used as adjunctive care for patients with superficial or minimally invasive tumors (stages 0, A, B1). Chemotherapy is indicated for patients at risk for tumor recurrence, including those with higher grade or several tumors, patients with coexisting urothelial atypia, and those with carcinoma in situ.

NURSING DIAGNOSIS	NURSING INTERVENTIONS	RATIONALE
	Administer or teach the patient to self-administer vitamins B_6 (pyridoxine) and C (ascorbic acid) and vitamin A retinoids as directed.	Systemic vitamins have shown some potential for reducing the risk of recurrence of superficial bladder tumors; although the pharmacologic mechanism remains unknown, vitamin therapy may bolster the body's immune response to urothelial cancer.[135]
	Administer hematoporphyrin-derivative therapy as directed.	Hematoporphyrin-derivative therapy is a prepared mixture of porphyrin that preferentially binds to neoplastic cells; when activated by white light, these porphyrins kill cells.[129,130]
	Prepare the patient for partial cystectomy as directed.	Partial cystectomy is the removal of part of the bladder and subsequent reclosure of the remaining bladder, avoiding the need for urinary diversion.
	Prepare the patient for radical cystectomy or radical cystoprostatectomy with incontinent or continent urinary diversion as directed.	Radical cystectomy is the removal of the bladder, perivesical fat, and regional lymph nodes; the prostate and part or all of the urethra are removed or spared as indicated.
	Prepare the patient for radiotherapy as directed.	External beam radiotherapy is used in conjunction with surgical tumor resection for bladder cancer. A single dose of 2,500 to 3,500 rad is given during surgery, and a follow-up dose of 3,000 to 4,000 rad of external beam therapy is given later. Intraoperative radiotherapy is useful for tumors in stages T_{is}, T_1, and T_2. External beam radiotherapy also may be used for palliation of advanced-stage tumors (D2 or T_4, M_1).
	Administer systemic chemotherapy before radical cystectomy or as palliative treatment for advanced-stage tumors as directed (Table 7-2).	Chemotherapy may be used to reduce the tumor before radical cystectomy or, in advanced-stage tumors (D2 or T_4, M_1), to reduce the tumor and associated symptoms.
	Administer immunotherapeutic agents, such as interferon inducer poly (I:C), streptococcal OK-432, or interleukin-2 (IL-2), as directed.	Immunotherapy agents are designed to intensify the body's immunologic response to malignant tumors; as of 1991 these agents were in clinical trials and had not been approved yet by the U.S. Food and Drug Administration.[134]
Altered patterns of urinary elimination related to bladder tumor and intravesical resection of tumors or chemotherapy	Advise the patient that urinary urgency and frequency may be caused or aggravated by bladder tumors and that treatment of these tumors is expected to alleviate these symptoms.	Bladder tumors cause vesical wall irritation sufficient to produce urinary frequency and urgency and sometimes urge incontinence.

→ > >

NURSING DIAGNOSIS	NURSING INTERVENTIONS	RATIONALE
	Advise the patient that administration of intravesical or systemic chemotherapy or immunotherapy will cause irritative voiding symptoms; reassure him that these effects are expected to be transient.	Intravesical chemotherapy kills neoplastic and some normal cells, causing bladder wall inflammation with consequent urinary urgency and frequency and urge incontinence among some patients.
	Advise the patient that radiotherapy is expected to produce irritative voiding symptoms; reassure the patient that these symptoms are expected to be transient.	Like chemotherapy, radiotherapy causes bladder inflammation and irritative voiding symptoms.
	Help the patient maintain an adequate fluid intake (at least 1,500 ml/day).	Fluids flush the urinary system and bladder, alleviating irritative symptoms by removing sediment from the bladder and reducing the likelihood of bacteriuria.
	Administer or teach the patient to self-administer urinary analgesic medications or anticholinergic/antispasmodic medications as directed.	Urinary analgesics reduce irritative voiding symptoms by unclear pharmacologic mechanisms; antispasmodic medications reduce irritative voiding symptoms and inhibit unstable bladder contractions.
	Teach the patient to void by a schedule (approximately q 2 h) during waking hours; teach the patient to avoid bolus intake of fluids with meals and to spread out his fluid intake during daytime hours (sipping beverages kept in a large container may be helpful). (See Fluid Intake: What, When, and How Much, page 303.)	A timed voiding schedule is used with or without antispasmodic medications to try to empty the bladder before a threshold volume is reached where unstable contractions occur. Fluid management strategies are designed to prevent bolus intake of fluids, which causes intense urgency and predisposes to incontinence, while ensuring adequate fluid intake.
	If a patient has established irritative voiding symptoms that persist for 6 months or longer after radiotherapy or chemotherapy has been completed, refer him to a urologist or nurse specialist for definitive management of the voiding dysfunction.	Established irritative voiding symptoms must be managed by a qualified physician or continence nurse specialist.
Pain related to urinary obstruction and retroperitoneal or bony metastasis	Assess pain for character, location, intensity, duration, and aggravating and alleviating factors.	Flank pain caused by obstruction typically is intense and localized to one side of the body. The pain is intensified by drinking fluids and is not relieved by a change in position or rest. In contrast, metastatic bone pain is dull, chronic, and localized to the long bones, pelvis, or spine. It is moderate to exquisitely intense and is relieved by position changes or rest.
	Prepare the patient for bladder tumor resection or partial or radical cystectomy as directed.	Resection of the bladder tumor relieves flank pain caused by obstruction by removing the source of obstruction.

NURSING DIAGNOSIS	NURSING INTERVENTIONS	RATIONALE
	Administer chemotherapy or radiotherapy as directed.	Radiotherapy or chemotherapy relieves bone pain by reducing or eradicating metastatic tumors; therapy may relieve flank pain by reducing the size of the tumor and thus relieving obstruction.
	Administer or teach the patient to self-administer analgesics or narcotic medications for pain.	Acute flank pain may require narcotic analgesia for pain relief; metastatic bone pain may be managed by analgesic or narcotic medications.
	Apply local heat to the flank for discomfort.	Local heat may relieve discomfort related to obstruction.
	Use nonpharmacologic maneuvers to help relieve pain, including restricting excessive movement and positioning to promote comfort.	Nonpharmacologic maneuvers are used in conjunction with analgesia to relieve pain related to obstruction or bony metastasis.
Altered tissue perfusion (peripheral, bladder) related to bladder cancer or radiotherapy-induced cystitis	Teach the patient to monitor his urine for evidence of hematuria; advise him to contact the physician promptly if excessive or unexpected bleeding occurs.	Hematuria may occur with bladder cancer and after transurethral tumor resection and intravesical chemotherapy; although hematuria typically is limited, significant bleeding may occur and requires prompt medical management.
	Reassure the patient that some hematuria is expected after transurethral resection of bladder tumors and intravesical chemotherapy; teach him to differentiate between the expected pink-tinged urine and bright red blood, which indicates excessive bleeding.	Pink-tinged urine is expected after chemotherapy or resection; bright red blood indicates excessive bleeding and requires prompt medical management.
	Monitor patient after procedures for significant hematuria; observe urine and monitor Hct, Hb, and vital signs; prepare patient for administration of formalin (1% to 10% solution) intravesically under regional or general anesthesia as directed.	A 1% to 10% formalin solution is prepared from a 37% formalin gas in sterile water. Typically, a 1% solution is instilled initially, followed by a 4% solution when bleeding is particularly severe. This treatment resolves significant, refractory hematuria.[134,135]
	Prepare the patient for a cystogram before instillation of the formalin.	A cystogram is necessary to detect vesicoureteral reflux; if reflux is present, Fogarty catheters are used to occlude the ureterovesical junction before instillation, protecting the upper urinary tracts from this irritative substance.
	Warn the patient that irritative voiding symptoms occur after instillation of formalin; maintain an indwelling catheter as directed.	Formalin irritates the bladder mucosa, and significant irritative voiding symptoms persist for a short period after instillation; a catheter may be used for drainage until these symptoms subside.

NURSING DIAGNOSIS	NURSING INTERVENTIONS	RATIONALE
Anticipatory grieving related to guarded prognosis in advanced-stage bladder tumors	Encourage the patient and family to talk about their feelings and concerns.	Open discussion of fears and feelings of distress is necessary before the patient and family can prepare for their potential loss.
	Keep the patient and family informed about the patient's plan of care and prognosis in consultation with the physician.	Accurate information helps the patient and family initiate and sustain the process of anticipatory grieving.
	Help the patient and family identify and obtain assistance to complete plans or arrangements for their potential loss.	Making a will and arranging for financial, spiritual, or other concerns help the patient and family cope as they prepare for a potential loss; these arrangements are also helpful following a death.
	Provide support for the patient's family, and encourage them to meet their own physical needs for nutrition, rest, and grieving during the patient's periods of crisis or intensive care.	Family members may neglect their own health in a misdirected attempt to care for the cancer victim; this only impedes the family members as they prepare for the potential loss of a loved one.
	Identify a strategy for contacting the family should death be likely or imminent.	Clearly identifying a way to contact the family should the patient face a crisis helps alleviate anxiety or guilt associated with leaving the patient to attend to personal needs.

5 EVALUATE

OUTCOME	DATA INDICATING THAT OUTCOME IS REACHED
Bladder cancer has been eradicated, and there are no metastases.	Imaging studies, pathologic analysis of biopsies, and endoscopic evaluation reveal absence of primary bladder tumors.
Patterns of urinary elimination have returned to premorbid parameters, *or* patient has established a new pattern of regular, complete bladder evacuation following creation of an ileal conduit or continent urinary diversion.	(1) The patient reports no irritative voiding symptoms, and his bladder diary demonstrates diurnal frequency q 2 h or less often with one or fewer episodes of nocturia. (2) The patient with a urinary diversion has no leakage with a self-intermittent catheterization program q 4-6 h. (3) The patient with an ileal conduit demonstrates complete urinary containment with the proper pouching system.
Flank pain has resolved.	The patient reports less or no flank pain; imaging studies show no obstruction.

OUTCOME	DATA INDICATING THAT OUTCOME IS REACHED
Bone pain has resolved.	The patient reports that bone pain is gone.
Hematuria has resolved.	Urinalysis and microscopic visualization reveal no red blood cells or visible blood in the urine.
Anticipatory grieving has been expressed, and steps have been taken to prepare for death in accordance with the patient's and family's wishes.	The patient and family recognize the guarded diagnosis and have devised strategies to make financial, legal, and other needed arrangements for a potential death; the patient and family express the feelings provoked by the guarded prognosis.

PATIENT TEACHING

1. Teach the patient the pathophysiology of cancer advancement and the significance of bladder cancer in particular. Emphasize that there are treatments that can arrest tumor growth or eradicate these malignancies.
2. Teach the patient the significance of recurrence of superficial tumors and the need for strict adherence to routine surveillance by endoscopy.
3. Teach the patient the relationship between hematuria, the recurrence of cancer, and the administration of intravesical chemotherapy or resection of bladder tumors. Teach the patient to recognize significant hematuria.
4. Teach the patient the names, actions, administration, and potential side effects of all medications, including antineoplastic agents, administered for bladder cancer.
5. Teach the patient about the process of radiotherapy and potential side effects, including stomatitis, altered appetite, and the potential for radiation cystitis.
6. Emphasize and reinforce the physician's teaching concerning the purpose, goals, and potential untoward effects of surgical procedures for bladder cancer.

CYSTECTOMY WITH ILEAL OR COLONIC CONDUIT

Cystectomy is the surgical removal of the bladder. Radical cystectomy, in men, is the surgical resection en bloc of the bladder, prostate, seminal vesicles, and pelvic peritoneum in men. In women, radical cystectomy involves removal of the bladder, pelvic peritoneum, urethra, uterus, broad ligaments, and anterior third of the vaginal wall. Because total urethrectomy is associated with significant morbidity in men, the distal urethra is left intact. A pelvic lymphadenectomy is also done during a radical cystectomy; the limits of this dissection are determined by the extent of probable involvement and the surgeon's preference.[163]

Since urine can no longer exit the body via the bladder, a urinary diversion (alternate site for urine elimination) is created. The most common form of urinary diversion is the ileal (Bricker) conduit.

The ileal conduit is created immediately after the cystectomy. A 15 to 20 cm segment of the terminal ileum is isolated from the fecal stream, along with its blood supply and mesentery. The distal end of this ileal

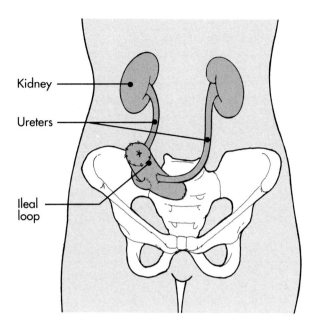

FIGURE 7-2
Urinary diversion (ileal conduit).

segment is brought out through the abdominal wall in the right lower quadrant and fashioned into a budded stoma. The ureters are anastomosed to the proximal end of the conduit in a freely refluxing manner, and the proximal end of the conduit is sutured closed. The conduit is designed in an isoperistaltic manner, serving as an exit route for urine rather than as a storage compartment.

Large bowel may be used as an alternative to the ileal conduit. In this case a segment of large bowel is

UNITED OSTOMY ASSOCIATION

Goal:	Advocacy and peer support for individuals coping with a urinary or gastrointestinal diversion
Address:	36 Executive Park Suite 120 Irvine, California 92714-6744
Contact:	National Office, 1-800-826-0826

used to form a conduit. The potential advantage of the large bowel conduit is the ability to implant the ureters into the conduit in a nonrefluxing manner. Unfortunately, because obstruction at the ureteroenteric junction is a common complication, the sigmoid conduit is only rarely used.

INDICATIONS

Invasive bladder cancer

CONTRAINDICATIONS

Superficial tumors amenable to less invasive procedures
Active inflammatory bowel disease

COMPLICATIONS

Infection
Hemorrhage
Urinary obstruction
Peristomal hernia
Stomal necrosis

PREPROCEDURAL NURSING CARE

NURSING DIAGNOSIS	NURSING INTERVENTIONS	RATIONALE
Knowledge deficit related to surgical procedure, goals, and potential untoward effects	Reinforce preoperative instruction, including a brief explanation of the procedure, its goals, potential untoward effects, and expected nursing care.	Preoperative anxiety diminishes the patient's ability to learn; repetition of instruction enhances learning and retention and reduces patient's anxiety about the procedure.
	Advise the patient that an extensive bowel preparation will be completed before urinary diversion.	Urinary diversion requires surgical reconstruction of a small segment of the terminal ileum; intensive preparation of the bowel is crucial to prevent bacterial infection from the normal bowel flora.

NURSING DIAGNOSIS	NURSING INTERVENTIONS	RATIONALE
	Advise the patient that an enterostomal (ET) nurse specialist will visit after surgery to help care for the urinary diversion and to teach him to care for his own conduit.	The ET nurse specialist teaches the patient to care for her ostomy and the peristomal skin; the ET nurse provides immediate postoperative care and ongoing care as the individual learns to manage and cope with a urinary diversion.
	Arrange for a preoperative visit from an individual with an ostomy.	A person with an ostomy can share experiences and provide insight into adjustment to a urinary diversion.
	Advise the patient that a nasogastric tube will be left in place until bowel sounds return.	Surgical manipulation of the bowel for urinary diversion causes transient paralytic ileus; a nasogastric tube is used to decompress the bowel, preventing vomiting and rupture of the reanastomosed bowel until peristalsis returns.
	Advise the patient that intravenous fluids will be administered until he can tolerate oral fluids.	Intravenous fluids maintain hydration and provide certain nutrients until peristalsis returns and the nasogastric tube is removed.
	Advise the patient that ureteral stents will be left in place until after discharge from the hospital.	Ureteral stents are left in place to prevent obstruction or rupture until the ureteroenteric junctions heal.
	Advise the patient that he will remain in the hospital for 7 to 10 days.	A 7- to 10-day hospital course typically is necessary to ensure recovery of peristalsis, essential education concerning ostomy care, and sufficient wound healing for discharge.
Potential for infection (systemic) related to surgical manipulation of the bowel	Administer intensive bowel preparation program as directed; continue the program for 2 to 3 days as directed.	Bowel preparation removes normal bacterial flora and fecal material from the intestinal tract before surgical manipulation.
	Administer antiinfective medications, including antibiotics and antifungal agents, as directed before surgery.	Antiinfective medications eradicate potential pathogens from the bowel before surgical manipulation.
Potential fluid volume deficit related to intensive bowel preparation	Provide clear liquids as feasible during bowel preparation until the night before surgery.	Clear liquids maintain hydration before surgery.
	Administer antiemetics as directed.	Bowel preparation may cause nausea and vomiting, rapidly depleting fluid and associated electrolytes; antiemetics suppress vomiting and symptoms of nausea.
	Administer intravenous fluids (under medical direction) before surgery if necessary.	Intravenous fluids may be necessary to maintain adequate hydration and to provide needed electrolytes before surgery.

POSTPROCEDURAL NURSING CARE

NURSING DIAGNOSIS	NURSING INTERVENTIONS	RATIONALE
Altered patterns of urinary elimination related to urinary diversion	Contain urinary output from the ileal conduit, using a pouching system with antireflux valve and spout; regularly assess the system for kinking or overfilling of the collection bag.	A pouching system is used to collect urinary output and to protect peristomal skin; kinked tubes or overfilled containers produce obstruction of urine by blocking outflow.
	Monitor urinary output for volume; if output falls precipitously, evaluate drainage from all tubes or drains.	Precipitous decline in urine output may indicate diminished renal function or (most likely) leak from reconstructed urinary system; urinary leak may cause increased drainage of urine from other tubes.
	Work with the ET nurse to provide an optimal pouching system.	As the stoma heals, its size decreases; the ET nurse helps monitor the stoma, changing the pouching system as indicated.
	Help the patient with pouching changes as appropriate.	The patient must be able to change the urinary pouch to perform self-care tasks with the new diversion.
Altered tissue perfusion (peripheral uroenteric) related to urinary diversion	Assess stoma for color and mucous secretions.	The stoma should be pinkish red and have a moist surface; a pale or dark color with drying of the surface may indicate necrosis of the conduit.
	Observe urinary output for evidence of excessive bleeding.	Bright red blood in the urine after surgery is unexpected and may indicate excessive bleeding; however, light red or pink-tinged urine will persist for the first week or 10 days after surgery.
	Monitor all surgical drains and dressings for bloody exudate.	Bleeding produces bright red output, indicating its probable source.
	Monitor hematocrit (Hct) and hemoglobin (Hb) for evidence of significant bleeding; compare data to preoperative levels.	Hct and Hb decline if there is postoperative hemorrhage.
	Monitor vital signs for indications of excessive blood loss.	Changes in vital signs (rapid pulse with increased blood pressure followed by declining blood pressure) indicate severe blood loss with impending hypovolemic shock.
Pain related to surgical trauma	Assess pain for its character, location, duration, and aggravating and alleviating factors.	Incisional pain is localized to the abdomen and is a dull, boring pain that may be aggravated by coughing and straining. Obstructive pain is intense and located in the flank; it is aggravated by fluid intake rather than coughing or movement.
	Administer analgesic or narcotic agents as directed.	These drugs temporarily relieve incisional or obstructive pain.

NURSING DIAGNOSIS	NURSING INTERVENTIONS	RATIONALE
	Report flank pain to the physician promptly; prepare the patient for temporary urinary diversion as directed.	Intense flank pain indicates obstruction that may require temporary urinary diversion or (in rare instances) reoperation.
	Splint the abdomen before pulmonary toilet; schedule analgesics so that the peak effect coincides with coughing and deep-breathing exercises.	Coughing and deep breathing aggravate incisional pain; splinting and giving analgesics before pulmonary toilet minimize this discomfort.
Impaired skin integrity related to urinary diversion, urinary leakage, presence of collection device, or surgical dressings	Regularly assess skin integrity at all drain sites and under surgical dressings and any tape.	Rashes or skin lesions are particularly likely on skin exposed to adhesives, urine, or other exudate.
	Routinely assess the peristomal skin for rashes or lesions.	Exposure to urine and elements of a pouching system increases the risk of monilial and other rashes.
	Teach the patient to dry the skin thoroughly with pouch changes.	Drying the skin completely helps prevent ammonia contact dermatitis or other lesions that result when skin is chronically exposed to urine or other exudate.
	Apply powder to the skin beneath the pouch with each change. (*Note:* Avoid powders with a cornstarch base.)	Powder helps protect the skin; cornstarch is avoided because it promotes the development of monilial rashes.
	Apply antifungal or antibacterial agents to the skin as directed.	Antiinfective creams or powders control specific lesions, such as a monilial rash.
	Apply vinegar to the peristomal skin if crystals from alkaline urine are noted.	Vinegar dissolves the alkaline salt crystals produced by very alkaline urine.
	Insert vinegar directly into the pouch two to four times a day, and administer ascorbic acid (250 mg qid) as directed.	Vinegar in pouch and daily doses of ascorbic acid reduce urinary pH in patients prone to alkaline crystal formation.
Body image disturbance related to urinary diversion	Provide the patient and family members opportunities to discuss the stoma and its meaning in their lives.	A urinary stoma and pouch can seriously damage a patient's body image; discussing the implications of an ileal conduit from the individual's perspective helps the nurse formulate specific strategies for coping with this change.
	Encourage the patient to participate in self-care tasks, such as pouch changes.	Participation in self-care assists with a positive adjustment to the presence of a stoma.
	Discuss potential problems associated with a urinary stoma (e.g., odor, leakage, and possible detection of the pouch under clothing), and help the patient devise specific strategies for managing or avoiding these problems.	Helping the patient think of preventive measures for socially embarrassing situations increases the patient's confidence as she participates in social events with a relatively new stoma.

➜ ❯ ❯

NURSING DIAGNOSIS	NURSING INTERVENTIONS	RATIONALE
	Help the patient contact the United Ostomy Association or other support/advocacy group as indicated (see box on page 222).	Advocacy groups provide the patient with strategies for coping with an ostomy based on shared experiences.
Altered sexuality patterns or sexual dysfunction related to cystectomy with urinary diversion	Allow the patient and partner to adjust to the impact of urinary diversion before addressing issues of sexuality.	In the immediate postoperative period, pain and altered patterns of urinary elimination are probably more immediate concerns than sexuality issues; however, it may be necessary to raise this issue eventually to help the patient resolve concerns related to sexuality.
	Advise a male patient that impotence may or may not occur, and if it does, it may be temporary or permanent; reassure him that impotence is a treatable condition.	Extensive surgical reconstruction may alter the neurovascular modulators that regulate erections, producing transient or chronic erectile dysfunction; pharmacologic measures, a vacuum erection device, or surgical treatments are available for affected patients (see Chapter 8).
	Advise a female patient that dyspareunia may occur as a temporary or ongoing problem following creation of a urinary or fecal ostomy.	Dyspareunia may occur following urinary diversion because of the formation of scar tissue (compromising vaginal elasticity), reduction of mucous secretions needed for lubrication, or discomfort related to proximate surgical reconstruction.
	Encourage the patient to express his or her feelings and concerns about sexual expression following urinary diversion; consult a sexual counselor as indicated to manage sexual dysfunction related to urinary diversion.	Urinary diversion may have a negative, neutral, or positive impact on perceptions of sexual attractiveness and expressions of sexuality; expressing feelings and concerns about sexuality helps the patient resolve negative feelings produced by a change in body image; complex or unresolved issues are managed by a qualified specialist.
	Help the patient overcome problems managing the urinary diversion (e.g., leakage, odor, problems with pouching).	Management problems exert a negative impact on the individual's sexuality.
	Reassure the patient and partner that normal sexual activity will not cause trauma to the ostomy.	Partners often fear engaging in intercourse with a partner who has a urinary stoma; the partner particularly fears traumatizing the stoma.

PATIENT TEACHING

1. Teach the patient the signs and symptoms of urinary tract infection with an ileal conduit.
2. Teach the patient to use a bedside urinary container at night.
3. Teach the patient to monitor the pH of the urine.
4. Teach the patient the importance of an adequate fluid intake (at least 1,500 ml per day).
5. Teach the patient the potential impact of particular foods on urinary odor. Specifically, instruct the patient that asparagus, fish, eggs, and spicy foods may temporarily create a pungent odor in the urine.
6. Teach the patient to empty the pouch before it is completely filled (complete filling increases the risk of pouch separation and leakage.
7. Teach the patient to stock supplies for pouch changes to avoid being caught without essential equipment.

CYSTECTOMY WITH CONTINENT DIVERSION

Recent advances in surgical reconstruction of the bowel have led to the development of techniques for building a continent reservoir for urine constructed of small or large bowel. Cystectomy is performed as described in the previous section, Cystectomy with Ileal or Colonic Conduit. In contrast, continent urinary diversion is constructed as an alternative to the incontinent ileal conduit.

A **Kock pouch** is a small bowel reservoir for urine that can be attached to the urethra or to a cutaneous stoma (Figure 7-3). The pouch is constructed of 17 cm of ileum for the efferent limb of the pouch, 22 cm for each of the two segments of the reservoir, and 17 cm for the afferent limb. The afferent and efferent limbs are used to provide urinary flow into the reservoir in a nonrefluxing manner, and the efferent limb is used as a continent nipple connected to the abdominal wall, requiring intermittent catheterization for emptying. The nipple valves are intussuscepted by inverting the ileum into the pouch, creating a telescoped segment of approximately 5 cm with a lip of ileum for anastomosis into the reservoir. The 22 cm ileal segments are detubularized and formed into a U-shaped reservoir that can hold 500 ml of urine or more.

An alternative application of the Kock pouch is the creation of a bladder substitute, or **hemi-Kock ileal reservoir**. In this case an afferent limb is constructed from a 17 cm ileal segment in a nonrefluxing manner to provide urinary inflow from the kidneys. In addition, the central reservoir is constructed and then attached to

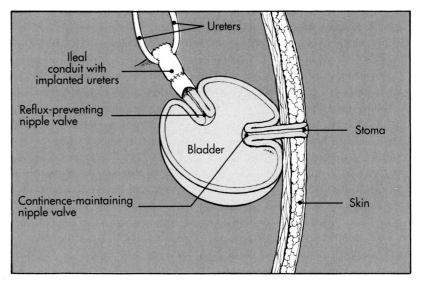

FIGURE 7-3
Kock pouch. (From Belcher, A: *Cancer Nursing,* St Louis, 1992, Mosby–Year Book.)

the preserved bladder base. Thus the urethral sphincter mechanism is used to maintain continence and the patient catheterizes the urethra or strain voids to empty the bladder. Clearly, one limitation of the hemi-Kock procedure is the inability to perform a radical cystectomy with prostatectomy, and patients with bladder cancer in or near the bladder base are not appropriate candidates for this procedure.[132]

A large bowel continent diversion is an alternate form of continent diversion. Large bowel has several potential advantages over small bowel. Because large bowel is less absorptive than ileum, the risk of metabolic disorders (including hypochloremic metabolic aci-

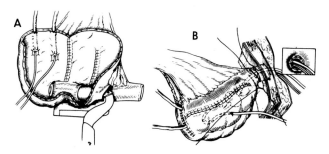

FIGURE 7-5
Mainz pouch. **A,** Staple fixation of the intussusception at the posterior wall of the ileocecal valve. **B,** The efferent loop is anastomosed to the abdominal wall. The preferred site of the Mainz group is the umbilicus. (From Thuroff J, Alker P, Riedmiller H, et al: *J Urol* 136:18, 1986; 140:285, 1988.)

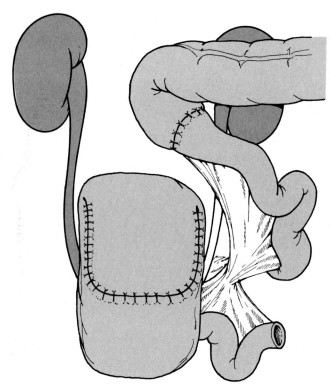

FIGURE 7-4
Indiana continent urinary reservoir.

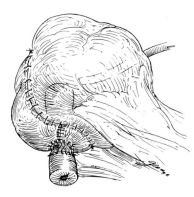

FIGURE 7-6
Continent right colonic urinary diversion developed at UCLA. (From Gillenwater et al, editors: *Adult and pediatric neurology,* ed 2, St Louis, 1991, Mosby–Year Book.)

dosis) is lessened. In addition, large bowel has a thicker, more muscular wall, enhancing the potential for implantation of the ureters in a nonrefluxing manner. However, because of large bowel's muscular walls, surgical repair must overcome the possible disadvantage of bolus contractions that have the potential to forcibly expel urine from the reservoir, producing dramatic urinary incontinence.

An **Indiana pouch** is created from the ascending colon, ileocecal valve, and terminal ileum (Figure 7-4). The colon is detubularized along its antimesenteric aspect to overcome the problem of high-pressure bolus contractions. The ureters are implanted into the walls of the colon in a nonrefluxing manner, and the ascending colon is folded over the colon and closed in a watertight fashion. The ileocecal valve forms the basic continence mechanism, which is strengthened or reinforced by plication of the bowel wall around the valve, reducing its diameter. This technique also assists in the

placement of an intermittent catheter for evacuation of urine from the reservoir.

Many other forms of continent urinary diversion have been used. A **Mainz pouch** uses 15 cm of cecum and ascending colon and 50 cm of terminal ileum (Figure 7-5). The colonic segment is detubularized and joined to a detubularized segment of ileum to form an intestinal plate. The ureters are brought into the pouch using a 5 cm submucosal tunnel located at the posterior tenia of the colon. The ileocecal valve is used as a continence mechanism, and the ileum is formed into a stoma, preferably at the umbilicus. A **UCLA pouch** uses the entire right colon, hepatic flexure, and about 14 cm of the terminal ileum (Figure 7-6). The colonic segment is detubularized along the anterior tenia to the level of the cecum, and the continent stoma is created by intussuscepting the terminal valve through the ileocecal valve. The valve is secured to the cecal wall, and the ureters are implanted into the pouch using a submucosal tunnel.[132]

INDICATIONS

Bladder cancer requiring cystectomy

Hostile neuropathic bladder dysfunction requiring urinary diversion

Certain cases of crippling interstitial cystitis

CONTRAINDICATIONS

Active inflammatory bowel disease

Unwillingness to engage in ongoing intermittent catheterization required for evacuation of the pouch

Inability to perform self-catheterization (e.g., poor dexterity or quadriplegia)

Congenital malformations of the bowel that make extensive reconstruction unfeasible

COMPLICATIONS

Small bowel pouches
  Incontinence
  Vesicoureteral reflux
  Ileoureteric junction obstruction
  Fistula
  Metabolic acidosis
  Electrolyte imbalances (rare)
  Vitamin B_{12} deficiency
  Prolonged diarrhea or bowel dysfunction
  Deterioration of renal function (rare)
Large bowel pouches*
  Incontinence
  Vesicoureteral reflux
  Ureteroenteric obstruction
  Fistula
  Diarrhea or bowel dysfunction
  Deterioration of renal function (rare)
*Small bowel may be used as supplemental material.

PREPROCEDURAL NURSING CARE

NURSING DIAGNOSIS	NURSING INTERVENTIONS	RATIONALE
Knowledge deficit related to surgical procedure, goals, and potential untoward effects	Reinforce preoperative instruction, including a brief explanation of the procedure, its goals, potential untoward effects, and expected nursing care.	Preoperative anxiety diminishes the patient's ability to learn; repetition of instruction enhances learning and retention and reduces anxiety related to the procedure.
	Advise patient that he will empty reservoir by intermittent catheterization or by strain voiding (only in certain cases when neobladder is attached to urethra).	Continent urinary diversions are designed to store urine at low pressures; they require catheterization for effective evacuation.
	Advise the patient that an ostomy tube will be left in the continent pouch for 2 to 4 weeks after surgery.	The continent diversion is placed on continuous drainage via an ostomy tube to prevent overdistention until wound healing is complete.
	Advise the patient that intravenous fluids will be administered after surgery until he can tolerate oral fluids.	Surgical reconstruction of the bowel causes temporary paralytic ileus, requiring nasogastric decompression; intravenous fluids maintain adequate hydration.
	Advise the patient that strenuous exercise and lifting of heavy objects are strictly forbidden for 30 to 45 days after surgery until wound healing is completed.	Strenuous exercise and lifting may compromise the continuity of a continent diversion; a period of 4 to 6 weeks is needed for thorough wound healing.

→ > >

NURSING DIAGNOSIS	NURSING INTERVENTIONS	RATIONALE
Potential for infection (systemic) related to surgical manipulation of the bowel	Administer intensive bowel preparation for 2 to 3 days before surgery as directed.	Bowel preparation cleanses the gastrointestinal tract of fecal material and normal flora that act as pathogens if exposed to the systemic circulation during surgical manipulation.
	Administer prophylactic antiinfective medications as directed.	Antibiotic and/or antifungal medications are administered to prevent potential systemic infection from normal bowel flora.
Potential fluid volume deficit related to intensive bowel preparation	Help the patient obtain oral fluids until the night before surgery.	Clear oral liquids maintain hydration during bowel preparation.
	Administer antiemetics as directed if nausea and vomiting occur.	Nausea and vomiting may occur during bowel preparation, causing rapid loss of fluids and associated electrolytes; antiemetic agents inhibit vomiting and suppress symptoms of nausea.
	Administer intravenous fluids as directed during bowel preparation.	Intravenous fluids maintain hydration and essential electrolytes when the patient cannot tolerate oral fluids.

POSTPROCEDURAL NURSING CARE

NURSING DIAGNOSIS	NURSING INTERVENTIONS	RATIONALE
Altered patterns of urinary elimination related to urinary diversion	Monitor ostomy drainage tube for volume of urinary output.	Urine is drained through an ostomy tube after surgery.
	Irrigate continent diversion q 2 h using sterile saline as directed (see Self-Irrigation for Reconstructed Bladders, page 310).	Irrigation removes excessive mucous secretions in the urine; these secretions can form clumps or strings that can obstruct the ostomy drainage tube; irrigation temporarily relieves this problem.
	Should urinary drainage decline or fail to reflect fluid intake, irrigate the ostomy tube first, then evaluate all other surgical or urinary drains (such as ureteral stents) and the surgical dressing. If these maneuvers fail to reveal the cause of compromised urinary drainage, consult the physician concerning evaluation for insufficient renal function.	Diminished urinary drainage following continent diversion is not an uncommon occurrence. By far the most common cause is occlusion with mucus, which can be reversed by irrigation. If the ureteroenteric junctions are obstructed, urinary drainage may be noted from an alternate drain, such as a surgical drain or ureteral stent. If all these maneuvers fail, the kidneys are evaluated for insufficient function.
	Help the patient attain an adequate fluid intake, typically in the form of parenteral fluids or total parenteral nutrition.	Fluid intake promotes urinary drainage and dilutes the urine, lessening the risk of mucous obstruction; parenteral fluids are administered until the nasogastric tube is removed.

NURSING DIAGNOSIS	NURSING INTERVENTIONS	RATIONALE
Altered tissue perfusion (peripheral uroenteric) related to cystectomy and continent urinary diversion	Monitor urinary output for evidence of excessive bleeding.	Some hematuria is expected after continent diversion—the urine should be light red or pinkish; a large volume of bright red urine with clots is unexpected and may indicate excessive bleeding.
	Monitor the surgical dressing and any other surgical drain for evidence of bleeding.	Bloody drainage from the incision line or other surgical drains may indicate excessive bleeding.
	Monitor the serum hematocrit (Hct) and hemoglobin (Hb) for evidence of bleeding; compare these values to preoperative data.	Hct and Hb decline if postoperative bleeding is significant.
	Monitor the vital signs for evidence of significant blood loss (rapid pulse with high blood pressure followed by declining pressure and evidence of hypovolemic shock); contact the physician promptly for evidence of significant bleeding.	Changes in vital signs signify dramatic blood loss, which requires rapid intervention.
	Regularly observe the urinary stoma for color and mucus; inform the physician immediately if evidence of compromised vascularity is noted.	The continent stoma should be red and moist with mucous secretions; a darkened, dry stoma indicates possible vascular compromise.
Pain related to cystectomy with continent urinary diversion	Assess pain for its location, character, duration, and aggravating and alleviating factors.	Incisional pain is a dull, boring pain in the midline of prolonged duration that is aggravated by movement or pulmonary toilet. Flank pain usually is very intense and limited to one side. Overdistention of the continent urinary diversion produces cramping abdominal pain, and gastric pains also may occur.
	Administer analgesic or narcotic agents as directed.	Narcotic or analgesic agents temporarily relieve incisional pain.
	Irrigate the continent diversion, and check surgical drains for urinary output; contact the physician promptly if abdominal cramps or flank pain is not rapidly relieved.	Abdominal cramping or flank pain indicates probable obstruction, requiring prompt reversal; a temporary urinary diversion may be required if irrigation or other measures fail to relieve discomfort.
	Administer antacids or antihistamines as directed.	Gastric discomfort is caused by acid secretions after surgery; antacids or antihistamines (cimetidine or others) relieve gastric discomfort and diminish the risk of peptic ulcers.

NURSING DIAGNOSIS	NURSING INTERVENTIONS	RATIONALE
Body image disturbance related to continent urinary diversion	Provide the patient and family members opportunities to discuss the stoma and its meaning in their lives.	A continent urinary diversion alters body image; discussing the implications of a continent stoma from the individual's perspective assists the nurse in formulating specific strategies for helping the patient cope with this change.
	Discuss potential management problems that may affect participation in social events (e.g., catheterization needs and the potential for leakage); help the patient identify strategies for managing any problems.	The ability to manage the continent stoma with minimal assistance and the ability to cope with potential problems are essential for the patient to deal positively with this major change in body image and self-care habits.
	Help the patient contact the United Ostomy Association or other support or advocacy group as indicated (see box on page 222).	Advocacy groups provide the patient with strategies for coping with an ostomy based on shared experiences.
Altered sexuality patterns or sexual dysfunction related to cystectomy with urinary diversion	Allow the patient and partner to adjust to the impact of continent diversion before addressing issues of sexuality.	In the immediate postoperative period, pain and altered patterns of urinary elimination are probably more immediate concerns than sexuality issues; however, it may be necessary to raise this issue eventually to help the patient resolve concerns about sexuality.
	Advise a male patient that impotence may or may not occur, and if it does, the problem may be temporary or permanent; reassure him that impotence is a treatable condition.	Extensive surgical reconstruction may alter the neurovascular modulators that regulate erections, producing transient or chronic erectile dysfunction; pharmacologic measures, a vacuum erection device, or surgical treatments are available for affected patients (see Chapter 8).
	Advise female patients that dyspareunia may occur as a temporary or ongoing problem following creation of a urinary or fecal ostomy.	Dyspareunia may occur after urinary diversion because of formation of scar tissue (which compromises vaginal elasticity), reduction of mucous secretions needed for lubrication, or discomfort related to proximate surgical reconstruction.
	Encourage the patient to express his or her feelings and concerns about sexual expression after continent diversion; consult a sexual counselor if indicated to manage sexual dysfunction related to urinary diversion.	Urinary diversion may exert a negative, neutral, or positive impact on perceptions of sexual attractiveness and expressions of sexuality; expressing feelings and concerns about sexuality helps the patient resolve negative fellings produced by a change in body image; complex or unresolved issues are managed by a qualified specialist.
	Help the patient overcome problems managing the continent diversion, including catheterization, mucus, and possible leakage.	Management problems have a negative impact on the individual's sexuality.

NURSING DIAGNOSIS	NURSING INTERVENTIONS	RATIONALE
	Reassure the patient and partner that normal sexual activity will not cause trauma to the ostomy.	Partners often fear engaging in intercourse with a partner who has a urinary stoma; the partner particularly fears traumatizing the stoma.

PATIENT TEACHING

1. Teach the patient the general nature and construction of their continent urinary diversion.
2. Teach the patient an appropriate catheterization and irrigation schedule in consultation with the physician.
3. Teach the patient specific strategies, including maintenance of adequate fluid intake and daily intake of 8 to 16 ounces of cranberry juice to minimize mucous production by the pouch.
4. Provide the patient with a medical-alert bracelet, and teach him to verbally instruct health care professional unfamiliar with continent urinary diversions to properly catheterize the continent stoma.

Prostate Tumors

Prostate cancer occurs as the result of primary or (in rare cases) metastatic tumors. Adenocarcinoma of the prostate is the commonest form of malignancy affecting men in the United States and the second most common cause of cancer-related deaths for this group.

Prostate carcinoma accounted for approximately 20% of all malignant tumors diagnosed in men in 1990 and 10% of all cancer-related deaths. Unsuspected or undiagnosed prostate adenocarcinomas were found in approximately 30% of all men over 50 years of age who died of unrelated causes.[152]

In rare cases the prostate is the site of other primary or secondary cancers. Rare occurrences of primary transitional cell carcinomas of the prostate, squamous cell carcinomas, and mucinous (colloid) carcinomas have been noted. The prostate also may be the site of invasive rhabdomyosarcomas or intraductal carcinomas.

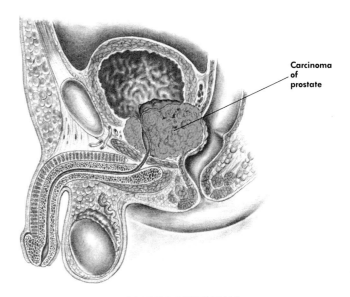

Carcinoma of prostate

PROSTATIC CARCINOMA

PATHOPHYSIOLOGY

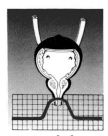

The pathophysiologic significance of prostate cancer lies in the tumor's propensity for local growth, invasion of adjacent structures, and metastasis to distant organ systems. Local invasion produces bladder outlet obstruction and obstructive uropathies; invasion of adjacent organs and distant metastasis may cause pain and ultimately death.

The cause of prostate adenocarcinoma remains unclear. A genetic predisposition has been suspected, although definitive evidence does not exist. Racial differences in the occurrence of adenocarcinoma of the prostate have been noted. Black men tend to have prostate adenocarcinoma at an earlier age with higher tumor stages and higher mortality than white men. In contrast, Native Americans, Oriental Americans, and Hispanics have a lower incidence of prostate cancer than either Caucasian or black Americans.[152]

Weak correlations have been noted connecting prostate cancer with sexually transmitted diseases,[171] serum levels of cadmium and zinc, dietary intake of fat,[131] and infection with specific viruses, including cytomegalovirus, herpes simplex virus type 2, and simian virus 40.[127,154,162]

The pathophysiology of malignant conversion to prostate adenocarcinoma remains unclear. Mutations within suppressor genes, unclear interactions with the hypothalamic-pituitary–Leydig cell hormonal axis, and a relationship with benign hyperplasia are thought to cause the development of prostatic adenocarcinoma, although the precise sequence of events is not known.

Prostate adenocarcinomas originate within the stroma of the gland. The tumor may appear as a firm, single or multifocal nodule. Typically these tumors originate in the posterior lobe near the outer margin of the stroma. As the tumor volume increases, it causes enlargement of the prostate gland and symptoms of bladder outlet obstruction.

Local invasion occurs as the tumor disrupts the prostatic capsule, through perineural spread or perivesical invasion. Denonvilliers' fascia is the first barrier to local expansion of prostate adenocarcinoma. After disruption of the prostatic capsule, the tumor often spreads to the fascial envelope surrounding the seminal vesicles and to the bladder base, causing bladder outlet and ureteral obstruction. Rectal invasion rarely occurs, presumably because of the strength of Denonvilliers' fascia in this area of the body. Intraurethral extension to the membranous urethra occurs in very advanced cases.

Metastatic spread occurs via lymphatic or vascular routes. Lymphatic metastasis involves the pelvic region, including the obturator nodes, hypogastrics, external iliacs, common iliacs, presacrals, presciatics, inguinals, and distant periaortic, mediastinal, and supraclavicular nodes. Distant organ metastasis most commonly involves the skeleton and the lungs, liver, adrenals, and kidneys.

Staging systems for prostate adenocarcinoma are used to determine options for care and as a general guideline for prognosis. A modified Jewett-Strong-Marshall system and the tumor, node, metastasis (TNM) system defined by the American Joint Committee on Cancer are common classification systems for prostate cancer.

The modified Jewett-Strong-Marshall system defines four basic stages of tumors, A through D. Stage A tumors are discovered inadvertently with transurethral or open resection for benign prostatic hypertrophy. Stage A1 tumors are noted on relatively few chips, whereas A2 tumors are more diffuse and have greater malignant significance. Stage B tumors can be detected on digital examination and are confined to the prostatic capsule. Stage B1 tumors have a nodule of 1.5 cm or less confined to one lobe of the gland; stage B2 tumors are multifocal, form a nodule larger than 1.5 cm, and involve most of a single lobe or induration of the prostate.

Stage C tumors appear to have spread beyond the prostatic capsule on clinical examination. As many as 50% of individuals with tumors in this stage have lymph node metastasis. Men with stage D tumors have distant organ metastasis. Stage D1 tumors are limited to the pelvic lymph nodes, and stage D2 tumors have spread to the bones, liver, or lungs.[152]

The TNM system for prostate carcinoma uses "T" for tumor, "N" for node, and "M" for metastasis. T_1 tumors are comparable to stage A malignancies, and T_2 tumors are comparable to stage B cancers. T_3 and T_4 tumors have spread beyond the prostatic capsule. The addition of the letter N to the descriptor indicates nodal involvement, and the letter M indicates distant organ metastasis.

In addition to staging systems, prostate adenocarcinomas are further classified by a grading system, which is used to determine the malignant potential of the tumor; the Gleason system is one of the most commonly used.[159] The Gleason system and other related grading systems are based on malignant cellular characteristics, glandular differentiation, cytologic atypia (atypical or aberrant cytologic characteristics), and nuclear abnormalities. Gleason defines grading scores up to 10, with scores of 2 through 4 indicating a well-differentiated tumor and scores of 8 through 10 defining poorly differentiated, aggressive tumors. With prostatic adenocarcinomas an individual may have two or more assigned grades representing different aspects of the tumor.

COMPLICATIONS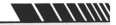

Bladder outlet obstruction
Ureteral obstruction
Pain
Lung dysfunction*
Liver dysfunction*
Bone dysfunction*
Death

*Related to metastasis.

HORMONAL THERAPY FOR PROSTATE CANCER

Estrogens (diethylstilbestrol, others)

Action: suppresses luteinizing hormone–inhibiting estrogen production

Side effects: risk of cardiovascular insult, peripheral edema, change in body habitus, gynecomastia, increased risk of thromboembolism

Antiandrogens (ketoconazole, aminoglutethimide, spironolactone, flutamide, megestrol acetate, cyproterone acetate, others)

Action: inhibits androgen synthesis or androgen action (competition for binding sites)

Side effects: nausea and vomiting, gynecomastia, hepatotoxicity, hypocalcemia

---

A PROSTATE SCREENING PROGRAM

Despite the high incidence of prostate cancer and related deaths among men in the United States, screening programs for men at risk remain scarce and poorly used. Cultural attitudes toward disorders of the male reproductive system may play a role in this phenomenon. A general lack of public education and awareness of the significance of prostate cancer and its prevalence in men over 40 years of age also exerts a profound influence.

A prostate screening program should be based on an evaluation of the local community and knowledge of the epidemiologic characteristics of the disease in the United States. Several screening modalities can be used. A digital examination performed by a urologist or trained nurse specialist is an excellent initial screening tool. Suspicious digital examination is further evaluated by transrectal prostatic ultrasound and transrectal or transperineal biopsy as indicated. Measuring the serum marker, prostatic-specific antigen, also serves as a screening method, possibly even before the onset of clinically apparent symptoms.

Educational seminars for prostate cancer are needed. These seminars should emphasize that men of any age may develop prostate cancer, although the risks increase after age 40. The audience should be told that the American Cancer Society recommends that all men over 40 years of age should have a digital rectal examination annually. The seminar should emphasize that the early stages of the disease are asymptomatic; fortunately, however, even early disease can be detected by digital rectal examination, increasing the probability of cure. The public also needs to be taught that voiding problems do not necessarily indicate cancer (obstructive symptoms are also caused by benign prostatic hypertrophy and other conditions). Nonetheless, obstructive voiding symptoms require prompt medical evaluation.

A screening program may be targeted to occur during Prostate Awareness Week (last week in September) or near some other significant date. The marketing plan for the program should be designed to inform all men in the local community and may include particular emphasis for at-risk groups, including men over 40 years of age and black men. A typical program will require a registration and sign area, general waiting room, screening waiting room, digital examination, and exit process, including provision of copies of results and private counseling with specific recommendations for follow-up and educational materials. The program is completed by a follow-up telephone call asking the patient and partner what follow-up he attained and what the results of this evaluation have revealed.

Urologic and other nurses are superbly equipped to coordinate prostate screening programs, which promote public health with regard to prostate cancer and provide the opportunity for early detection and cure for individuals in the community.

From Sueppel[175] and Wilkinson and Retzer.[179a]

DIAGNOSTIC STUDIES AND FINDINGS

Diagnostic test	Findings
Transrectal prostatic ultrasound	Hypoechogenic area or nodule; increased volume of prostate gland may be noted
Serum prostate-specific antigen (PSA)	Elevated (>2.5 ng/ml) (mild elevation of PSA ≤ 10 ng/ml may be noted with BPH)
Serum alkaline phosphatase	Elevated with advanced disease
Intravenous pyelogram/urogram (IVP/IVU)	Evidence of obstructive uropathy at the level of the bladder outlet or ureterovesical junction
Radionuclide bone scan	Bony metastasis
Plain x-rays of bones	Bony metastasis
Chest x-ray	Lung metastasis
Abdominal computed tomography (CT)	Occasionally used to detect metastasis to the pelvis, sternum, or vertebral column not evident on radionuclide bone scan; may reveal significantly enlarged lymph nodes
Magnetic resonance imaging (MRI)	The role of MRI in the evaluation of prostate cancer; it has potential applications in detecting bone metastasis and the extent of local tumor spread
Lymphangiography	Lymphatic node metastasis

MEDICAL MANAGEMENT

GENERAL MANAGEMENT, CHEMOTHERAPY, AND RADIOTHERAPY

External beam radiotherapy to prostate

Implantation of interstitial iodine-125 (^{125}I) radioactive seeds

Implantation of gold-198 seeds combined with external beam radiotherapy

Implantation of interstitial iridium-192 seeds

Exogenous estrogens to arrest tumor growth (see box on page 235).

Antiandrogenic agents (see box on page 235).

Luteinizing hormone–releasing hormone (LH-RH) agonists

Chemotherapeutic agents for metastatic disease

Radiotherapy to bony metastasis as palliation for pain

SURGERY

Radical prostatectomy for en bloc resection of localized tumor

Pelvic lymphadenectomy (primarily a staging procedure)

Channel transurethral prostatic resection for nearly complete or acute urinary retention

Orchiectomy as an alternative to hormone therapy

Transurethral resection of the prostate (TURP) with neodymium YAG (yttrium-aluminum-garnet) laser ablation of localized tumor

1 ASSESS

ASSESSMENT	OBSERVATIONS
Prostate	Digital examination reveals asymmetric posterior lobe enlargement and specific hard nodules or induration
Pelvic lymph nodes	Pelvic lymph nodes may be enlarged, matted, and hardened on palpation
Pain	Flank pain may be associated with obstruction and bone pain with metastasis
Urinary retention	Diurnal urinary frequency, nocturia, diminished force of urinary stream, postvoid dribbling, and feelings of incomplete bladder emptying
Sexual dysfunction	Erectile dysfunction or impaired libido

2 DIAGNOSE

NURSING DIAGNOSIS	SUBJECTIVE FINDINGS	OBJECTIVE FINDINGS
Altered protection related to prostate cancer with potential for local growth, invasion of adjacent structures, and metastasis to distant organ systems	Complains of symptoms of urinary retention or (in advanced cases) flank pain or bone pain	Digital exam of prostate reveals asymmetric enlargement with firm nodules or induration of gland; urinary stream is poor with prolonged voiding time and significant postvoid residual volume; flank pain or bone pain is associated with clinical evidence of advanced (metastatic) disease
Altered patterns of urinary elimination related to prostate gland enlargement causing bladder outlet obstruction	Complains of feelings of urinary retention (diminished force of stream, postvoid urinary dribble, diurnal frequency, nocturia, feelings of incomplete bladder emptying)	Voiding diary demonstrates diurnal frequency greater than 12 h, nocturia more than one episode per night, urinary residual volume >100 ml or 25% of total bladder capacity; observation of urinary stream demonstrates poor stream with prolonged voiding time
Diarrhea related to external beam or interstitial radiotherapy, postradiation proctitis	Complains of frequent, loose, watery stools with or without discomfort of the bowel	Bowel elimination patterns reveal frequent elimination; serum electrolytes may be altered
Pain related to metastasis of prostate cancer to bone	Complains of dull, boring bone pain aggravated by movement or exertion	Chronic bone pain correlates with evidence of skeletal metastasis
Anxiety related to diagnosis of cancer and uncertainty of prognosis or treatment modalities	Expresses fear or uncertainty about diagnostic or therapeutic procedures for prostate cancer	The patient exhibits denial of the presence or significance of cancer and refuses to undergo diagnostic or therapeutic procedures because of denial or fear

→ > >

NURSING DIAGNOSIS	SUBJECTIVE FINDINGS	OBJECTIVE FINDINGS
Anticipatory grieving related to advanced-stage prostate carcinoma with guarded diagnosis	Patient and family express distress and fear about the patient's prognosis	Objective clinical evidence is consistent with advanced-stage cancer with guarded prognosis
Sexual dysfunction related to radical prostatectomy, hormonal therapy for prostate carcinoma	Reports loss of libido or erectile dysfunction	Nocturnal screening evaluation of erectile function demonstrates objective evidence of impotence

3 PLAN

Patient goals

1. Prostate cancer will be eradicated and there will be no metastasis.
2. Urinary elimination patterns will return to premorbid parameters.
3. Metastatic bone pain will be prevented or resolved.
4. Bowel elimination patterns will return to premorbid parameters.
5. Expressions of anxiety about diagnosis and prognosis are replaced by a realistic understanding of the tumor's stage and the likely prognosis.
6. Patient and family will be able to express their grief and begin to prepare for patient's possible death.
7. Sexual dysfunction will be resolved, and the patient and his partner will have a mutually satisfying relationship.

4 IMPLEMENT

NURSING DIAGNOSIS	NURSING INTERVENTIONS	RATIONALE
Altered protection related to prostate cancer with potential for local growth, invasion of adjacent structures, and metastasis to distant organ systems	Advise the patient with evidence of asymmetric prostate enlargement, nodules, or induration on digital examination to seek prompt evaluation and care from a urologist.	Asymmetric prostate enlargement, nodules, or induration may indicate cancer of the prostate gland; evaluation and biopsy are indicated.
	Advise the patient with an abnormal prostatic ultrasound to seek or continue medical evaluation for possible prostate cancer.	Hypoechogenic areas on prostate ultrasound justify further investigation to determine whether prostatic cancer is present.
	Prepare the patient for radical prostatectomy as directed (see Radical Prostatectomy, page 243).	Radical prostatectomy is used to remove prostate malignancies contained within the capsule.
	Prepare the patient for external beam radiotherapy for invasive or advanced prostate cancer as directed.	External beam radiotherapy is used to impede or eradicate prostate cancer and metastatic sites to the bone or lymph nodes.

NURSING DIAGNOSIS	NURSING INTERVENTIONS	RATIONALE
	Advise the patient undergoing external beam radiotherapy that he may experience side effects, including diarrhea, nausea and vomiting, suppressed appetite, and cystitis.	External beam radiotherapy affects rapidly proliferating cells, including tumor cells and normal components of the gastrointestinal and bladder mucosa; symptoms of diarrhea, altered appetite, nausea, and cystitis may occur when the bowel or bladder mucosa is compromised.
	Prepare the patient for interstitial radiation therapy as directed.	Interstitial radiation therapy uses radiated seeds to deliver radiation to the prostate.
	Advise the patient that interstitial radiation therapy may cause symptoms of diarrhea, proctitis, and irritative voiding symptoms.	Interstitial radiation therapy attacks rapidly proliferating malignant and normal cells near and inside the prostate gland.
	Prepare the patient for transurethral resection of the prostate with neodymium YAG laser resection of focal tumors.	Laser resection of tumors may play a role in the management of early stage tumors.
	Administer chemotherapy as directed for invasive or metastatic prostate cancer.	Chemotherapy is used to inhibit or eradicate advanced prostate malignancies.
	Advise the patient that chemotherapy may cause side effects, including nausea, vomiting, suppressed appetite, and alopecia.	Chemotherapy, like radiotherapy, attacks both neoplastic and normal cells that reproduce rapidly.
Altered patterns of urinary elimination related to prostate gland enlargement causing bladder outlet obstruction	Advise the patient to void on a regular basis, approximately q 2 h; teach the patient to double void to maximize bladder evacuation.	Routine voiding and double voiding may reduce residual urinary volumes and increase regular bladder evacuation.
	Teach the patient a fluid management program, emphasizing intake of an adequate volume of fluid over a 24-h period (at least 1,500 ml) while avoiding drinking large volumes of fluid with meals (see Fluid Intake: What, When, and How Much, page 303).	A fluid management program is designed to ensure adequate fluid intake while avoiding rapid consumption of fluids over a brief period, which predisposes the patient to acute urinary retention.
	Administer alpha blocking agents (e.g., prazosin, terazosin, or doxazosin) as directed.	Alpha blocking agents inhibit alpha adrenergic tone in the prostatic urethra, reducing urinary retention related to prostatic carcinoma.
	Prepare the patient for radical prostatectomy as directed (see Radical Prostatectomy, page 243).	Radical prostatectomy obliterates bladder outlet obstruction through resection of the prostate and its capsule.
	Prepare the patient for channel transurethral resection of the acutely obstructive prostate as directed.	Transurethral resection of the prostate may be used to relieve severe or acute urinary retention related to prostate tumor growth.

→ > >

NURSING DIAGNOSIS	NURSING INTERVENTIONS	RATIONALE
Diarrhea related to external beam or interstitial radiotherapy, postradiation proctitis	Advise patient to reduce intake of fatty or spicy foods during periods of diarrhea.	Fatty or spicy foods irritate the bowel, increasing diarrhea.
	Help the patient ensure an adequate fluid intake during periods of diarrhea; emphasize fluids that contain essential electrolytes (e.g., Gatorade).	Diarrhea causes rapid excretion of water and electrolytes from the body; fluids containing essential electrolytes are particularly important to offset losses caused by diarrhea.
	Administer antidiarrheal agents as directed.	Antidiarrheal agents slow motility to offset fluid losses produced by diarrhea.
Pain related to metastasis of prostate cancer to bone	Evaluate pain for location, character, intensity, duration, and alleviating and aggravating factors.	The pain produced by skeletal metastasis from prostate cancer is dull and boring and located in affected bones; the pain typically is intense and chronic and is aggravated by exertion and movement.
	Administer analgesics as directed to relieve pain.	Narcotic agents may be used for bone pain in certain cases; however, in many instances nonsteroidal antiinflammatory agents or analgesics may offer more effective relief from skeletal discomfort.
	Provide local heat as indicated.	Local application of heat temporarily relieves bone pain.
	Restrict excessive movement or exertion if bone pain is severe or if the risk of pathologic fracture is significant.	Excessive movement or exertion aggravates skeletal pain caused by bony metastases.
	Administer systemic radiotherapy or chemotherapy as directed.	External beam radiotherapy may be used to palliate (reduce the size and associated pain of) skeletal metastases.
Anxiety related to diagnosis of cancer and uncertainty of prognosis or treatment modalities	Reassure the patient that prostate cancers are typically relatively slow growing and treatable.	Prostate tumors are amenable to various treatments; the tumors often are discovered incidentally on transurethral resection for benign prostatic hyperplasia or during a screening evaluation before local invasion or metastasis.
	Explain or reinforce explanation of all diagnostic or therapeutic procedures; emphasize the goal of the procedure and its role in the patient's treatment program; include family members in teaching whenever possible.	Anxiety is intensified by a lack of knowledge of therapeutic or diagnostic procedures, and explanation of the procedures is likely to reduce this anxiety; repetition of explanations and sharing teaching with family members further reduce anxiety stemming from failure to recall information after initial teaching.

NURSING DIAGNOSIS	NURSING INTERVENTIONS	RATIONALE
Anticipatory grieving related to advanced-stage prostate carcinoma with guarded prognosis	Encourage the patient and family to talk about their feelings and concerns.	Open discussion of feelings of distress and fear is necessary before the patient and family can prepare for possible loss of a loved one.
	Keep the patient and family up-to-date on the patient's plan of care and prognosis in consultation with the physician.	Accurate information helps the patient and family initiate and sustain the process of anticipatory grieving.
	Help the patient and family identify and obtain assistance in completing plans or arrangements for a possible death.	Making a will and arranging for financial, spiritual, or other concerns help the patient and family cope as they prepare for a possible loss; these arrangements are also helpful following a death.
	Provide support for the patient's family, and encourage them to meet their own physical needs for nutrition, rest, and grieving during the patient's periods of crisis or intensive care.	Family members may neglect their own health in a misdirected attempt to care for the cancer victim; this only impedes the family members as they prepare for the possible death of a loved one.
	Identify a strategy for contacting the family should death be likely or imminent.	Clearly identifying a way to contact the family should the patient face a crisis helps alleviate anxiety or guilt associated with leaving the patient to attend to personal needs.
Sexual dysfunction related to radical prostatectomy, hormonal therapy for prostate carcinoma	Offer the patient and his partner the opportunity to discuss concerns about sexual dysfunction.	Concerns about sexual dysfunction may be subjugated to more pressing issues such as pain or control of invasive tumor; however, once these issues are successfully managed, issues of sexual dysfunction become significant.
	Reassure the patient that erectile dysfunction related to surgical or other therapy is treatable.	Erectile dysfunction is reduced by the use of nerve-sparing radical prostatectomy procedures or by subsequent treatment using surgical or pharmacologic means.
	Inform the patient who undergoes radical prostatectomy or surgical orchiectomy that infertility is expected.	Radical prostatectomy or surgical orchiectomy alters the male reproductive system, eliminating the ability to produce viable sperm.
	Help the patient and his partner obtain care from a urologist or sexual counselor as indicated.	Sexual dysfunctions, including erectile dysfunction, infertility, ejaculatory dysfunction, and altered libido, are treated by a qualified specialist.

5 EVALUATE

PATIENT OUTCOME	DATA INDICATING THAT OUTCOME IS REACHED
Prostate cancer has been eradicated, with no metastasis.	Clinical evaluation, imaging studies, and pathology reports indicate absence of primary prostate adenocarcinoma; serum tumor markers (PSA, alkaline phosphatase) have returned to normal levels.
Urinary elimination patterns have returned to premorbid parameters.	Diurnal voiding frequency returns to q 2 h or less often, and nocturia falls to one episode or none per night; postvoid residual volume falls to less than 25% of total bladder capacity or 100 ml.
Metastatic bone pain has been prevented or has resolved.	The patient reports relief from chronic pain related to bony metastasis and is knowledgeable about a specific strategy for managing this pain should it recur; *or,* prostate cancer has been eradicated or slowed before spreading to skeletal sites.
Bowel elimination patterns have returned to premorbid parameters.	Diarrhea has resolved; stool consistency has returned to normal, and frequency of bowel movements has returned to premorbid patterns (typically every day or every other day).
The patient's anxiety about the diagnosis and prognosis have been replaced by a realistic understanding of the tumor's stage and likely prognosis.	The patient and his family can accurately identify the stage of the prostate cancer and the goals of the treatment plan.
The patient and family have begun the grieving process and are preparing for possible death of a loved one.	The patient and family talk about feelings related to the possible death of the patient with a guarded prognosis and prepare for this potential loss in accordance with their wishes.
Sexual dysfunction has resolved, and the patient and his partner have a mutually satisfying relationship.	Erectile dysfunction is managed and the ability to engage in intercourse has been restored; other sexual dysfunctions, including discord in an intimate relationship and diminished libido, have been identified and treated in consultation with a qualified specialist.

PATIENT TEACHING

1. Teach the patient the pathophysiology of prostate cancer and the significance of local invasion and metastasis to distant sites.
2. Teach the patient the goals and purpose of all therapeutic and diagnostic evaluations and how they fit into his treatment plan.
3. Teach the patient the names, dosage, administration, and potential side effects of all hormonal or chemotherapeutic agents used to treat prostate cancers.
4. Teach the patient the route of administration, schedule, goals, and potential side effects of external beam or interstitial radiotherapy.
5. Teach the patient the symptoms of potential recurrence of local disease (urinary retention with frequency, nocturia, and diminished force of stream with feelings of incomplete bladder emptying) if the prostate is not removed via radical prostatectomy.
6. Teach the patient strategies for managing and reducing bone pain related to skeletal metastasis.

RADICAL PROSTATECTOMY

Radical prostatectomy is the surgical removal of the prostate, seminal vesicles, and prostatic capsule followed by reanastomosis of the urethra to the bladder. Different surgical approaches and variations of this basic resection can be used, depending on the patient's tumor and the surgeon's familiarity with and preference for a given approach or technique. The most commonly used approaches are the suprapubic or retropubic, perineal, and transcoccygeal. Specific techniques have been described to minimize two significant potential complications of radical prostatectomy: impotence and incontinence. A nerve-sparing technique has been described that is designed to reduce the incidence and severity of erectile dysfunction following prostatectomy.[177] Malizia and his associates[157] described a technique for preserving the smooth muscle of the bladder neck, thus reducing the risk of incontinence. The patient is placed in a supine position for a perineal prostatectomy. The patient is placed prone in a jackknife position with tape for spreading the buttocks when performing a transcoccygeal prostatectomy.

Lymphadenectomy may also be performed for prostate cancer. The patient typically is placed in a gentle Trendelenburg's position. The bladder is filled with saline, lifting the peritoneum above the incision. The pelvis is entered through a midline or Pfannenstiel incision, and the pelvic lymph nodes are exposed and dissected. This procedure may be performed following radical prostatectomy.[140]

INDICATIONS

Prostate cancers contained within the capsule (stages A1, A2, B1, and B2)

CONTRAINDICATIONS

Advanced stage lesions that have penetrated the capsule (stages C, D1, and D2)

COMPLICATIONS

Impotence (erectile dysfunction)
Incontinence
Infection
Separation of urethra and bladder

PREPROCEDURAL NURSING CARE

NURSING DIAGNOSIS	NURSING INTERVENTIONS	RATIONALE
Knowledge deficit related to surgical procedure, goals, and potential untoward effects	Reinforce preoperative instruction, including a brief explanation of the procedure, its goals, potential untoward effects, and expected nursing care.	Preoperative anxiety diminishes the patient's ability to learn; repetition of instruction enhances learning and retention and reduces anxiety.
	Advise the patient that radical prostatectomy requires bowel preparation before surgery and a low-residue diet afterward to maximize healing of the bladder-urethral anastomosis.	Bowel preparation prevents infection if the bowel is entered during the prostatectomy; a low-residue diet prevents disruption of the urethrovesical anastomosis from straining to defecate.
	Remind the patient that a catheter will be left in the urethra after surgery and that it may be removed 10 to 14 days later.	The catheter ensures bladder drainage as the urethrovesical junction heals.
	Advise the patient that incontinence or erectile dysfunction may occur after radical prostatectomy; remind him that the first, crucial goal of prostatectomy is complete removal of the cancer.	Complete resection of the prostate carcinoma is the essential goal for radical prostatectomy; certain cases may require more extensive resection, increasing the risk of postoperative impotence or incontinence.

→ > >

NURSING DIAGNOSIS	NURSING INTERVENTIONS	RATIONALE
	Reassure the patient that postoperative complications of erectile dysfunction or incontinence are treatable.	Stress incontinence from sphincter damage and impotence respond to several management strategies; care is undertaken by a qualified specialist.

POSTPROCEDURAL NURSING CARE

NURSING DIAGNOSIS	NURSING INTERVENTIONS	RATIONALE
Altered tissue perfusion related to potential for disruption of newly created ureterovesical anastomosis	Monitor the Foley catheter q 1-2 h during the immediate postoperative period for patency and for bright red blood with clots.	Bright red blood with clots may indicate excessive bleeding from the surgical site; this may lead to occlusion of the catheter, causing disruption of the urethral-to-bladder anastomosis.
	Monitor the hematocrit (Hct), hemoglobin (Hb), and vital signs for evidence of excessive bleeding after radical prostatectomy.	Hct and Hb show a decline when compared to preoperative values if significant bleeding occurs; the vital signs will also change if blood loss is severe (i.e., rapid pulse and high blood pressure followed by slowed pulse and declining pressure).
	Administer anticholinergic/antispasmodic medications as directed for bladder spasms.	Bladder spasms (uncontrolled contractions of the detrusor muscle) may occur after radical prostatectomy, potentially compromising urethrovesical integrity when they are severe; anticholinergic medications inhibit these spasms.
	If the catheter becomes dislodged, notify the physician immediately; do not try to replace it without consulting the physician.	The urethral catheter rarely becomes dislodged, but attempts to reinsert it are avoided, because misdirected or traumatic attempts may disrupt the urethrovesical anastomosis.
	Provide the patient with a low-residue diet for the first several weeks after surgery as directed.	A low-residue diet softens the stool, preventing the need to strain to defecate; this diminishes the risk of disrupting the urethrovesical anastomosis before adequate wound healing.
	Administer stool softeners as directed.	Stool softeners also help soften the stool, reducing the need to strain to defecate.
	Avoid enemas during the immediate postoperative period.	Enemas may disrupt the healing urethrovesical anatomy.
Altered patterns of urinary elimination related to radical prostatectomy	Monitor the Foley catheter for evidence of occlusion.	Occlusion of the catheter causes bladder overdistention and unstable detrusor contractions, with leakage around the catheter.

NURSING DIAGNOSIS	NURSING INTERVENTIONS	RATIONALE
	Administer anticholinergic/antispasmodic medications as directed.	Antispasmodic/anticholinergic medications inhibit unstable contractions while the catheter is in place, preventing leakage around the catheter.
	Advise the patient that some dribbling incontinence may occur after the catheter is removed.	This leakage typically is caused by stress incontinence related to reconstruction of the sphincter after radical prostatectomy.
	Teach the patient to perform pelvic muscle exercises after the catheter has been removed (see Pelvic Muscle Exercises, page 304).	Pelvic floor muscle exercises minimize or eradicate stress incontinence by strengthening the periurethral muscles, thus improving urethral sphincter closure.
	Administer or teach the patient to self-administer alpha sympathomimetics as directed.	Alpha sympathomimetics reduce or ablate stress incontinence by improving smooth muscle tone in the urethra and by stimulating the alpha adrenergic receptors of the rhabdosphincter.
	If the patient has persistent stress incontinence that is not resolved by pelvic exercises or pharmacotherapy, help him consult a continence specialist.	Postprostatectomy stress incontinence is amenable to several management options; care is provided by a qualified specialist.
Pain related to radical prostatectomy	Assess pain for its location, duration, character, intensity, and alleviating and aggravating factors.	Incisional pain is characterized by a dull, boring discomfort in the suprapubic, perineal, or coccygeal (rectal) area; spasms may produce a sharp, cramping pain of short duration that is relieved by urinary leakage; dull, chronic abdominal discomfort may be caused by constipation after prostatectomy.
	Administer or teach the patient to self-administer analgesic or narcotic agents for postoperative incisional pain.	Analgesic or narcotic agents temporarily relieve incisional pain.
	Administer antispasmodic/anticholinergic medications for bladder spasms as directed.	Antispasmodic/anticholinergic agents inhibit the unstable detrusor contractions that cause pain related to bladder spasms.
	Administer stool softeners as directed; maintain a low-residue diet after radical prostatectomy.	A low-residue diet and stool softeners prevent constipation and associated lower abdominal discomfort.
	Combine pharmacologic therapy with other measures to relieve discomfort.	Pharmacologic agents temporarily relieve discomfort; the patient's comfort is best achieved by using these agents along with nonpharmacologic measures (e.g., minimizing environmental noise and distractions and positioning the patient properly).

Testicular Tumors

Testicular tumors are the product of primary tumors that arise from the components of the testis and its appendages. Testicular cancer also develops through metastasis of primary tumors from distant organs.

Testicular malignancies are relatively uncommon, occurring in approximately two to three men per 100,000 each year. These tumors often occur in young men between 25 and 35 years of age. The most common form of testicular tumor is the seminoma (germ cell tumor), which arises from the germinal elements of the testicular parenchyma. Seminomas account for 90% to 95% of all primary malignancies. The remaining 5% to 10% of primary testicular tumors are largely non-germ cell malignancies (Leydig cell and Sertoli cell tumors and gonadoblastomas). Metastatic tumors of the testes are particularly uncommon, although metastatic tumors arising from leukemias, lymphomas, prostate carcinomas, and lung, renal, or gastrointestinal tumors have been described.

Several types of tumors arise from the germinal elements of the testis. Seminomas account for 30% to 40% of all germ cell tumors. They are further divided into anaplastic, classic (typical), and spermatocytic tumors. Seminomas arise from the germ cells that line the seminiferous tubule. Anaplastic, classic, and spermatocytic cell tumors are distinguished by their cytologic characteristics. Embryonal cell tumors account for approximately 20% of germ cell tumors. They are particularly aggressive tumors that arise from the adult or infantile forms (also called endodermal sinus tumors). A *teratoma* consists of more than one layer of germinal cell elements. Teratomas account for approximately 5% of all germ cell tumors and often are loculated, with cells resembling endodermal, ectodermal, and mesodermal structures. A *choriocarcinoma* is a relatively aggressive tumor consisting of syncytiotrophoblastic and cytotrophoblastic cells. Carcinoma in situ tumors are relatively rare, but when they do occur, they frequently involve both testes. In addition, mixed cell tumors account for almost 40% of all germ cell malignancies.

Non–germ cell tumors arise from the nongerminal, supportive structures of the testis. Leydig cell tumors are the most common; they occur during childhood and young adulthood. Sertoli cell tumors are extremely rare, accounting for less than 1% of all testicular tumors. Gonadoblastomas are also quite rare, comprising less than 0.5% of all testicular cancers.[164]

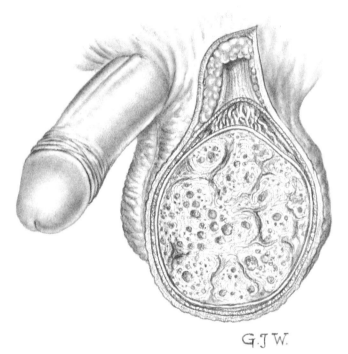

G.J.W.

TESTICULAR TUMOR

PATHOPHYSIOLOGY

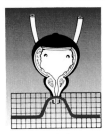

The pathophysiologic significance of testicular cancer arises from its propensity for local growth, invasion of adjacent structures, and metastasis to distant organs. Testicular tumors initially grow to crowd out the normal parenchyma. The tunica albuginea covering the testis serves as an initial barrier to tumor spread. After the tumor crosses the albuginea or invades the epididymis via the testicular tubules, it spreads to the spermatic cord, scrotum, or contralateral testis.

Metastasis from testicular tumors may spread via lymphatogenous or hematogenous routes. During normal embryogenesis, the testis migrates to the scrotum from the abdomen, but the lymph nodes remain in the abdomen. In adult men, the nodes draining the testes range from paraaortic chains from T1 to L4, although most are located near the renal hilum. Thus lymphatic metastasis from right-sided testicular tumors is more likely to involve the precaval, preaortic, right common iliac, and right external iliac nodes rather than more proximate pelvic nodes. Likewise, nodal metastasis from the left testis is to the preaortic, left common iliac, and left external iliac nodes.[164]

Distant organ metastasis primarily involves the structures of the retroperitoneum, lungs, liver, brain, and bones. Choriocarcinomas are particularly prone to hematogenous spread; the lungs are the most common site of metastasis from a choriocarcinoma.[153]

Staging systems for testicular tumors are used to determine treatment options and to provide clues to prognosis. A three-stage clinical system (A through C) for testicular cancers is commonly used.[169] Stage A tumors are limited to a single testis. Stage B tumors have spread beyond a single testis; B1 tumors involve a testis and retroperitoneal lymph nodes, and B2 tumors involve a node that is larger than 2×6 cm on computed tomography (CT) imaging. Stage C tumors have metastasized to lymph nodes above the diaphragm or to solid abdominal organs. The American Joint Committee for Cancer Staging has applied a TNM system to testicular cancer.[164,169] In this system "T" indicates primary tumor, "N" indicates node, and "M" indicates metastasis. T_1 tumors are limited to the testis, T_2 tumors have broken through the tunica albuginea or extended into the epididymis, T_3 malignancies have invaded the spermatic cord, and T_4 tumors have invaded the scrotum. T_{is} is a special indicator denoting intratubular cancer (carcinoma in situ) and T_x tumors are not yet classified. The addition of the letter "N" indicates nodal metastasis; N_1 indicates microscopic evidence of nodal metastasis in the absence of gross evidence, N_2 signifies grossly apparent nodal spread, N_3 indicates extranodal disease, and N_4 denotes extensive, unresectable retroperitoneal disease. The addition of M_1 to the system indicates metastasis to distant organs.

COMPLICATIONS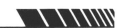

Infertility
Anemia
Obstructive uropathy*
Pulmonary dysfunction*
Weight loss, chronic nausea and vomiting*
Bone pain*
Death

*Related to metastatic disease.

DIAGNOSTIC STUDIES AND FINDINGS

Diagnostic test	Findings
Testicular ultrasound	Hypoechogenic region, indicating tumor
Serum alpha-fetoprotein (AFP)	Elevated with nonseminomatous testicular tumors
Serum beta human chorionic gonadotropin (beta-HCG)	Elevated with nonseminomatous tumors and occasionally elevated with seminomas
Serum lactic acid dehydrogenase (total serum LDH), isoenzyme I	Elevated with nonseminomatous tumors and occasionally with seminomas
Chest x-ray	Lung metastasis
Abdominopelvic computed tomography (CT scan)	Larger nodal metastasis; retroperitoneal or abdominal metastatic tumors

MEDICAL MANAGEMENT

GENERAL MANAGEMENT, RADIOTHERAPY, AND CHEMOTHERAPY

Systemic chemotherapy for eradication of early-stage tumors (seminomas, possibly nonseminomas) and for palliation of advanced tumors with metastatic disease.

Low-volume external beam radiotherapy for early-stage seminomas and patients with limited retroperitoneal lymphatic spread

SURGERY

Inguinal exploration with delivery of the testis into the surgical field (for **suspected** testicular tumor)

Radical orchiectomy (for confirmed testicular malignancy)

Open retroperitoneal lymphadenectomy or partial lymphadenectomy

Laparoscopic retroperitoneal lymph node dissection

1 ASSESS

ASSESSMENT	OBSERVATIONS
Testicular consistency	Painless mass in one or both hemiscrotums; a hydrocele also may be noted
Lymph nodes	Supraclavicular, scalene, and inguinal nodes may be enlarged
Chest	Gynecomastia may be noted (this is particularly common with Sertoli cell and Leydig cell tumors)
Pain	Back pain may indicate retroperitoneal mass, and flank pain may indicate obstructive uropathy
Abdomen	Abdominal mass may be noted
Breathing patterns	Mild dyspnea, chronic cough, and hemoptysis may be noted with pulmonary metastasis
Nutritional status	Weight loss and nausea and vomiting are present with gastrointestinal metastasis or advanced disease

2 DIAGNOSE

NURSING DIAGNOSIS	SUBJECTIVE FINDINGS	OBJECTIVE FINDINGS
Altered protection related to testicular cancer with potential for local growth, invasion of adjacent structures, and metastasis to distant organ systems	Notes painless testicular enlargement (typically unilateral) with sensation of pressure	Testicular mass with or without hydrocele
Fluid volume deficit related to vomiting or diarrhea resulting from radiotherapy, chemotherapy, or gastrointestinal metastasis	Complains of nausea, vomiting, and intolerance of food	Signs of dehydration; laboratory values may show diminished levels of serum electrolytes; weight loss and poor nutrition
Pain related to tumor metastasis	Complains of lower back, flank, or bone pain	Lower back pain is chronic and aggravated by movement; bone pain is dull, boring, chronic, and aggravated by movement, typically is located in an extremity or near a joint, and may be intense.
Anxiety related to diagnosis of cancer and uncertainty of prognosis or treatment modalities	Expresses fear or uncertainty about diagnostic or therapeutic procedures for testicular cancer	Exhibits denial of the presence or significance of testicular cancer and refuses to undergo diagnostic or therapeutic procedures because of denial or fear
Anticipatory grieving related to advanced-stage testicular carcinoma with guarded prognosis	Patient and family express distress and fear concerning the prognosis	Objective clinical evidence is consistent with advanced-stage cancer with guarded prognosis
Sexual dysfunction (infertility) related to treatments required for testicular cancer	States fear of infertility following eradication of testicular cancer.	Laboratory semen analysis reveals depressed sperm count or abnormal morphology or motility.
Body image disturbance related to testicular cancer and its impact on sexual function, sexuality	Expresses feelings of loss or worthlessness as a man or as an individual	Behavior is consistent with anger or depression; statements of self-degradation or worthlessness are noted

→ › ›

3 PLAN

Patient goals

1. Testicular cancer will be eradicated, and there will be no evidence of metastasis.
2. Pain will be eradicated or controlled.
3. Weight loss will be reversed, and laboratory values will indicate adequate nutritional intake.
4. Hydration and electrolyte balance will be maintained.
5. Expressions of anxiety about diagnosis and prognosis will be replaced by a realistic understanding of the tumor's stage and the likely prognosis.
6. Grieving will be expressed, and preparations for a potential death will be made in accordance with the patient's and family's wishes.
7. Sexual dysfunction (infertility) will be addressed or resolved.
8. Negative perceptions of body image will be resolved.

4 IMPLEMENT

NURSING DIAGNOSIS	NURSING INTERVENTIONS	RATIONALE
Altered protection related to testicular cancer with potential for local growth, invasion of adjacent structures, and metastasis to distant organ systems	Prepare the patient for inguinal exploration as directed.	Inguinal exploration is used to confirm clinical suspicion of testicular malignancy.
	Reinforce surgical teaching, that inguinal exploration will be expanded into radical orchiectomy if indicated (see Radical Inguinal Exploration and Orchiectomy, page 255).	Radical orchiectomy is used to remove the primary tumor when cancer has been confirmed.
	Prepare the patient for external beam radiotherapy as directed.	External beam radiotherapy is used for low-stage seminomas and limited-volume retroperitoneal nodal metastasis. Radiotherapy is applied to the retroperitoneal nodes to the level of the diaphragm for stage A seminomas; a more extensive field for radiotherapy may be used for B2 tumors (including the mediastinum and supraclavicular areas).[164]
	Advise the patient undergoing radiotherapy that he may experience side effects, including nausea, loss of appetite, urinary urgency, and diarrhea with rectal sensitivity.	Radiotherapy affects rapidly proliferating tumor cells and normal cells, including those lining the urinary bladder and gastrointestinal tract.
	Administer systemic chemotherapy for testicular cancer as directed.	Chemotherapy is used to treat higher-stage seminomas (B2 and C); combination therapy typically is used.
	Advise the patient that chemotherapy may cause side effects, including nausea and vomiting, loss of appetite, and immunosuppression with consequent increased susceptibility to infection and alopecia.	Chemotherapy affects rapidly reproducing tumor cells and normal cells, including those lining the gastrointestinal and urinary systems and hair cells; chemotherapeutic agents also affect the white blood cells and their precursors in the bone marrow.

NURSING DIAGNOSIS	NURSING INTERVENTIONS	RATIONALE
	Prepare the patient for retroperitoneal lymph node dissection as directed.	Lymph node dissection is used for treatment and staging; open surgery or laparoscopic approaches may be used (see page 256).
	Administer multiple-agent systemic chemotherapy for the patient with high-stage testicular cancer.	Survival rates using primary chemotherapy are dramatically greater than traditional surgical debulking procedures with subsequent chemotherapy (70% versus 43%).[169]
	Help the patient undergoing chemotherapy, especially multiple-agent therapy for advanced disease, to attain adequate nutrition; provide small, frequent meals.	Symptoms of nausea, vomiting, and appetite suppression often compromise nutritional status; frequent small meals following the patient's taste preferences, with emphasis on chilled, nonspicy, or fatty foods, maximize tolerance of foods.
	Administer nutritional supplements or total parenteral nutrition as directed.	Nutritional supplements are used when food intolerance is severe enough to cause serious starvation, further decreasing the body's protective mechanisms.
	Advise the patient of the crucial need to keep all follow-up appointments and to follow diagnostic procedures.	Routine surveillance after successful treatment of a testicular malignancy is every 3 months for 2 years, then every 6 months for 5 years, and annually after the fifth-year anniversary; follow-up evaluations are crucial because of the significant risk of tumor recurrence.
Fluid volume deficit related to vomiting or diarrhea resulting from radiotherapy, chemotherapy, or gastrointestinal metastasis	Help the patient ensure an adequate fluid intake (at least 1,500 ml/day).	Fluid intake maintains hydration, particularly with losses from vomiting or diarrhea.
	Provide the patient with electrolyte fluids.	Fluids rich in essential electrolytes are particularly important when fluid losses are accompanied by electrolyte loss from diarrhea or vomiting.
	Administer antiemetic or antidiarrheal agents as directed.	Antiemetic agents inhibit vomiting and reduce symptoms of nausea; antidiarrheal agents reduce diarrhea, causing greater conservation of fluids and associated electrolytes.
	Administer intravenous fluids or total parenteral nutrition as directed.	Intravenous fluids or total parenteral nutrition ensures adequate nutrition when oral fluid intake is inadequate.
	Administer chemotherapy as directed with nutritional support as required for chronic vomiting with food intolerance.	Chronic intolerance of food may occur as a result of gastrointestinal metastasis; chemotherapy is used to reduce or eradicate metastatic disease, and nutritional support is administered as indicated.

→ › ›

NURSING DIAGNOSIS	NURSING INTERVENTIONS	RATIONALE
Pain related to tumor metastasis	Assess pain for its location, character, duration, and aggravating and alleviating factors.	Scrotal pain classically is absent with a testicular tumor. Bone pain is characterized as dull, boring, and chronic and is aggravated by excessive movement or strenuous exercise. Bone pain is localized to the extremities, back, or joints. Retroperitoneal pain from nodal metastasis is characterized as a chronic ache in the lower back that is relatively unaffected by rest.
	Administer or teach the patient to self-administer analgesic or narcotic agents.	Narcotic or analgesic agents (e.g., nonsteroidal antiinflammatory drugs) temporarily relieve bone or back pain.
	Administer chemotherapy or radiotherapy as directed.	Chemotherapy or radiotherapy may relieve metastatic pain by reducing the tumor and thus related discomfort.
	Provide local heat to the back as indicated.	Local application of heat may temporarily relieve back discomfort.
Anxiety related to diagnosis of cancer and uncertainty of prognosis or treatment modalities	Provide opportunities for the patient to express feelings of anxiety and fear related to the suspicion of cancer.	Testicular cancer typically affects young men, who may feel particularly unable to cope with the reality of a potentially life-threatening disease.
	Help the patient contact supportive friends and family members.	Cultural attitudes may prevent a young man from aggressively seeking support from family or close friends; assistance with mobilizing social support systems is helpful.
	Carefully explain all diagnostic and therapeutic procedures, emphasizing their role in the treatment of cancer.	Anxiety may cause resistance to potentially painful procedures; careful explanation helps refocus the patient on the need for these procedures in his treatment plan.
Anticipatory grieving related to advanced-stage testicular carcinoma with guarded prognosis	Encourage the patient and family to talk about their feelings and concerns.	Open discussion of feelings of distress and fear is necessary before the patient and family can prepare for the possible loss of a loved one.
	In consultation with the physician, provide the patient and family with up-to-date information about the patient's plan of care and prognosis	Accurate information helps the patient and family to initiate and sustain the process of anticipatory grieving.
	Help the patient and family identify and obtain assistance to complete plans or arrangements for a possible death.	Making a will and arranging for financial, spiritual, or other concerns helps the patient and family cope as they prepare for a potential loss; these arrangements are also helpful following a death.

NURSING DIAGNOSIS	NURSING INTERVENTIONS	RATIONALE
	Provide support for the patient's family, and encourage them to meet their own physical needs for nutrition, rest, and grieving during the patient's periods of crisis or intensive care.	Family members may neglect their own health in a misdirected attempt to care for the cancer victim; this strategy only impedes the family members as they prepare for the possible death of a loved one.
	Identify a means of contacting the family should death be likely or imminent.	Clearly identifying a way to contact the family should the patient face a crisis helps alleviate anxiety or guilt associated with leaving the patient to attend to personal needs.
Sexual dysfunction (infertility) related to treatments required for testicular cancer	Advise the patient that testicular cancer and its treatment will alter fertility *potential;* reassure him that this does not necessarily lead to infertility.	Testicular cancer alters fertility potential, but advanced surgical management, chemotherapy, and radiotherapy have dramatically improved the chance of maintaining the potential to father children following successful ablation of cancer.
	Advise the patient to discuss fertility concerns with his urologist.	Options for preserving sperm have increased with relatively recent advances in our understanding of reproductive physiology and technology for sperm freezing; the patient's urologist is best qualified to review these options.
	If the patient has abnormal results on semen analysis after recent treatment for testicular cancer, reassure him that fertility potential may improve significantly with time; instruct him to consult his urologist or a fertility specialist.	Sperm production is suppressed by several components of cancer treatment; sperm count, viability, and motility may improve as the effects of chemotherapy, radiotherapy, and compromised nutrition subside; evaluation and care by the patient's urologist or a urologist who specializes in male infertility are indicated.
	If the patient has retrograde ejaculation after retroperitoneal lymph node dissection, advise him that treatment options are available, including pharmacologic therapy and electroejaculation stimulation; refer the patient to his urologist or a male infertility specialist for definitive care.	Retrograde ejaculation is the misdirection of sperm into the bladder rather than out from the urethra; it is caused by bladder neck incompetence. The condition is treatable, and care is provided by a qualified specialist (see Chapter 9).
Body image disturbance related to testicular cancer and its impact on sexual function, sexuality	Provide the patient with opportunities to discuss his feelings about body image changes before, during, and after treatment for testicular cancer.	Testicular cancer affects the male reproductive system, altering a basis of gender identity; this represents a profound threat to body image, often in a young man attempting to discover and establish his identity as an adult male in society.

→ > >

NURSING DIAGNOSIS	NURSING INTERVENTIONS	RATIONALE
	Gently remind the patient that gender identity and value as an adult male are based on several factors rather than simply the biologic potential to reproduce; continue to offer realistic information about the potential for preserving fertility after cancer treatment.	Sexuality and role identity for humans rely on more than biologic function; anxiety generated by a threat to body image often leads to a loss of this realization.
	Reassure the patient who experiences alopecia and weight loss while undergoing radiotherapy or chemotherapy that these changes are temporary and can be reversed after therapy has been completed.	Body image disturbance is intensified by the alopecia and loss of muscle mass (and athletic prowess) stemming from chemotherapy or radiotherapy.
	Refer the patient to a qualified counselor if he has persistent, unresolved issues related to body image disturbance.	Anxiety and fear related to body image disturbance are expected in a patient with testicular cancer; however, inadequate coping patterns or prolonged depression indicates the need for professional counseling.

5 EVALUATE

OUTCOME	DATA INDICATING THAT OUTCOME IS REACHED
Testicular cancer has been eradicated and there is no evidence of metastasis.	Clinical evaluation, pathology reports, and imaging studies show no primary tumor or metastatic disease.
Pain has been eradicated or controlled.	Bone or lower back pain is absent or has been alleviated.
Hydration and electrolyte balance are maintained.	There are no clinical signs of dehydration, and oral intake is adequate (at least 1,500 ml/day); serum electrolyte values are within normal limits.
Expressions of anxiety about the diagnosis and prognosis have been replaced by a realistic understanding of the tumor's stage and the likely prognosis.	The patient can describe the tumor's stage and the treatment program; expressions of anxiety are supported by an understanding of the disease and its treatment.

OUTCOME	DATA INDICATING THAT OUTCOME IS REACHED
Grieving is expressed, and preparations for possible death are being made in accordance with the patient's and family's wishes.	Expressions of grieving are noted, and a realistic plan of action for impending or possible death is formulated.
Sexual dysfunction (infertility) has been addressed or resolved.	Semen analysis reveals an adequate sperm count and normal morphology and motility, *or* the patient has sought assistance from an infertility specialist.
Negative perceptions of body image have been resolved.	Negative perceptions of body image are absent, *or* the patient has sought help from a professional counselor.

PATIENT TEACHING

1. Teach all young men to perform self testicular examination on a monthly basis (see Testicular Self-Examination, page 312).
2. Teach the patient the names, dosage, administration, and potential side effects of chemotherapeutic drugs and specific strategies for minimizing side effects.
3. Teach the patient undergoing radiotherapy about the common side effects of therapy and specific strategies for minimizing these effects.
4. Teach the patient with a history of testicular cancer to examine the remaining testis monthly.

RADICAL INGUINAL EXPLORATION AND ORCHIECTOMY

Radical inguinal orchiectomy is the surgical approach for diagnosis and treatment of testicular cancer. This procedure is different from simple orchiectomy in that it provides better control of vascular and lymphatic channels and allows simplified placement of a prosthetic device if indicated. The incision is made just above and parallel to the inguinal ligament. The spermatic cord is identified and isolated at the level of the pubic tubercle, and the testis is delivered into the surgical field with traction on the spermatic cord and inversion of the scrotum. The testis is inspected and palpated, and then the testis and epididymis are removed, along with the coverings. The vas deferens is ligated separately from the spermatic cord so that lymphadenectomy can be performed without having to mobilize the tethered segment of the vas deferens. A testicular prosthesis may be placed in the affected hemiscrotum after orchiectomy.[148]

RETROPERITONEAL LYMPHADENECTOMY

Retroperitoneal lymphadenectomy is the surgical resection of nodal metastases produced by a primary testicular tumor.

Thoracoabdominal retroperitoneal lymphadenectomy is the excision of lymph nodes and solid tumor from the diaphragm to the transversalis fascia and abdominal musculature on the anterior and ipsilateral side; the psoas muscle, quadratus lumborum, and anterior spinous ligament posteriorly; and the contralateral renal hilum and ureter. The incision extends from the eighth or ninth rib to the epigastric area of the abdominal wall near the umbilicus.[166]

A **modified retroperitoneal lymph node dissection** uses a more limited area for resection, resulting in less risk of retrograde ejaculation and infertility.[166]

A newer approach for retroperitoneal lymph node dissection is **laparoscopic node dissection.** This technique involves inserting an endoscopic instrument through a tiny incision in the umbilicus to visualize and resect nodes. A video monitoring system is attached to the laparoscope, and working ports of the instrument are used to resect the affected nodes. The technique allows nearly incision-free node dissection and marked reduction in the risk of retrograde ejaculation. The role of laparoscopic surgery in limited node dissection is under evaluation.[136]

INDICATIONS

Staging and therapy for selected testicular tumors

CONTRAINDICATIONS

Advanced-stage tumors more amenable to primary chemotherapy

Early-stage tumors with no evidence of nodal involvement

COMPLICATIONS

Infection
Pneumonia
Intraoperative hemorrhage
Retrograde ejaculation and infertility
Impotence (rare)

PREPROCEDURAL NURSING CARE

NURSING DIAGNOSIS	NURSING INTERVENTIONS	RATIONALE
Knowledge deficit related to surgical procedure, goals, and potential untoward effects	Reinforce preoperative instruction, including a brief explanation of the procedure, its goals, potential untoward effects, and expected nursing care.	Preoperative anxiety diminishes the patient's ability to learn; repetition of instruction enhances learning and retention and reduces anxiety.
	Advise the patient that fertility potential may be altered by extensive lymphadenectomy but that treatment is available for this problem.	Retrograde ejaculation may occur after full thoracoabdominal lymphadenectomy, but pharmacotherapy and electroejaculation stimulation therapy can help patients overcome related infertility.
	Provide an opportunity for the patient to discuss sperm banking with his urologist before surgery.	Sperm banking is a potential means of promoting fertility in the face of retroperitoneal lymphadenectomy and the associated risk of infertility.

POSTPROCEDURAL NURSING CARE

NURSING DIAGNOSIS	NURSING INTERVENTIONS	RATIONALE
Altered tissue perfusion related to laparoscopic node dissection	Monitor the patient's vital signs every hour for the first night after laparoscopic node dissection.	Because of the limited view of the surgical field during laparoscopic node dissection, inadvertent nicking of a blood vessel is possible; significant bleeding causes rapid pulse followed by declining pulse and blood pressure with subsequent hypovolemic shock unless quick intervention occurs.
	Monitor hematocrit (Hct) and hemoglobin (Hb); compare postoperative values with preoperative data.	Hct and Hb decline with more subtle bleeding.
	Administer parenteral fluids or blood as directed.	Rapid bleeding may be replaced by transfusion until surgical repair is completed.
Pain related to surgical trauma	Assess pain for its location, character, duration, and alleviating or aggravating factors.	The incision for retroperitoneal lymphadenectomy may be extensive, involving the anterior abdominal wall and thorax; thus incisional pain may be intense.
	Administer narcotic agents as directed.	Narcotic agents temporarily relieve incisional pain.
	Help the patient relieve his pain by non-pharmacologic means (e.g., minimizing environmental noise, positioning the patient properly, and limiting excessive movement).	Nonpharmacologic pain relief measures complement the effects of narcotics by maximizing factors that reduce discomfort and avoiding maneuvers that exacerbate pain.
Ineffective airway clearance related to thoracoabdominal incision and related pain	Help the patient with pulmonary toilet after surgery.	Pulmonary toilet is routinely done after surgery; it is particularly emphasized after thoracoabdominal incision, because postoperative pain is aggravated by coughing and deep-breathing exercises.
	Splint the patient's chest during pulmonary toilet.	Splinting the chest with a pillow reduces the discomfort caused by pulmonary toilet.
	Schedule pulmonary toilet so that these maneuvers are done near peak action of analgesia.	The discomfort associated with pulmonary toilet is more tolerable when narcotic agents are near their peak action.

PATIENT TEACHING ■

1. Teach the patient pulmonary toilet techniques before surgery, and emphasize their importance during the postoperative period.
2. In cases involving extensive lymphadenectomy, provide the patient with information about sperm banking or other alternatives to manage infertility caused by postoperative retrograde ejaculation.

CHAPTER 8

Male Sexual Dysfunction

Erectile Dysfunction (Impotence)

Erectile dysfunction, or impotence, is the failure to produce or sustain tumescence of sufficient rigidity for vaginal penetration and fertilization of an ovum. The term impotence is synonymous with erectile dysfunction; however, it is used cautiously, since it often has pejorative connotations.

Both psychogenic and organic factors contribute to erectile dysfunction. Treatment is aimed at restoring normal erectile and orgasmic function or mimicking the erect penis by injecting a drug into the phallus or through the use of mechanical or surgically implanted devices.

Sexual dysfunction in the male may be noted anytime after the onset of puberty. The incidence of erectile dysfunction increases with age. The incidence of men who seek treatment for erectile dysfunction during the fourth decade of life is 1.5% of the general population; by the seventh decade of life, the incidence has risen to 25% of all men. Although the aging process does not inevitably lead to impotence, sexual activity does generally decrease with age because of a variety of social, cultural, and physical factors. A survey of men revealed that 88% of sexually active males under 20 years of age engage in intercourse at least once each week. During the fourth decade of life, the proportion of men reporting intercourse at least once a week declined to 80%. During the sixth decade of life, only 50% of the men surveyed reported intercourse on a weekly basis; by the seventh decade, only 25% had intercourse each week.[192]

The relative incidence of impotence from psychogenic versus organic causes has received great attention. Some investigators have reported that 90% to 95% of cases of impotence are the result of psychogenic causes.[192,193] However, recent data using more sophisticated diagnostic techniques reveal a greater percentage of men whose erectile dysfunction has organic as well as psychogenic components.[192]

PATHOPHYSIOLOGY

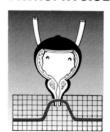

A wide variety of organic conditions may cause or be associated with impotence. Within this discussion only some of the more commonly encountered organic causes of impotence are considered.

A number of disease processes are associated with erectile dysfunction. These medical disorders may affect the physiologic processes of erection directly, or they may suppress sexual drive without causing true impotence. The psychosocial implications of illness, particularly a chronic condition, may alter a man's self-image and profoundly affect his sexual identity and sexual behaviors. To understand and treat this complex problem, the nurse or physician must have an understanding of the underlying influences affecting erectile function in each individual.[192]

Endocrine problems may affect male sexual function by altering normal function of the hypothalamic-pituitary-gonadal hormonal axis. The typical result of this problem is hypogonadism, which is potentially reversible. The range of hypogonadism is significant and includes cases of mildly impaired libido and incidences of overt eunuchoidism requiring long-term hormonal replacement.[194]

The severity of impotence related to endocrine disorders is based on the age of onset and related symptoms that influence any medical decision to attempt to establish or restore potency in an affected male. Complete prepubertal gonadotropic failure may be expressed as hypogonadotropic eunuchoidism, Kallmann's syndrome, or a specific luteinizing hormone–follicle-stimulating hormone disorder. In all of the above conditions, a failure of the production and propagation of gonadotropins is noted prepubertally and persists throughout the patient's lifetime. Abnormal growth patterns, a high-pitched voice, and a lack of secondary sex characteristics are associated with hypogonadism, leading to impaired sexual function and infertility. Kallmann's syndrome is associated with significant mental retardation, which may affect the medical approach to treatment of impotence.[192,194]

Partial prepubertal gonadotropic failure produces symptoms similar to those of delayed puberty that actually do stem from an identifiable hormonal deficit rather than from normal developmental processes. These males have significantly decreased testosterone levels arising from a deficiency in the production of follicle-stimulating hormone (FSH) and luteinizing hormone (LH), or luteinizing hormone only.[192]

Selective postpubertal hypogonadism is associated with a loss of testosterone production and a gradual loss of beard and body hair, declining libido, and resultant impotence and infertility. The eunuchoid aspects of this condition are not as prominent as those associated with prepubertal hypogonadism.

Panhypopituitarism causes erectile dysfunction and a number of other hormonal imbalances. The condition is caused by a lesion that renders the pituitary or hypothalamus functionless or by surgical or traumatic ablation.

Several congenital syndromes cause erectile dysfunction along with other medical problems. Prader-Willi syndrome causes neonatal hypotonia, mental retardation, obesity, and hypogonadism. Laurence-Moon-Biedl syndrome is an autosomal recessive disorder that results in retinitis pigmentosa, polydactyly, renal anomalies, cryptorchidism, and erectile dysfunction. Familial cerebellar ataxia is also associated with hypogonadism, along with ataxic movements and neural deafness. Other syndromes associated with hypogonadism and

impotence include Klinefelter's syndrome, Noonan's syndrome, and Ullrich's syndrome.

Any disease or drug that produces hyperprolactinemia also interferes with the hypothalamic-pituitary-gonadotropic axis and causes erectile dysfunction. Medical conditions associated with hyperprolactinemia include certain hormone-producing tumors, endocrine disorders, and a number of drugs such as estrogen compounds and psychotropic drugs.

Other endocrine-based disorders involving the thyroid or adrenal glands may affect erectile function. Castration has been used since antiquity to decrease libido and ultimately ablate normal male sexual function.[192,194]

Chronic heart disease has been associated with impotence, which may be attributed to the disease processes involved and to the use of certain antihypertensive drugs or digitalis preparations. Men with heart disease that is reasonably well controlled should consider sexual activity reasonably safe. In many of these men, erectile dysfunction may be prevented by prudent counseling. Sexual dysfunction may be complicated by the use of antihypertensive or antidepressant medications. Digoxin may also adversely affect sexual function by reducing LH and testosterone levels in the body while raising estradiol. Among those men who undergo heart transplant, erectile dysfunction is a potential complication that may be associated with postoperative immunosuppressions.[192]

Erectile dysfunction is relatively common among men who have chronic renal insufficiency and renal failure. Multiple factors contribute to the problem, related both to the disease process itself and to the use of dialysis as a treatment modality. Impotence is a result of Leydig's cell abnormalities with concomitant decreases in the production of testosterone. Hyperprolactinemia and hyperparathyroidism may further complicate the situation. Erectile dysfunction may worsen after the start of dialysis. Many problems in erectile dysfunction are resolved by renal transplant, although transient impotence may be noted in patients who have ligation of the internal artery to provide a blood supply for the transplanted kidney.

Kass and his associates[184] studied a group of men with chronic obstructive pulmonary disease and found that 19% had problems with sexual function. The incidence of impotence in these men was largely attributed to psychosocial aspects of the disease rather than primary organic sexual dysfunction.

Several neurologic conditions are associated with erectile dysfunction. The presence of erectile dysfunction in spinal cord injury is influenced by the level of the lesion, the presence of spinal shock, and the "completeness" of the injury. Following a traumatic injury to the spinal cord, all erectile activity of the penis is inhib-

COMMONLY USED TESTS FOR NOCTURNAL PENILE TUMESCENCE (IN THE EVALUATION OF ERECTILE DYSFUNCTION)

Snap gauge device

A disposable device is attached to the midshaft of the penis by a Velcro strap; the device contains three pressure bands that break at increasing pressures, evaluating the rigidity of a single tumescent episode.

Advantages

1. The procedure is noninvasive and painless.
2. The device is inexpensive and disposable.
3. Simple application is easily taught for home use.
4. Monitoring can be done over several nights, possibly improving the validity of results.

Nocturnal penile tumescence (NPT) monitor

An analog or computer-based monitor provides continuous monitoring during sleep; strain gauges filled with silicone or mercury are placed at the base of the penis and just below the corona.

Advantages

1. The procedure is noninvasive and painless.
2. The system allows evaluation of the number and duration of tumescent episodes per night and quantitative evaluation of the increase in penile circumference at the base and corona (no data are provided on rigidity).

Rigiscan monitor

A computer-based penile tumescence monitor records penile tumescence much as the NPT monitor does; however, the Rigiscan monitor also provides information on the rigidity of tumescent episodes.

Advantages

1. This system combines the advantages of the NPT monitor and snap gauge evaluation.
2. Data are obtained on the number and duration of tumescent episodes, the change in circumference of the penile shaft, and the rigidity of individual erections.

*The clinical significance of nocturnal penile tumescence testing remains controversial. Test results presuppose that erectile activity occurs during sleep unless organic impotence is present. However, difficulty with sleep or anxiety-provoking dreams may interfere with erectile activity in the absence of organic dysfunction.

---

ited. The generation of posttraumatic erections is typically associated with cessation of spinal shock. The period of time after which erectile activity reappears following spinal cord injury is highly variable, ranging from 24 hours to 18 months.

Two types of erection are observed in men with spinal cord injury: reflexogenic erections, which are mediated by spinal cord centers, and psychogenic erections, which are mediated by supraspinal sexual centers. The incidence of erections among men with spinal cord injuries is 63.5% to 94%, but the incidence of consistently successful erections is 23% to 33%.[192] The relatively low rate of successful potency among men with spinal cord injuries is largely the result of the characteristics of reflexogenic erections, which are relatively brief and respond to a variety of tactile sensations, rendering penile response significantly altered from previous brain-centered control of sexual response.

Ejaculation is relatively rare among men with a spinal cord injury. Ejaculation requires smooth coordination between autonomic and somatic impulses. The likelihood of orgasm among patients with complete spinal cord injuries is 3% to 19.7%. Lower spinal cord injury is correlated with an increased likelihood of ejaculation but a relatively low incidence of erections (24.2%).[192]

Multiple sclerosis is another neurologic condition associated with male sexual dysfunction.[193] Demyelination of the lateral horns of the lumbar spinal cord is theorized to be the critical underlying organic explanation for impotence among these men. Approximately 91% of men with multiple sclerosis have significant sexual dysfunction.

Epilepsy involving the parietal lobes of the brain is

associated with a higher incidence of impotence than other forms of the disease.[193] In most cases the relative contribution of antiseizure medications to sexual dysfunction is negligible. Many men experience continuing desire for sex with inability to sustain or maintain erections, and fewer experience a loss of libido.

Diabetes mellitus is a causative factor in the development of erectile dysfunction because of a complex interplay of psychologic and organic factors. Erectile dysfunction may be noted near the time a diagnosis of diabetes is established; the diagnosis contributes to psychosocial factors (alterations in self-image and anxiety related to chronic disease) and physiologic factors resulting from insulin deficiency. Sexual dysfunction is generally resolved after the condition is regulated with exogenous insulin.

Later problems related to sexual function in the diabetic male have an insidious onset and are generally progressive. Hormonal factors have been theorized but are not supported by objective evidence. Diabetic neuropathies are often implicated in the genesis of impotence among diabetic men based on indirect evidence linking autonomic nervous abnormalities. Vascular compromise associated with diabetic angiopathy may influence potency by affecting the arterial blood supply of the cavernous bodies of the penis.[192,194]

Various vascular disorders may also lead to male sexual dysfunction by adversely affecting the vascular component of erections. Aortoiliac occlusion leads to erectile impairment in approximately 70% of affected men. Arteriosclerosis is connected with an increased incidence of erectile dysfunction, although a causal link is not always apparent. Peripheral arterial insufficiency most commonly occurs in men over 40 years of age, so other factors of aging may exert an influence. However, it is known that arteriosclerosis is the most common cause of occlusion of the penile artery, which may lead to erectile insufficiency, and that as many as 40% to 50% of men with diagnosed peripheral arterial disease report sexual dysfunction if questioned closely.[192,194]

Many drugs have been associated with erectile dysfunction. Duration, frequency, and dosage of the drug affect the likelihood of impotence or loss of libido and secondary erectile dysfunction. It is essential to assess the use of all drugs including prescribed, over-the-counter, and recreational agents a man may be using.

Endocrine drugs are used in a variety of hormonal abnormalities and may be used to treat cancer. Any exogenous estrogens or progestins ultimately result in impotence if given in sufficient dosages. Anabolic steroids may suppress endogenous steroid levels and cause impotence when the drug is discontinued.

Antihypertensive drugs, particularly the alpha- and beta-adrenergic blocking agents, are associated with impotence, although the exact mechanism of sexual dysfunction may be more closely related to a loss of libido than to lowering of systemic arterial blood pressure.[75] The following antihypertensive drugs are associated with male sexual dysfunction: clonidine (Catapres), guanethidine (Ismelin), hydralazine (Apresoline), monoamine oxidase inhibitors, methyldopa (Aldomet), phentolamine (Regitine), propranolol (Inderal), and reserpine (Serpasil).

Two cardiac agents, digoxin and disopyramide, are commonly linked to male sexual dysfunction. Disopyramide is an antiarrhythmic agent with parasympathetic properties that may contribute to erectile difficulties.[192]

The diuretic agents chlorthalidone and spironolactone may cause loss of libido and erectile dysfunction in a few instances. Hydrochlorothiazide is also linked to sexual dysfunction.

Psychoactive drugs affect the central nervous system in many ways that are poorly understood. A significant number of these drugs, including sedatives, amphetamines, antidepressants, and antipsychotic agents, may cause impotence, presumably because of their effects on the central nervous system. The precise mechanisms by which this side effect occurs are not completely understood. These drugs include weight reduction drugs (diethylpropion and phentermine hydrochloride), antidepressant agents (amitriptyline and monoamine oxidase inhibitors), antianxiety/sedative agents (benzodiazepines and glutethimide), and lithium carbonate.

Anticholinergic agents such as propantheline are known to cause impotence as a side effect. Antiparkinson drugs are linked to erectile dysfunction and delayed ejaculation. The immunosuppressive agents are associated with impotence, but the underlying mechanism may be related to chemically induced psychogenic factors and general alterations in metabolism. Indomethacin is related to impotence arising from its antiprostaglandin effects. Metronidazole suppresses libido by some unknown process.[192]

A number of recreational drugs also affect male sexual function. Alcohol has been known to heighten desire while adversely affecting performance. Alcoholism is particularly associated with an increased incidence of impotence. Tobacco use has been linked to erectile dysfunction in several recent studies. Nicotine may cause impotence by causing vasoconstriction of the penile arteries, although the phenomenon requires further study to establish a causal link. Other drugs connected with male sexual dysfunction include amphetamines, barbiturates, opiates, cannabis (the active component of marijuana), and cocaine.[192,194]

A comprehensive discussion of the drugs that affect male sexual function is beyond the scope of this chapter. Inserts in packages of individual drugs are an excellent source for assessing sexual dysfunction as a caus-ative agent when impotence is a problem. However, nurses must be aware that overzealous cautions regard-ing potential sexual dysfunction are not indicated, since such counseling may itself increase performance anxiety and exacerbate impotence.

Certain surgical procedures of the abdomen, thorax, and genital area may result in temporary failure of erec-tile function; prostatectomy and ileostomy or colostomy are particularly likely to result in alterations in male sexual function. Of all the forms of prostatectomy, open surgery using a perineal approach is the most likely to produce impotence. Transurethral resection of the prostate, the most common approach to prostatectomy, should not result in impotence but is associated with retrograde ejaculation. An open, communicative rela-tionship with the patient, including anticipatory guid-ance of expected postoperative potency, is associated with a dramatically reduced likelihood of complaints of erectile dysfunction following the procedure.[192]

Any extensive surgical procedure involving the lower abdomen may lead to the inadvertent destruction of nerves or blood vessels that supply the cavernous bodies in the penis. The incidence of erectile dysfunc-tion is particularly high in men who undergo ileostomy or colostomy with the attendant alteration in body im-age. Thus sexual dysfunction in these men may have psychogenic and organic components.

Erectile dysfunction may also arise from local disor-ders of the penis such as priapism, Peyronie's disease, and abnormal leakage of blood from the corpora caver-nosa. Priapism is a prolonged, painful erection caused by the blockage of blood flow from the corpora cavern-osa. Underlying causes may be primarily traumatic, neurogenic, vascular, or neoplastic. Some men experi-ence idiopathic episodes of priapism, although the con-dition has been tentatively linked to alcohol and drug use often noted among these men. Peyronie's disease is an abnormal lateral curvature of the penis that is most likely to occur during the fifth and sixth decades of life. The etiology is unclear; curvature is caused by fibro-elastic plaques that form in the penis. The plaques may regress spontaneously, or they may persist despite var-ious treatment methodologies. Impotence often accom-panies Peyronie's disease and may be related to abnor-mal blood flow through the corpora cavernosa. Mechan-ical defects of the corpora cavernosa may result in low intracavernous pressure, which causes insufficient ri-gidity for penetration. Potency is restored by surgical repair of the defect.

VASCULAR DISORDERS

Erectile dysfunction also can be caused by vascular dis-orders that interfere with the mechanical processes needed to engorge the cavernous bodies. The advent of dynamic infusion cavernosometry and cavernosography has greatly enhanced our understanding of the signifi-cance and prevalence of vascular disorders that contrib-ute to erectile dysfunction.

Arterial disorders cause erectile dysfunction when the inflow is insufficient to engorge the cavernous bod-ies. Disorders of the major arteries supplying the pelvis and penis affect the internal pudendal, iliac, and ab-dominal aorta. Arteriosclerosis, diabetic angiopathy, pelvic trauma, cigarette smoking, and pelvic steal syn-drome may cause insufficient arterial inflow and erec-tile dysfunction (Table 8-1).

Venous outflow disorders may contribute to erectile dysfunction when they allow excessive outflow of blood from the cavernosal bodies (Table 8-1). The cause of "venous leak" remains unclear; local trauma, incompe-tence of the venous valves, and fibrosis from Peyronie's disease or other causes have been implicated.

COMPLICATIONS

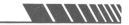

Infertility (inability to effectively inseminate fe-male for fertilization)
Shame, humiliation, and social isolation
Dysfunctional intimate relationships

Table 8-1

EVALUATION OF NEUROVASCULAR SOURCES OF IMPOTENCE

Type of impotence	Presenting symptom	Response to pharmacologic stimulation
Neuropathic impotence	Inability to initiate erection	Effective erection (patient may be hyper-sensitive to vasodilators)
Arterial impotence	Inability to attain erection	Ineffective or no erection
Venous impotence	Inability to sustain erection	Erection is achieved, but duration is brief

From Lue.[189]

DIAGNOSTIC STUDIES AND FINDINGS

Diagnostic Test	Findings
Serum endocrine evaluation	Serum testosterone: below normal with testicular failure Serum follicle-stimulating hormone, luteinizing hormone: elevated with testosterone insufficiency, depressed with primary pituitary disorder Serum prolactin: elevated levels suppress testosterone production Thyroid hormones (T_3, T_4): elevated or suppressed with specific disorders of the thyroid (indirectly compromises erectile dysfunction)
Penile Doppler ultrasound	Abnormal penile blood flow or pelvic steal syndrome (does not evaluate subtle inflow abnormalities that may compromise erectile activity)
Duplex ultrasonography	Evaluation of specific penile arteries (used to evaluate more subtle inflow abnormalities)
Penile angiography	Detailed evaluation of arterial vasculature for patients who are candidates for revascularization surgery
Nocturnal penile tumescence	Evaluation of psychogenic versus organic erectile dysfunction (presence of nocturnal tumescence episodes may indicate psychogenic dysfunction, whereas absence of such episodes may indicate an organic cause) (see box, page 260)
Dynamic infusion cavernosometry, cavernosography (DICC)	Differentiation of neuropathic and vascular impotence; provides detailed evaluation of arterial inflow abnormalities, venous leak (including identification of leakage from specific veins) (Figure 8-1, page 264), and abnormal compliance of sinusoidal system of cavernous body (see Chapter 3)
Sacral-evoked and genitocerebral-evoked potential testing	Nonspecific tests for impotence that demonstrate subtle neuropathy of the pelvic region, which may contribute to erectile dysfunction

MEDICAL MANAGEMENT

GENERAL MANAGEMENT AND PHARMACOLOGY

Replacement therapy for endocrine abnormalities

Intracavernous injection or transdermal application of vasodilators to induce penile erection (see box on page 264)

Administration of yohimbine alkaloid (see box on page 264)

Vacuum erection device to mechanically produce erection

SURGICAL THERAPY

Implantation of a penile prosthesis

Incision of Peyronie's plaques

Venous ligation procedure

Arterial revascularization procedure with or without venous ligation

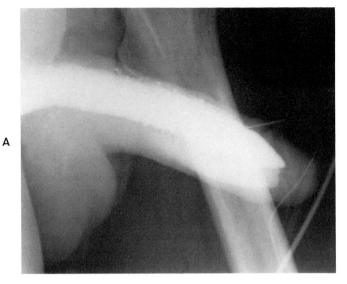

A

B

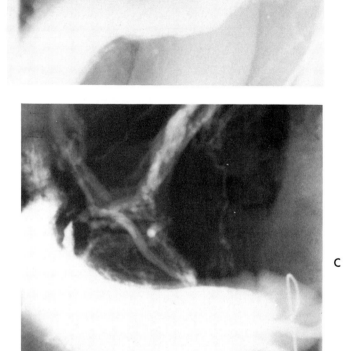

C

FIGURE 8-1
Cavernosography is used to locate specific venous leaks. **A,** Minimal leakage from dorsal vein is seen above corpora cavernosa filled with contrast. **B,** Leak in cavernosal veins. **C,** Massive leakage of cavernosal veins and into spongiosum.

PHARMACOLOGIC DILATORS FOR ERECTILE DYSFUNCTION

Injectable agents

Papaverine*
Phentolamine*
Prostaglandin E_1* (PGE_1)

Side effects

Fibrotic penile lesions (particularly with papaverine)
Priapism (prolonged, painful erection that can damage tissue unless reversed)
Discomfort at injection site (particularly with PGE_1)
Hepatoxicity (rare complication associated with use of papaverine)

Transdermal agent

Nitroglycerin paste

Side effects

Cardiac effects (dysrhythmias, palpitations)
Headache
Absorption by sexual partner (with accompanying headache) rarely occurs

*Dosage and administration are determined by the physician.

YOHIMBINE THERAPY FOR ERECTILE DYSFUNCTION

Pharmacologic action

Adrenergic blocking agent of limited duration; may stimulate erection by vasodilatory effect

Dosage and administration

6 mg tid, PO

Side effects

Fluid retention (stimulates release of antidiuretic hormone)
Diaphoresis
Nausea and vomiting

DRUGS ASSOCIATED WITH ERECTILE DYSFUNCTION

Antihypertensive agents

Sympatholytics (alpha-methyldopa, clonidine)
Alpha-adrenergic blocking agents (prazosin, phenoxy-benzamine)
Beta-adrenergic blocking agents (propranolol, atenolol)
Vasodilators (hydralazine)
Diuretics (spironolactone, other thiazides)

Psychotropic agents

Major tranquilizers/antipsychotics (chlorpromazine, thioridazine)
Antidepressants (imipramine, amitriptyline)
Antianxiety agents (diazepam, chlordiazepoxide)

Illicit or abused substances

Alcohol   Heroin
Cocaine   Nicotine
Narcotics

Hormonal agents

Androgens   Estrogens
Antiandrogens

Anticholinergic agents

Propantheline   Methantheline bromide

Antacids: Cimetidine

Cardiac agents: Digoxin

From Wein AJ, van Arsdalen KN: Drug induced male sexual dysfunction, *Urol Clin North Am* 15(1):23, 1988.

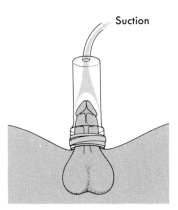
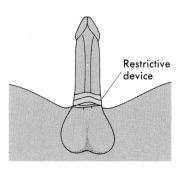

FIGURE 8-2
Vacuum erection device.
(From Beare P and Myers J: *Principles and practice of adult health nursing,* St Louis, 1990, Mosby—Year Book.)

1 ASSESS

ASSESSMENT	OBSERVATIONS
Erectile dysfunction	Patient reports difficulty attaining or sustaining erections; pharmacologically induced erection is of insufficient duration or rigidity for effective vaginal penetration
Dysfunctional relationship	Patient reports difficulties in relationship with significant other stemming from erectile dysfunction
Low self-esteem	Patient reports negative feelings of self-worth related to erectile dysfunction

→ › ›

2 DIAGNOSE

NURSING DIAGNOSIS	SUBJECTIVE FINDINGS	OBJECTIVE FINDINGS
Sexual dysfunction related to erectile dysfunction	Reports difficulty attaining an erection, difficulty sustaining an erection to complete intercourse, or erections of insufficient rigidity for effective vaginal penetration	Tumescence is not induced by pharmacologic stimulation, or induced or observed erections are of poor duration and rigidity for effective vaginal penetration
Altered sexuality patterns related to erectile dysfunction	Reports difficulty maintaining intimate relationships, at least partly because of erectile dysfunction	Patient has undergone an alteration in his principal significant relationship (separation, divorce from partner or spouse) or has a history of inability to establish a lasting relationship
Situational low self-esteem related to erectile dysfunction	Expresses negative feelings of self-worth and guilt or shame associated with erectile dysfunction	Self-worth has been impaired by erectile dysfunction

3 PLAN

Patient goals

1. Erectile dysfunction will be resolved.

2. Significant relationships will be maintained or initiated.
3. Self-esteem will return to premorbid level.

4 IMPLEMENT

NURSING DIAGNOSIS	NURSING INTERVENTIONS	RATIONALE
Sexual dysfunction related to erectile dysfunction	Refer the patient with documented psychogenic erectile dysfunction to a qualified therapist.	Increased knowledge of the physiologic basis of erectile dysfunction has improved the identification and successful management of psychogenic impotence; specific techniques to help the individual with erectile dysfunction are managed by a qualified specialist.
	Identify specific drugs that create or exacerbate erectile dysfunction, and help the patient alter his medication regimen (in consultation with the physician).	Specific medications increase the risk of erectile dysfunction in certain patients even though they produce no ill effects in others; changing a specific medication regimen may alleviate or eradicate the problem without the need for more invasive interventions (see box on page 265).
	Administer or teach the patient to self-administer hormone replacement therapy as directed.	Disorders of the hypothalamic pituitary-gonadal axis may reduce libido and cause erectile dysfunction; replacement hormone therapy is indicated to restore or attain erectile function.

NURSING DIAGNOSIS	NURSING INTERVENTIONS	RATIONALE
	Teach the patient to self-inject pharmacologic erection agents as directed (see Self-Injection for a Pharmacologic Erection Program, page 311); involve the patient's partner in this instruction whenever possible.	Pharmacologic erection therapy involves stimulating an erection by self-injection of drugs used for this purpose; the patient is taught to self-inject a vasodilator or a combination of agents; the dosage, route, and frequency of administration are determined by the physician.
	Teach the patient to recognize and manage priapism.	Priapism is a serious, untoward effect of self-injection therapy; sustained erection for longer than 4 to 6 hours after injection causes pain and eventual tissue necrosis unless promptly reversed. Irrigation with an alpha-adrenergic sympathomimetic drug in a hospital emergency department may be required to reverse priapism.
	Teach the patient specific strategies to reduce the risk of priapism, including proper dosage and administration of injectable drugs and administration of oral alpha-adrenergic agonists as directed.	The risk of priapism is reduced by proper administration of erection-stimulating medications. Overdosage and too-frequent injection significantly increase the incidence of priapism. Oral adrenergic agonists, administered under the physician's direction, may reduce the severity of priapism and prevent a trip to the hospital emergency department.
	Teach the patient to self-administer nitroglycerin paste as directed; involve the patient's partner in this instruction whenever possible.	Nitroglycerin paste is administered transdermally to produce local vasodilation and tumescence.
	Teach the patient specific side effects of transdermal nitroglycerin paste, including the risk of priapism and the risk of inadvertent absorption by the patient's partner, which can result in a headache.	Priapism and inadvertent absorption by the patient's partner are potentially serious side effects of transdermal vasodilator therapy.
	Teach the patient to self-administer oral agents (e.g., yohimbine) as directed.	Yohimbine may enhance the generation, rigidity, and duration of tumescence through its adrenergic blocking properties, which produce its "aphrodisiac"-like effects.
	Help the patient select and learn to use a vacuum erection device; involve the patient's partner whenever possible.	A vacuum erection device is designed to mechanically shunt blood into the cavernous bodies and trap the blood there until intercourse has been completed; the device is made up of a vacuum pump mechanism to shunt blood into the penis and a constrictive ring to prevent rapid loss of the erection (see Figure 8-2 on page 265).

NURSING DIAGNOSIS	NURSING INTERVENTIONS	RATIONALE
	Help the patient choose the best device for his needs.	The ideal vacuum device has a pump that is easy to manipulate and a safety valve that prevents introduction of excessive negative pressure. The constriction device should be relatively easy to manipulate and pliable, allowing it to be worn without discomfort. The constriction device must also provide sufficient venous compression to maintain an adequate erection for several hours.
	Teach the patient to avoid the risk of ischemia of the penis associated with misuse of the device.	Wearing the constrictive ring for too long a time has the potential to cause ischemia and to damage the penis; consult the physician and manufacturer's instructions to determine the maximum length of time a constriction device may be worn.
	Prepare the patient for surgical implantation of a penile prosthesis as directed (see Implantation of a Penile Prosthesis, page 270).	A penile prosthesis is a surgically implanted device that is placed into the cavernosal bodies to mimic tumescence. Semirigid devices maintain a continuous erect state; and inflatable devices can be manipulated to mimic a flaccid or erect state.
	Prepare the patient for venous ligation or arterial revascularization to manage vasculogenic impotence.	Revascularization procedures minimize or reverse arterial insufficiency or venous leaks; the goal of surgery is to restore the ability to attain and sustain an adequate erection using psychogenic stimulation or to restore sufficient vascular competence for self-injection therapy.
Altered sexuality patterns related to erectile dysfunction	Involve the patient and his partner in care whenever possible.	Erectile dysfunction has a great potential to disrupt intimate relationships because of its adverse effects on sexual expression; enlisting both partners in care assists in communication and provides an opportunity for shared problem solving.
	Provide opportunities for the patient's partner to express her feelings about the patient's erectile dysfunction, both in his presence and in private as indicated.	Erectile dysfunction affects both patient and partner; medical management of the problem should involve both partners.
	Refer the couple to a qualified counselor when indicated.	Significant discord related to erectile dysfunction (usually coexisting with other issues) is managed by a qualified counselor.

NURSING DIAGNOSIS	NURSING INTERVENTIONS	RATIONALE
Situational low self-esteem related to erectile dysfunction	Provide the patient with opportunities to discuss his feelings about erectile dysfunction; emphasize his worth and the availability of medical treatment for this problem.	Erectile dysfunction often causes feelings of low self-esteem and inadequate performance as "a man"; reassurance of the individual's worth, coupled with definitive action to correct or overcome erectile dysfunction, helps the patient reverse his situational low self-esteem.
	Help the patient identify and participate in a support group as indicated.	A support group for erectile dysfunction provides the patient with an opportunity to share his experiences with others and to identify strategies for coping with and overcoming low self-esteem.
	If the patient manifests clinically significant depression related to erectile dysfunction, refer him to a qualified mental health specialist.	Erectile dysfunction may cause serious depression and mental duress in susceptible patients; mental health disorders caused by erectile dysfunction are managed by a qualified specialist.

5 EVALUATE

PATIENT OUTCOME	DATA INDICATING THAT OUTCOME IS REACHED
Erectile dysfunction has resolved.	Erections obtained by psychogenic, pharmacologic, mechanical, or surgical means are of sufficient rigidity and duration for successful vaginal penetration.
Significant relationships have been maintained or initiated.	The married patient maintains a mutually satisfying relationship.
Patient's self-esteem has returned to premorbid level.	Patient relates a return of feelings of self-worth comparable to his premorbid state; he reports feeling that he has confronted and overcome his problems related to erectile dysfunction.

PATIENT TEACHING

1. Provide the patient with basic information about the numerous factors that contribute to erectile dysfunction. Explain that although one factor may predominate in an individual case, dealing with all alterable factors maximizes the likelihood of reversing the dysfunction.
2. Teach the patient undergoing endocrine therapy to self-administer medications whenever feasible. Teach the patient to be alert for side effects of these agents.
3. Teach the patient to self-inject vasodilators using clean technique. Emphasize the crucial importance of proper preparation, storage, and administration of injectable drugs and the potentially fatal risks associated with sharing needles or using a contaminated needle. Teach the patient to use appropriate barrier techniques (i.e., condom) to prevent transmission of any sexually transmitted disease. Remind the patient that injection *does* compromise skin integrity.
4. Teach the patient to seek prompt medical treatment

should a pharmacologically induced erection last for longer than 6 hours.

5. Teach the patient undergoing self-injection therapy to inspect the penile shaft frequently for signs of scarring from overinjection. If he notes such scarring, he should temporarily stop injecting the drug and seek medical advice before restarting injection therapy.

6. Teach the patient how to put on, remove, and clean a vacuum erection device. Teach him to inspect the skin regularly for signs of ischemia, such as discolored skin, from excessively long application of a constriction device or improper use of the vacuum mechanism.

IMPLANTATION OF A PENILE PROSTHESIS

A penile prosthesis is a device implanted into the cavernous bodies to restore erectile function. There are two basic types of devices: semirigid and inflatable. Semirigid devices are composed of two rods, typically constructed of silicone, that are implanted into the corporal bodies and maintain a continuous state of erection (Figure 8-3). A **Small-Carrion implant** has a silicone exterior and a silicone sponge inside; a **Jonas prosthesis** consists of silicone over silver wires; and a **Finney implant** is hinged to assist with concealment.

Inflatable implants differ from semirigid devices in their ability to mimic a flaccid as well as an erect state. A **Scott inflatable prosthesis** consists of dual rods that are filled with fluid from an abdominal reservoir (Figure 8-4). A **two-piece inflatable prosthesis** works on the same principle as the Scott device but combines the pump and reservoir into a single device to reduce the risk of mechanical complications. A **one-piece inflatable system** uses smaller baffling systems within each implanted rod to provide erect and flaccid states (Figure 8-5).

Other devices use a cable surrounded by plastic bodies to attain an erection. The erection is attained by shortening the cable, causing the plastic bodies to collapse together and thus produce penile rigidity (Figure 8-6).

Penile prostheses are implanted through a distal penile, scrotal, or penoscrotal incision. A pelvic incision is required for placement of an abdominal reservoir. General or spinal anesthesia commonly is used.

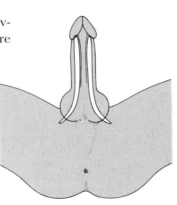
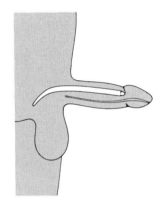

FIGURE 8-3
Semirigid intrapenile prosthesis.
(From Beare P and Myers J: *Principles and practice of adult health nursing,* St Louis, 1990, Mosby–Year Book.)

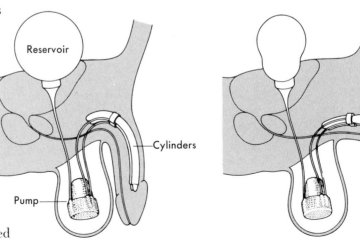

Reservoir

Cylinders

Pump

FIGURE 8-4
Scott inflatable penile prosthesis.
(From Beare P and Myers J: *Principles and practice of adult health nursing,* St Louis, 1990, Mosby–Year Book.)

INDICATIONS

Erectile dysfunction not amenable to pharmacologic or mechanical management

Erectile dysfunction in a patient who cannot tolerate or refuses nonsurgical management options

CONTRAINDICATIONS

Inflatable devices are avoided in patients unable to manipulate the inflation-deflation mechanism

Semirigid devices are preferred in patients with urethral strictures, prostate disorders, or noninvasive carcinomas

COMPLICATIONS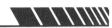

Infection
Erosion
Mechanical failure

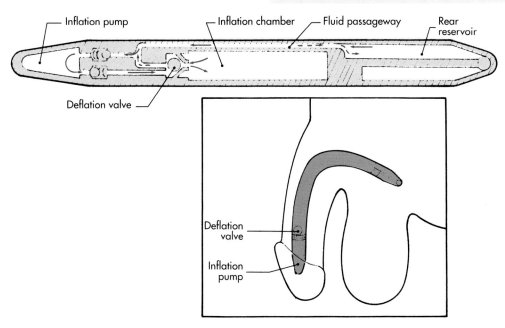

FIGURE 8-5
One-piece inflatable penile prosthesis.

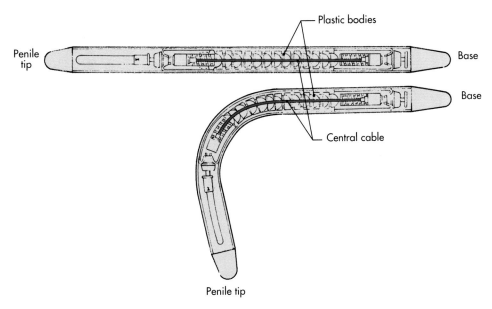

FIGURE 8-6
One-piece prosthesis with central cable that shortens plastic bodies to produce erection.

PREPROCEDURAL NURSING CARE

NURSING DIAGNOSIS	NURSING INTERVENTIONS	RATIONALE
Knowledge deficit related to surgical procedure, goals, and anesthesia	Reinforce the surgeon's explanation of the procedure, its goals, and potential untoward effects; review expected nursing care following surgery.	Anxiety before surgery reduces retention of knowledge; repeating instruction increases learning and retention.
	Explain to the patient that a Foley catheter may be placed during surgery, and that it will be removed shortly after the procedure.	A Foley catheter may be inserted during surgery for urinary drainage; it is removed shortly after surgery because neither the bladder nor the urethra is entered, and thus retention does not commonly occur.
	Advise the patient that his scrotum and penis will be tender and bruised, but that incisional pain will be minimal compared to more invasive procedures; reassure him that pain will be aggressively managed.	A scrotal hematoma will persist for several weeks after implantation of a prosthesis; the area will be tender to touch and to pressure, although nonnarcotic analgesics typically provide effective pain relief after the immediate postoperative period.
Potential for infection related to surgical incision and manipulation	Meticulously prepare the scrotal area before surgery as directed.	Shaving the scrotal and perineal area and an antiseptic soap scrub minimize the risk of intraoperative or postoperative infection.
	Obtain urine culture as indicated; report any infections to the physician before surgery.	Bacteriuria or other infections are eradicated *before* surgery to reduce the risk of postoperative infection of the penile prosthesis.
	Administer antiinfective medications as directed before surgery.	Bacterial infection is a serious complication of implantation of a penile prosthesis; antiinfective medications reduce this risk.

POSTPROCEDURAL NURSING CARE

NURSING DIAGNOSIS	NURSING INTERVENTIONS	RATIONALE
Potential for infection related to surgical incision, manipulation, and presence of prosthetic device	Monitor the patient for signs of wound infection (e.g., purulent exudate, fever, or urethral discharge).	Infection in the surgical site is a serious complication of implantation surgery; explantation may be required if the infection reaches the prosthetic device.
	Administer antiinfective medications as directed.	Systemic antibiotics reduce the risk of postoperative infection.
	Advise the patient of the long-term risk of infection of a penile prosthesis; consult the physician, and teach the patient to obtain prophylactic antibiotic therapy before invasive procedures as directed.	Infection may occur as late as several years after implantation of a penile prosthetic device; prophylactic antibiotic therapy may reduce this risk.

NURSING DIAGNOSIS	NURSING INTERVENTIONS	RATIONALE
Pain related to surgical trauma	Assess pain for location, character, duration, and aggravating and alleviating factors.	Incisional and scrotal pain are expected after implantation of a penile prosthesis; in rare cases urinary retention will cause lower abdominal or suprapubic discomfort; prolonged pain may occur as an idiopathic condition (diabetics are particularly susceptible) or as a sign of infection.
	Administer analgesic or narcotic medications as directed.	Narcotics and analgesics temporarily relieve incisional and scrotal pain.
	Insert an indwelling catheter, or straight catheterize the patient for urinary retention as directed.	Catheter drainage of the bladder relieves the discomfort caused by urinary retention.
	Elevate the scrotum, and remove constrictive clothing as indicated.	Pressure and a dependent scrotal position exacerbate incisional and scrotal pain.
Altered skin integrity (potential) related to presence of penile prosthesis	Ask the physician how long the patient should refrain from intercourse.	Abstinence from coitus is required to allow time for complete wound healing.
	Teach the patient with an inflatable device how to inflate and deflate the device.	Regular manipulation of the inflatable prosthesis promotes formation of a fibrous covering over the prosthesis, which is necessary for optimum wound healing.
	Warn the patient that having intercourse too soon may compromise skin integrity and wound healing.	Premature stress on the prosthesis may impair wound healing and, in severe cases, cause erosion of the device through the skin.
	Teach the patient how to monitor the penis for signs of prosthetic erosion; explain that the skin will appear translucent, and that the device may be partly visible beneath the penile skin.	Erosion is an extremely rare complication of modern prostheses; nonetheless, it represents a serious complication that may require explantation.

PATIENT TEACHING ▪▪▪▪▪▪▪▪▪▪▪▪▪▪▪▪▪▪▪▪▪▪▪▪▪▪▪▪▪▪▪▪▪▪

1. Teach the patient how to manipulate the prosthesis (inflate for erection and deflate for flaccidity) *before* surgical implantation; reinforce this instruction after the surgery.
2. Teach the patient how to monitor the prosthesis for signs of infection or erosion.
3. Explain the ongoing risk of infection, and help the patient obtain prophylactic antibiotics before invasive procedures.
4. Teach the patient to conceal the device under his clothing as indicated; recommend relatively loose-fitting pants and jockey shorts rather than boxer shorts.

ARTERIAL REVASCULARIZATION/VENOUS LIGATION PROCEDURES

Arterial revascularization procedures are designed to restore sufficient arterial inflow to the corporal bodies for adequate tumescence. Surgical procedures requiring direct arterial anastomosis have not been widely used in the United States and have not met with consistent success in other countries. However, the **Virag procedures** have met with greater success. The Virag procedures arterialize veins in the penis, in contrast to the traditional methodologies, which involve artery-to-artery anastomosis. The Virag V procedure is an end-to-side anastomosis of the epigastric artery to the deep dorsal vein with a shunt between the vein and the cavernous body. The success of this procedure (defined as the number of patients able to attain and sustain psychogenically induced erections) is as high as 60%.[182]

Venous ligation procedures are designed to relieve excessive venous runoff ("leak") during tumescence to increase the individual's ability to sustain an erection. The procedures typically include removal of the deep dorsal vein of the penis and its direct branches that empty into the internal or external pudendal veins. Plication of the penile suspensory ligament may be combined with ligation to further compress venous outflow from the dorsal penile vein. Selection of individual veins is determined by results of cavernosography and cavernosometry.[188]

Although vascular reconstructive procedures have enjoyed only limited success, further surgical experience and refinements in techniques are likely to enhance the role of these procedures in the management of erectile dysfunction.

CHAPTER 9

Infertility

Infertility is the inability of a couple to achieve fertilization and pregnancy. *Sterility* is the complete inability to reproduce, and *subfertility* is the failure to achieve pregnancy in a reasonable time frame, although the potential for conception remains realistic. The terms infertility and subfertility are used synonymously. The description *primary infertility* applies to couples who have never produced a child; *secondary infertility* applies to those who have had a child but cannot achieve fertility again despite engaging in unprotected sexual intercourse for a reasonable period. A urologist provides primary management for male aspects of infertility, and a gynecologist manages female infertility; however, a nurse sees the infertile couple as a single unit with specific care needs. This chapter discusses the nursing management of an infertile couple and common procedures for achieving or reversing elective sterilization.

Approximately 15% of all married couples experience difficulty with reproduction. Normally conception is attained within 1 year of the instigation of unprotected sexual intercourse. Couples who cannot achieve a pregnancy after this period are appropriate candidates for fertility evaluation and care, if they wish to seek assistance.[200]

Infertility typically is attributable to physiologic abnormalities, although cultural, religious, or psychologic variables may contribute to or cause the condition. For approximately 30% of infertile couples, the man's system is the predominant contributing factor; a dysfunction in the woman is predominant in 40% to 50% of cases; and in the remaining 20% to 30%, both partners are found to be subfertile. Careful evaluation reveals a physiologic cause in approximately 85% to 90% of affected couples, and 50% to 60% of these achieve pregnancy with appropriate management.[199]

Male Factor Infertility

Male factor infertility occurs when the man's reproductive system is affected by physiologic factors that reduce the likelihood of conception. Male factor subfertility may be an isolated problem or may coexist with disorders of the woman's reproductive system.

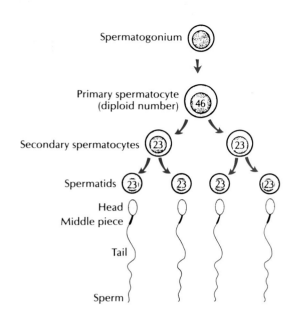

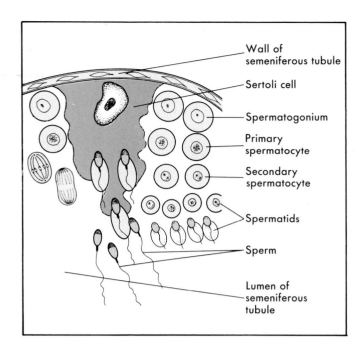

FIGURE 9-1
Male factor infertility. (From Bobak I et al: *Maternity and gyne-cologic care: the nurse and the family,* ed 4, St Louis, 1989, Mosby–Year Book.)

PATHOPHYSIOLOGY

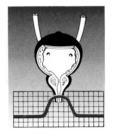

Infertility in men arises from a variety of sources. Childhood or congenital disorders may contribute to infertility in the adult. Chromosomal disorders such as Klinefelter's syndrome predispose the individual to infertility. Cryptorchidism (failure of one or both testes to descend) may impair the fertility of the affected testis, particularly if spontaneous descent or surgical repair is not completed until late childhood or adolescence. Mumps orchitis may damage the testicular parenchyma, producing testicular hypotrophy and depressed spermiogenic function. Cystic fibrosis may result in infertility caused by anomalies of the reproductive tract (e.g., absence of the epididymis) or ciliary disorders.

Endocrine disorders also affect a man's fertility potential. Late-onset puberty may be either a variant of normal or a serious hormonal disorder. Similarly, early-onset puberty may be entirely normal or a precocious puberty caused by adrenogenital syndrome, leading to subfertility (Table 9-1).

Exposure to toxins may suppress spermiogenisis transiently or permanently. Prenatal exposure to diethylstilbestrol (DES) increases a man's risk of epididymal cysts and cryptorchidism. Environmental toxins in the workplace, including radiation, excessive heat, or specific chemicals, have been linked to depressed sperm production. Certain drugs also affect spermiogenesis

(Table 9-2). These medications typically have a transient effect on sperm production or motility.

Surgical procedures also can affect fertility. Unilateral orchiectomy for testicular cancer affects the total sperm count, and bilateral orchiectomy, of course, renders a man sterile. Retroperitoneal lymph node dissection for staging and treating testicular cancer may impair fertility, causing retrograde ejaculation. Bladder neck surgery, including Y-V plasty, bladder neck incision, and sphincterotomy, also causes retrograde ejaculation. Prostatectomy produces infertility; transurethral, open, or radical prostatectomy causes retrograde ejaculation and interrupts the reproductive tract. Vasectomy commonly is performed for purposeful interruption of the reproductive tract to prevent fertilization and pregnancy. Occasionally it also is performed to eliminate the chance of epididymitis in susceptible males. Surgery of the pelvis may affect fertility potential through inadvertent changes in the neurologic or vascular supply of the testes.

Complications caused by chronic illness influence fertility potential. Diabetic neuropathy may cause retrograde ejaculation or impair spermiogenesis. Recurrent respiratory infections may be the result of ciliary deficiency disorders that are reflected in the cilia of the epididymis. Recurrent epididymitis may cause scarring and stenosis of the epididymis or vas deferens, blocking normal transport of sperm to the ejaculatory ducts for expulsion. Insufficient renal function affects several or-

Table 9-1

ENDOCRINE DISORDERS AFFECTING MALE FERTILITY POTENTIAL

Hypothalamic disorders
  Kallmann's syndrome
Pituitary disorders
  Panhypopituitary syndrome (result of trauma, surgery, or radiation)
  Hypogonadotropic hypogonadism (low serum follicle-stimulating hormone [FSH], luteinizing hormone [LH], or testosterone levels)
  Growth hormone (GH) insufficiency
Testicular disorders
  Hypergonadotropic hypogonadism (elevated serum FSH and LH with suppressed testosterone levels)
  Idiopathic hygonadism
Hyperprolactinemia
Adrenal disorders
  Adrenal insufficiency
  Adrenogenital syndrome
  Congenital adrenal hyperplasia
Hypothyroidism (rare)

Table 9-2

MEDICATIONS AFFECTING MALE FERTILITY POTENTIAL

Anabolic steroids
Cimetidine
Antiinfective agents
  Nitrofurantoin
  Sulfasalazine
  Metronidazole (may suppress libido)
Chemotherapeutic drugs
Illicit drugs
  Ethanol (excessive intake or alcoholism)
  Cannabis
  Monoamine oxidase
  Amyl nitrite, butyl nitrate
  Ethyl chloride
  Methaqualone
  Barbiturates
  Hallucinogens

gan systems, including the testicular parenchyma. Sickle cell anemia also affects fertility potential, possibly because of adverse effects on the blood supply of the testes. Liver disease, morbid obesity, and other systemic diseases may affect reproductive functioning through impaired fertility, diminished libido, or erectile dysfunction.

Acute illness often has a transient effect on fertility potential. Acute bacterial or viral illness that causes fever and malaise may impair sperm production, although the effect is not immediate. Because of the time factor involved in sperm production and maturation, the effects of an acute, febrile illness are reflected in semen samples obtained 2½ to 3 months after the illness.

Testicular torsion also affects fertility potential by cutting off or reducing the blood supply to the testis. In some individuals this can affect spermiogenesis within 6 hours; in most males, spermiogenesis is adversely affected or arrested after 12 hours (see Chapter 4).

Behavioral and cultural influences also affect fertility potential, as when the timing or frequency of intercourse frustrates conception. Not uncommonly, couples may have intercourse too frequently or too seldom to achieve conception. Some couples are unaware of the physiology of the woman's ovulatory cycle and its influence on the potential for fertilization of a viable ovum. The frequency and timing of intercourse also may be influenced by cultural traditions or personal or religious considerations. Although most infertility problems are attributed to physiologic determinants, cultural, psychologic, or religious considerations may exacerbate or cause infertility.

Varicocele may be another factor affecting fertility, although the effect varies. Varicocele is a condition manifested by several dilated veins in one or both hemiscrotums. The left testicle is more susceptible to this condition than the right one, because the left testicular veins drain against higher hydrostatic pressure. Varicocele may cause pain and pressure in the affected testis, and it affects sperm motility and production in as many as 65% to 70% of sexually active males.[197,198]

COMPLICATIONS

  Anxiety, distress
  Shame
  Dysfunction of intimate relationship

INTERPRETING DATA FROM SEMEN ANALYSIS

Pattern 1: Normal semen analysis

Evaluate for "female factor"
Obtain more sensitive tests for spermiogenic function
   Sperm penetration assay (SPA)
   In vitro sperm migration through cervical mucus
Normal SPA, in vitro migration test: reevaluate "female factor"
Abnormal SPA, in vitro migration test: reevaluate "male factor"
   Scrotal exploration with testicular biopsy
   Testicular vasography
   Venography for testicular venous reflux
   Transrectal ultrasonography of accessory sex organs

Pattern 2: Azoospermia

Centrifuge sample to verify absence of sperm
Postejaculate urine analyzed for sperm (retrograde ejaculation)
Azoospermia confirmed
   Serum FSH (if more than three times normal, prognosis is guarded)
   Suppressed FSH
     Obtain LH, prolactin values
     Elevated prolactin: obtain values for adrenocorticotropin hormone (ACTH), thyroid-stimu-
     lating hormone (TSH), and growth hormone (GH)
Seminal fructose (evaluates ductal patency)
Testicular vasography and biopsy

Pattern 3: Multiple abnormal seminal factors

Abnormal FSH (proceed as outlined under Pattern 2)
Low ejaculate volume (evaluate for retrograde ejaculation)
Abnormal viscosity
Abnormal motility (asthenospermia)
   Positive agglutination test indicates inflammation
   Pyospermia indicates inflammation
   Endocrine test abnormalities indicate hypoandrogenic state
   Diminished sperm concentration versus polyzoospermia (hyperconcentration of sperm)

From Lipshultz et al.[198]

DIAGNOSTIC STUDIES AND FINDINGS

Diagnostic Test	Findings
Endocrine evaluation	
Follicle-stimulating hormone (FSH)	Elevated in testicular failure; if more than three times normal, indicates significant gonadal dysfunction (primary testicular failure)
Luteinizing hormone (LH)	Obtained in selective cases; may be subnormal with pituitary dysfunction; minimal elevation may be noted with primary testicular failure
Prolactin	Elevated with pituitary dysfunction
Urinalysis/24-hour collections	Elevated urinary 17-ketosteroids; dihydroepitestosterones (DHEAs) noted with congenital adrenal hyperplasia
Semen analysis[198] (see box above)	*Volume:* (nl. 1-5 ml) may be suppressed with infertility; *sperm density:* (nl. >20 million/ml, or total count >50 million to 60 million) reduced in infertility; *viscosity:* significance of abnormal viscosity in infertility remains unclear; *motility and forward progression:* (evaluated within 2 h of collection; normal is at least 2 on a scale of 0-4) impaired with infertility; *agglutination:* increased clumping of sperm indicates inflammation or immunologic disorder; *pyospermia:* (normally absent) white blood cells in semen may indicate inflammation or immunologic disorder; *morphology:* (normal is at least 60% or more normal cells) abnormal cells indicate primary testicular dysfunction

DIAGNOSTIC STUDIES AND FINDINGS—cont'd

Diagnostic Test	Findings
Testicular biopsy	Distinguishes ductal obstruction from parenchymal dysfunction
Vasography (typically combined with testicular biopsy)	Ductal obstruction causing oligospermia or aspermia
Sperm penetration assay (SPA)	Used to determine fertilization potential for assisted in vitro fertilization procedures; quantifies potential for ovum penetration with or without zona stripping
Mucus migration test	Objective comparison of sperm movement in an in vitro setting; quantifies motility
Venography	Testicular venous reflux, indicating "subclinical" varicocele
Transrectal ultrasound	Abnormal anatomy of accessory sex organs (seminal vesicles, vas deferens); spermatocele or obstruction

MEDICAL MANAGEMENT

GENERAL MANAGEMENT AND DRUG THERAPY

Endocrine replacement therapy for hypothyroidism, hypogonadotropic hypogonadism, congenital adrenal hyperplasia, hyperprolactinemia

Antiinfective drugs for pyospermia or positive semen culture results

Alpha sympathomimetic drugs for retrograde ejaculation

Electroejaculation stimulation for retrograde ejaculation

Sperm washing for immunologic infertility or retrograde ejaculate obtained by electroejaculation stimulation technique (wash-up technique may be used as adjunct to select most viable spermatozoa)

Clomiphene or tamoxifen for idiopathic oligospermia

Human chorionic gonadotropin (HCG) with or without human menopausal gonadotropin (HMG) for idiopathic oligospermia

Testolactone (Teslac) for idiopathic oligospermia

Gonadotropin-releasing hormone (GnRH) for idiopathic oligospermia

In vitro fertilization or intrauterine insemination for immunologic abnormalities (antisperm antibodies or hostile cervical environment)

Steroids for antisperm antibodies

Kallikrein* for impaired sperm motility

Pentoxifylline* for idiopathic oligospermia (under investigation)

Scrotal hypothermia for idiopathic oligospermia or varicocele

Microinjection techniques (adjunctive to in vitro fertilization techniques)

*Not approved by the U.S. Food and Drug Administration for this use.

MEDICAL MANAGEMENT—cont'd

SURGERY

Repair of varicocele

Vasovasostomy for reversal of vasectomy or repair of intrinsic ductal obstruction

Epididymovasostomy for epdidymal obstruction

Resection of the ejaculatory ducts

Table 9-3

THERAPY OPTIONS FOR MALE FACTOR ENDOCRINE-RELATED INFERTILITY

Hypothyroidism
  Agent: Levothyroxine
  Dosage: Dosage and frequency determined by endocrinologist
  Potential side effects: Irritability, insomnia, nausea, diarrhea, weight gain, heat intolerance, leg cramps

Leydig cell failure with testosterone deficiency
  Agent: Testosterone cypionate
  Dosage: 200 mg twice weekly
  Potential side effects: Urticaria at injection site, postinjection induration

Hypogonadotropic hypogonadism
  Agents: Combination therapy: Human chorionic gonadotropin (HCG)/human menopausal gonadotropin (HMG)
  Dosage: HCG: 2,000 IU three times weekly
          HMG: 75 IU three times weekly
  Potential side effects: Headache, irritability, fatigue, arterial thromboembolism

Congenital adrenal hyperplasia
  Agents: Hydrocortisone (cortisol) or other agents as directed
  Dosage: Dosage and frequency determined by endocrinologist
  Potential side effects: Vertigo, headache, decreased glucose tolerance, nausea, increased appetite, ulcer disease, osteoporosis, diminished skin thickness, bruising

Hyperprolactinemia
  Agent: Bromocriptine
  Dosage: 5-10 mg/day
  Potential side effects: Dizziness, headache, orthostatic hypotension, nausea, urinary frequency, diuresis, fatigue, nasal congestion

From Lipshultz et al.[198]

Table 9-4

ALPHA SYMPATHOMIMETIC AGENTS FOR RETROGRADE EJACULATION

Agent: Pseudoephedrine (available in over-the-counter preparations such as Sudafed or Sudafed S.A. capsules, and others)
Dosage: Sudafed: 30-60 mg before intercourse
  Sudafed S.A. capsules: 1 capsule before intercourse
Potential side effects: Irritability, insomnia, urinary retention, exacerbation of hypertension
Agent: Phenylephrine (available in over-the-counter preparations such as Dexatrim without caffeine, Neo-Synephrine, and others)
Dosage: Dexatrim without caffeine: 1 tablet before intercourse
Potential side effects: Irritability, insomnia, urinary retention, exacerbation of hypertension
Agent: Imipramine (Tofranil)
Dosage: 25 mg tid
Potential side effects: Drowsiness, dry mouth, urinary retention, exacerbation of hypertension

---

Table 9-5

TREATMENT OPTIONS FOR IDIOPATHIC OLIGOSPERMIA

HCG
Combination HMG/HCG
Clomiphene citrate
Tamoxifen
Testolactone
GnRH
Pentoxifylline
Steroids

1 ASSESS

ASSESSMENT	OBSERVATIONS
Endocrine disorders	Precocious genital development or delayed development with hypogonadotropic hypogonadism; gynecomastia, feminization of male body habitus with hyperprolactinemia, signs of congenital adrenal hyperplasia, or hypothyroidism may be present
Testicular abnormalities	Small or missing testis; painful testis noted with orchitis or testicular torsion
Epididymal disorders	Pain with epididymitis; absence of epididymis; cystic enlargement or fibrosis noted with chronic infection and subsequent obstruction
Varicocele	Engorgement of the pampiniform plexus (resembling a bag of worms) may be noted; subtle enlargement may be noted with Valsalva maneuver while patient is standing
Prostate or seminal vesicle disorders	With prostatitis, boggy enlargement of the prostate and tenderness are noted on digital examination; absence of seminal vesicles or enlargement is noted with obstruction or infection

2 DIAGNOSE

NURSING DIAGNOSIS	SUBJECTIVE FINDINGS	OBJECTIVE FINDINGS
Sexual dysfunction related to male factor infertility	Individual or couple reports inability to conceive a child after a reasonable period of unprotected sexual intercourse	Conception is not achieved after 1 year of anticipatory (unprotected) intercourse
Knowledge deficit related to optimum techniques for attaining pregnancy	Couple reports uncertainty about techniques for maximizing likelihood of conception	Couple uses ineffective or suboptimal techniques to attain conception
Low self-esteem, situational related to infertility	Couple reports feelings of uncertainty about their performance or in the stability of their relationship	Stated feelings or behaviors reveal feelings of self-degradation or worthlessness related to infertility

3 PLAN

Patient goals

1. Conception will be achieved.
2. The couple will learn effective techniques to maximize the likelihood of conception.
3. The couple will regain feelings of self-worth.
4. The marital relationship will remain intact and positive.

➜ ❯ ❯

4 IMPLEMENT

NURSING DIAGNOSIS	NURSING INTERVENTIONS	RATIONALE
Sexual dysfunction related to male factor infertility	Help the patient identify and remove or minimize exposure to known gonadotoxins, environmental factors, or medications that reduce fertility potential.	Environmental, chemical, or pharmacologic factors may cause or exacerbate infertility; eliminating these factors is expected to increase fertility potential.
	Teach the patient to apply scrotal hypothermia.	Scrotal hypothermia may have a positive effect on spermiogenesis.
	Teach the patient to self-administer thyroxine replacement drugs for hypothyroidism as directed.	In rare cases hypothyroidism may render a man infertile; replacement therapy may restore normal fertility potential without further intervention.
	Administer or teach the patient to self-administer testosterone cypionate as directed.	Isolated testosterone deficiency (Leydig cell failure) is managed by exogenous hormone replacement (Table 9-3, page 280).
	Administer or teach the patient to self-administer human menopausal gonadotropin (HMG), human chorionic gonadotropin (HCG), gonadotropin-releasing hormone (GnRH), or a GnRH analog as directed.	Hypogonadotropic hypogonadism is managed by pituitary stimulation with HMG, HCG, GnRH, or a GnRH analog (Table 9-3).
	Administer or teach the patient to self-administer glucocorticoid drugs for congenital adrenal hyperplasia as directed.	The relationship between congenital adrenal hyperplasia and infertility remains uncertain; if this condition causes infertility, corticosteroid replacement therapy is expected to improve fertility potential (Table 9-3).[200]
	If the patient has hyperprolactinemia, help him consult a neurosurgeon as directed.	Hyperprolactinemia may be idiopathic or may occur as the result of a prolactin-secreting tumor[198]; resection of the tumor is expected to reverse hyperprolactinemia and improve fertility potential.
	Administer or teach the patient to self-administer bromocriptine as directed.	Bromocriptine improves fertility potential among men with idiopathic hyperprolactinemia (Table 9-3); kallikrein, if approved for use in the United States, may improve fertility potential for men with hyperprolactinemia.
	Administer or teach the patient to self-administer immunosuppressive agents as directed.	Immunosuppressive drugs may be given over a brief period to manage very high serum levels of sperm-agglutinating antibodies.
	Monitor the individual closely for side effects of immunosuppressive therapy, including aseptic necrosis of the hip.	Immunosuppressive therapy is used only in highly selective cases over a limited period of time because of the potential for serious side effects.[200]

NURSING DIAGNOSIS	NURSING INTERVENTIONS	RATIONALE
	Administer or teach the patient to self-administer alpha sympathomimetic drugs as directed. Prepare the patient for electroejaculation stimulation therapy as directed (see Special Procedure: Electroejaculation Stimulation).	Alpha sympathomimetic agents tighten the smooth muscle of the bladder neck, decreasing the risk of retrograde ejaculation (Table 9-4, page 280). Electroejaculation stimulation therapy is used to attain a viable sperm specimen in men with retrograde ejaculation who are poor candidates for or do not respond to alpha sympathomimetic drugs.
	Administer or teach the patient to self-administer antiinfective medications as directed.	Antiinfective drugs are used for men with infection in the semen noted as pyospermia and culture-proven pathogens.
	Administer or teach the patient to self-administer medical agents for idiopathic oligospermia as directed.	Idiopathic oligospermia may be amenable to one or a combination of agents; therapy is empiric and based on previous experience and careful consideration of potential contributing factors (Table 9-5, page 280).
	Prepare the patient for varicocele ligation as directed.	Ligation of a clinically significant varicocele improves spermiogenesis and fertility potential by reducing the temperature of the affected testis; the role of ligation or subclinical varicoceles remains controversial.[197]
	Prepare the patient for vasovasostomy as directed (see Special Procedure: Vasovasostomy/Vasoepididymostomy).	Vasovasostomy is the surgical repair of obstruction of the vas deferens; this obstruction typically occurs after vasectomy but may arise from congenital or acquired disorders.
	Prepare the patient for epididymovasostomy as directed (see Special Procedure: Vasovasostomy/Vasoepididymostomy).	Epididymovasostomy is the surgical creation of a direct anastomosis between the epididymis and the vas deferens; it is indicated to correct obstruction of the epididymis resulting from congenital, acquired (infectious), or iatrogenic causes.
	Prepare the patient for resection of the ejaculatory ducts as directed.	Ejaculatory resection is performed selectively for patients with azoospermia, low semen volume, and absent fructose in the semen; the procedure is performed from a transurethral approach.
	Prepare the patient for sperm retrieval methods in conjunction with intrauterine insemination (IUI), in vitro fertilization (IVF), and related special techniques (see In Vitro Fertilization, page 295).	The sperm is obtained through special techniques when IUI, IVF, or other special procedures for fertilization are used.
Knowledge deficit related to optimum techniques for attaining pregnancy	Teach the couple the basic principles of reproduction, including the menstrual cycle, events that accompany ovulation, and optimal frequency for intercourse.	The frequency and timing of intercourse may exacerbate or cause infertility in certain cases.

→ ❯ ❯

NURSING DIAGNOSIS	NURSING INTERVENTIONS	RATIONALE
	Help the couple seek cultural solutions for culturally related habits that influence the frequency and timing of intercourse.	Typically, cultural remedies for infertility problems can be identified to resolve frequency and timing issues that reduce fertility potential.
Low self-esteem, situational related to infertility	Encourage both partners to express their feelings about infertility, both individually and together; reassure them that these feelings are common and neither negative nor positive.	Expressing their feelings allows the couple to identify issues related to low self-esteem and to cope with these feelings rather than blindly responding to them.
	Help the couple address and attain medical care for infertility issues as indicated.	Seeking medical care for issues related to infertility provides an opportunity to aggressively and jointly pursue a positive solution to a legitimate health problem.
	Refer the couple with significant self-esteem disorders to a qualified counselor.	Significant self-esteem problems affecting the individual and couple are best managed by a specialist.

5 EVALUATE

PATIENT OUTCOME	DATA INDICATING THAT OUTCOME IS REACHED
Conception has been achieved.	Pregnancy has been attained and sustained, producing a viable infant.
The couple is knowledgeable about effective techniques to maximize the likelihood of conception.	The couple accurately relates the events of the menstrual cycle and the timing of ovulation; they can accurately state the basic principles of timing and frequency of intercourse.
The partners have regained their feelings of self-worth.	Individually and together, the two acknowledge feelings of positive self-evaluation and identify specific actions to resolve infertility problems.
The marital relationship has remained intact and positive.	Individually and together, the partners express their resolve to maintain the relationship and to resolve infertility problems together.

PATIENT TEACHING

1. Teach the couple about the menstrual cycle and the significance of ovulation.
2. Teach the patient and partner the names, dosage, administration, and side effects of all medications.
3. Emphasize the importance of following the appropriate regimen and of follow-up care, including repeated diagnostic evaluations, to the success of fertility care.
4. Instruct the patient in the purpose, general procedure, and goals of all diagnostic and therapeutic procedures.

ELECTROEJACULATION STIMULATION

Electroejaculation stimulation (EES) is a technique in which a controlled electrical current is applied to the pudendal plexus to attain ejaculation (Figure 9-2). The patient is prepared for the procedure by catheterization or urination to empty the bladder. A special solution is infused into the bladder that supports the viability of spermatozoa. An anal probe is gently inserted into the anus, and an electrical current is applied until ejaculation occurs; any semen ejaculated in an antegrade fashion is harvested into a container. The probe is withdrawn and the bladder catheterized to obtain the retrograde ejaculate. The specimen is spun and subjected to a swim-up technique that separates viable spermatozoa. The concentrated "semen" is then exposed to the woman's ovum via IUI, IVF, or a related procedure.

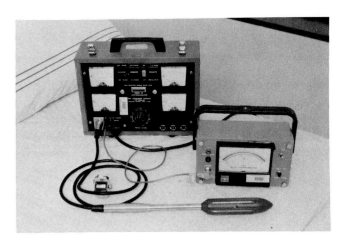

FIGURE 9-2
Electroejaculation stimulation equipment.

INDICATIONS

Retrograde ejaculation caused by retroperitoneal lymph node dissection
Ejaculatory disorder caused by spinal injury, multiple sclerosis, spina bifida, or other neurologic disorders

CONTRAINDICATIONS

Human immunodeficiency virus (HIV) infection
Retrograde ejaculation amenable to pharmacotherapy

COMPLICATIONS

Autonomic dysreflexia
Burning of the anal mucosa

PREPROCEDURAL NURSING CARE

NURSING DIAGNOSIS	NURSING INTERVENTIONS	RATIONALE
Knowledge deficit related to procedure, its goals, and potential untoward effects	Reinforce preprocedural teaching provided by the urologist, including the type of anesthesia used (if any); outline expected nursing care during and after the procedure.	Anxiety before a medical procedure reduces the efficiency of learning and retention of knowledge; repeating preprocedural teaching enhances other instruction.
	Consult the nurse anesthetist or anesthesiologist about the choice of anesthesia.	General anesthesia or systemic, intravenous anesthesia is required for a patient with normal sensation or for a patient with a spinal injury with partly preserved sensations.
	Advise the patient that a nurse or other health care professional milks the urethra for antegrade semen during the procedure.	Antegrade semen is collected and added to the concentrated specimen obtained from the retrograde ejaculate for insemination of the woman.
	Teach the patient to alkalinize the urine 24 h before EES.	Alkalinization with oral sodium bicarbonate pills enhances sperm viability.

→ → →

NURSING DIAGNOSIS	NURSING INTERVENTIONS	RATIONALE
Autonomic dysreflexia (potential) related to electrostimulation and distention of the anal sphincter	Advise the patient with a spinal injury that autonomic dysreflexia is a potential side effect of the procedure.	Autonomic dysreflexia may be a side effect of anal distention caused by placement of the probe and/or application of the electrical current to the sympathetic plexus.
	Assess the patient's relative risk of autonomic dysreflexia. A patient with a relatively high thoracic lesion is at particular risk, as is any patient with a history of autonomic dysreflexia. Consult the physician about using alpha antagonists or other antidysreflexia medications before EES.	Autonomic dysreflexia is managed by prophylactic administration of an alpha sympathomimetic antagonist to prevent episodes of hypertension.
	Monitor blood pressure throughout the procedure; use an electronic monitor to obtain rapid, repetitive measurements as indicated.	Autonomic dysreflexia causes hypertension as a side effect of massive sympathetic firing; regular, rapid blood pressure monitoring is indicated to detect and promptly reverse potentially dangerous hypertension.
	Monitor blood pressure after the procedure as indicated; encourage the patient who has received alpha blocking drugs during EES to drink fluids and to lie back if he feels dizzy.	Alpha blocking agents may cause hypotension after the procedure when the stimuli producing autonomic dysreflexia are discontinued.

POSTPROCEDURAL NURSING CARE

NURSING DIAGNOSIS	NURSING INTERVENTIONS	RATIONALE
Fatigue related to EES procedure	Allow the patient to rest after EES.	Temporary fatigue is common after this procedure, particularly among men with a spinal injury who do not undergo the procedure with anesthesia.

PATIENT TEACHING ▪▪▪▪▪▪▪▪▪▪▪▪▪▪▪▪▪▪▪▪▪▪▪▪▪▪▪▪▪▪▪

1. If the man has a spinal injury, teach him how to obtain a urine specimen for culture before the procedure. Explain that a sterile urine is crucial for insemination of the woman.
2. Teach the man with a spinal injury the significance of a bladder management program in determining the quality and viability of sperm. Encourage the patient with an indwelling urethral catheter to explore an alternative bladder management program before electroejaculation stimulation in consultation with his urologist.
3. Teach the patient who is prone to autonomic dysreflexia to rest and drink beverages after EES to minimize the potential for hypotension and fatigue, which sometimes develop after the procedure when antihypertensive medications are used.

V ASOVASOSTOMY/ VASOEPIDIDYMOSTOMY

A *vasovasostomy* is an end-to-end surgical anastomosis of the vas deferens. The anastomosis is achieved using a microsurgical technique; the obstructed or fibrotic segment of the vas deferens is resected, and sperm cells are identified in the segment of the tubule to be rejoined. A *vasoepididymostomy* is the anastomosis of the epididymis and vas deferens, bypassing an obstruction of the terminal ductus. Both procedures are done through a small scrotal incision.[196]

INDICATIONS

Obstruction of the epididymis caused by infection, fibrosis, or congenital defects
Reversal of a vasectomy

CONTRAINDICATIONS

None

COMPLICATIONS

Fibrosis of the anastomotic site
Infection

PREPROCEDURAL NURSING CARE

NURSING DIAGNOSIS	NURSING INTERVENTIONS	RATIONALE
Knowledge deficit related to the procedure, its goals, and potential untoward effects	Reinforce the urologist's preprocedural teaching; discuss anticipated nursing care.	Anxiety before a medical procedure reduces the efficiency of learning and retention of knowledge; repeating this teaching increases the efficiency of learning.
	Consult the physician about the type of sedation or anesthesia to be used for the vasovasostomy or vasoepididymostomy.	Vasovasostomy or vasoepididymostomy typically is performed on an outpatient basis using local anesthesia and systemic sedation.
	Advise the patient that the scrotal incision is relatively small.	In most cases a scrotal incision of about 2.5 to 3 cm is used for the procedure.[196]

POSTPROCEDURAL NURSING CARE

NURSING DIAGNOSIS	NURSING INTERVENTIONS	RATIONALE
Altered tissue perfusion (peripheral) related to surgical reconstruction of the ductus deferens and/or epididymis	Advise the patient that he will need to remain at home for 1 week after the procedure; vigorous exercise should be avoided for 4 weeks after surgery, and sexual intercourse is avoided for 2 weeks.	Activity is limited following surgery to prevent disruption of the delicate surgical anastomosis.

NURSING DIAGNOSIS	NURSING INTERVENTIONS	RATIONALE
Pain related to scrotal surgery	Provide the patient with a scrotal support.	The scrotal support minimizes pain caused by scrotal jostling after surgery.
	Teach the patient to self-administer analgesic medications as directed.	Analgesics temporarily relieve postoperative discomfort.

PATIENT TEACHING

1. Advise the patient to obtain a semen analysis every 2 months after surgery or until conception has been achieved to evaluate the physiologic effects of the surgery.

Female Factor Infertility

Female factor infertility occurs when the woman's reproductive system is affected by physiologic factors that reduce the likelihood of conception. Female factor subfertility may exist as an isolated factor or may coexist with disorders of the man's reproductive system.

PATHOPHYSIOLOGY

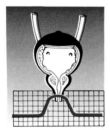

Female factor infertility is a multifaceted problem that may arise from several sources, although often one factor predominates. Ovulatory dysfunction is responsible for as many as 25% of cases involving primarily female factor infertility.[199] Many conditions can affect the ovulatory cycle. Intensive exercise and stress may affect ovulation, as may prolonged malnutrition arising from eating disorders such as anorexia nervosa or bulimia.

Disorders of the endocrine system affect a woman's ovulatory cycle when they affect the hypothalamic-pituitary-ovarian axis. Primary anovulation syndromes are associated with partial or total arrest of the development of secondary sex characteristics, anovulation, and amenorrhea. Congenital disorders (e.g., Prader-Willi, Kallmann's, and Laurence-Moon-Bardet-Biedl syndromes) and genetic disorders (e.g., Turner's syndrome, testicular feminizing syndrome, or poly X genetic states) lead to primary anovulation with abnormal feminization of the body habitus. A congenital central nervous system defect such as hydrocephalus or disorders affecting the hypothalamus also may alter fertility potential in women.

Acquired conditions also may affect the hypothalamic-pituitary-ovarian system. Tumors of the hypothalamus or central nervous system or infection of the brain or pituitary may affect the endocrine functions of this axis. Sheehan's syndrome is the result of postpartum pituitary hemorrhage and necrosis from severe hypertension and bleeding during labor and delivery. It is a rare cause of infertility and amenorrhea. Iron deposits in the pituitary from thalassemia or other diseases causing hemosiderosis can suppress the secretion of follicle-stimulating hormone (FSH) and luteinizing hormone (LH) from the pituitary, causing infertility.

Hypersecretion of prolactin by the pituitary causes an abnormally short feedback loop, suppressing the release of gonadotropin-releasing hormone (GnRH). Hyposecretion of GnRH causes suppression of luteinizing hormone release from the pituitary and failure of normal progestin secretion in the ovary, with follicular atresia. Hyperprolactinemia may result from drugs that block the synthesis or binding of dopamine or from agents that act as serotonin agonists. A pituitary macroadenoma causes markedly increased prolactin, and a diagnostic evaluation is indicated even when other reasons for elevated serum prolactin are detected.

Primary ovarian dysfunction leads to infertility by affecting the ovulatory/menstrual cycle. Primary ovarian failure is detected by elevation of FSH and LH in the serum with low estradiol levels, whereas secondary

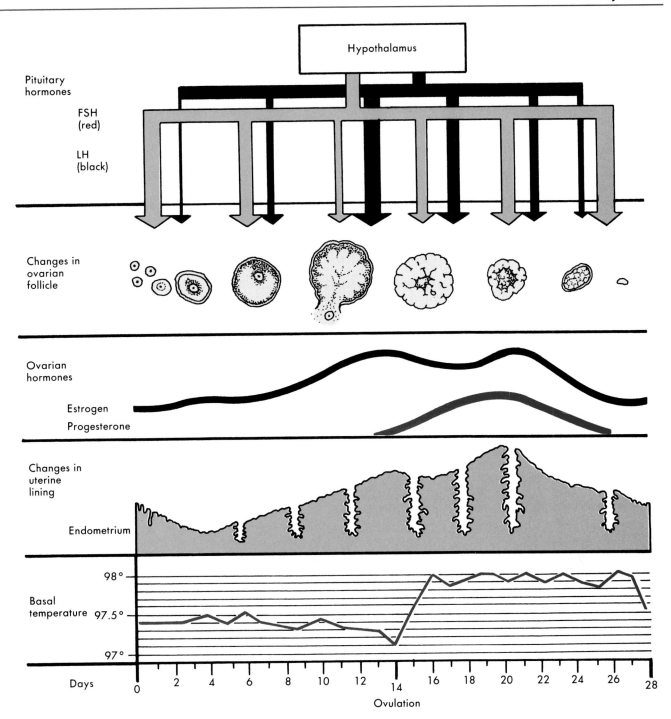

FIGURE 9-3
Female factor infertility. (From McCance K and Huether S: *Pathophysiology: the biological basis for disease in adults and children,* St Louis, 1990, Mosby–Year Book.)

failure (arising from the hypothalamus and pituitary) is manifested as low serum levels of estradiol in combination with depressed FSH and LH levels. Women with deficiencies of specific steroidogenic enzymes experience primary anovulation and abnormal development of a female body habitus. Other women experience an unexplained defect in FSH and LH receptors in the ovary, causing primary anovulation with elevated FSH and LH production but diminished estradiol produc-

tion. Swyer's syndrome is a defect of the embryogenesis of the ovary. Dysgenesis is caused by a failure of the spermatogonia to migrate to the genital ridge. The resulting ovaries are unable to secrete estradiol or form follicles for ovulation.

Secondary causes of ovarian failure include multicystic ovarian disorders (Stein-Leventhal syndrome) and marked obesity. Tumors or hemorrhage may produce ovarian failure with anovulation and infertility.

Autoimmune disorders reduce fertility potential when they affect the ovaries. Ovarian failure also can arise from metabolic disorders (e.g., hypothyroidism, liver disease, renal insufficiency, or hypersecretion of androgens from the adrenal glands), tumors, or excessive ingestion of androgenic steroids. Chemotherapy or environmental toxins also can disrupt the ovulatory cycle, producing infertility.

Disorders of the pelvic organs (uterus, fallopian tubes, and adjacent structures) also affect the potential for fertility in women. Obstruction of the fallopian tubes, which can be caused by a variety of disorders, influences the transport of ova from the ovary to the uterine wall. Obstruction can be caused by congenital malformation of the fallopian tube, submucosal leiomyoma, polyps, or proximal or distal blockage caused by inflammation (salpingitis). Disorders of tubal transport also affect fertility potential. Common causal disorders include agglutination of the tubular fimbriae, adhesions, or peritubular cysts. Sexually transmitted infection can lead to pelvic inflammatory disease and scar-

ring of the tubular system or inflammation of the cervix, uterus, or ovaries. Endometriosis and structural defects of the uterus also affect fertility potential when they compromise tubular patency, transport, or the ovum's ability to implant into the uterine wall. Submucosal myomas, bicornuate or septate uterus, hypoplasia caused by endocrine disturbance, and pelvic inflammatory disease affect fertility when they frustrate the potential for implantation and pregnancy.

The inlet to the uterus, the cervix, is a source for infertility when obstruction or inflammation prevents fertilization by sperm. A history of abnormal Pap smear, postcoital bleeding, cryotherapy, conization, or in utero exposure to diethylstilbestrol (DES) may indicate a cervical source for infertility. Specific obstructive lesions of the cervix occur, such as polyps, pedunculated fibroids, or congenital atresia. Alterations in the cervical mucus, possibly arising from infection caused by *Chlamydia* or *Ureaplasma* organisms or from surgical ablation of the endocervical glands, also may predispose a woman to infertility.

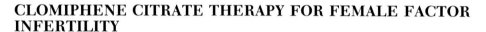

Table 9-6

CLOMIPHENE CITRATE THERAPY FOR FEMALE FACTOR INFERTILITY

Dosage and actions
50 mg daily for 5 days (dosage and schedule of administration are determined by a gynecologic specialist); precise pharmacologic activity is unknown; drug probably stimulates pituitary to release gonadotropins to stimulate estrogens

Side effects
Hot flashes, emotional lability, depression, bloating, visual changes, increased incidence of twins

From Martin.[199]

DIAGNOSTIC STUDIES AND FINDINGS

Diagnostic Test	Findings
Endocrine evaluation	
Follicle-stimulating hormone (FSH)	Elevated with ovarian failure, suppressed with pituitary or hypothalamic disorder
Luteinizing hormone (LH)	Elevated with ovarian failure, suppressed with pituitary or hypothalamic disorder, suppressed with hyperprolactinemia
Prolactin	Elevated with hyperprolactinemia; tumor suspected with marked elevation
Estradiol	Suppressed with endocrine disorder
Endometrial biopsy	Obtained within 1 to 2 days of LH surge; detects inadequate progestin production and ovulation
Basal body temperature (BBT)	Indirect evidence of luteinization noted in biphasal body temperature surge of 0.5° to 0.8° during last 2 weeks of cycle (not definitively diagnostic)
Ultrasonography of pelvis	Dominant follicle; ovulation detected by disappearance of preovulatory follicle (more specific than BBT)
Postcoital (Sims-Huhner) test	Fewer than five highly motile spermatozoa in the upper cervix; inadequate spinnbarkeit and arborization suggest secretory defect
Immunologic compatibility evaluation	(See Male Factor Infertility, page 278)
Evaluation of cervical mucus	Thickening of cervical mucus with tacky character and loss of crystalline fern pattern on drying within 24 hours of ovulation

DIAGNOSTIC STUDIES AND FINDINGS

Diagnostic Test	Findings
Hysterosalpingogram	Scheduled after menstruation and before ovulation to detect anatomic defects of the uterus and tubes, as well as polyps, tumors, or proximal or distal tubular stenosis; an oil- or water-based dye is infused into the uterine cavity through the cervix (The choice of dye depends on the goals of the examination. The oil-based contrast offers greater subsequent pregnancy rates with generally better imaging; water-based contrast materials offer greater comfort, better imaging of rugae, and diminished retention when a granuloma is present.)
Ureterotubal insufflation (Rubin's test)	Carbon dioxide is insufflated into the fallopian tubes; inability to insufflate is noted with obstruction
Laparoscopy	Used to examine uterine contour and to detect tubular abnormalities, including agglutinated fimbriae, peritubular cysts, endometrial lesions, tumors, and masses
Cervical culture	Bacterial infection of the cervical mucus

MEDICAL MANAGEMENT

GENERAL MANAGEMENT AND DRUG THERAPY

Guarded diagnosis with limited evaluation with marked elevation of FSH resistant to pharmacotherapy (adoption and other alternatives should be discussed)

Embryo or egg donation

Clomiphene citrate therapy

Supplementation of clomiphene citrate with estrogen, corticosteroids, and human chorionic gonadotropin (HCG)

Therapy with human menopausal gonadotropin (HMG) in combination with HCG

Therapy with gonadotropin-releasing hormone (GnRH) or its analogs

Progestin injections

Antiinfective medications for pelvic inflammatory disease

Therapy with danazol for endometriosis

Therapy with GnRH and gestrinone for endometriosis*

Intrauterine insemination

In vitro fertilization (IVF) with embryo transfer

Ovum transfer

Gamete intrafallopian tube transfer (GIFT)

SURGERY

Reversal of tubal ligation or reconstruction of obstructed fallopian tube

Surgical or laser resection of endometrial lesions

*The U.S. Food and Drug Administration has not yet approved the use of these agents to treat endometriosis.

1   ASSESS

ASSESSMENT	OBSERVATIONS
Ovulatory patterns	Frequency of ovulatory/menstrual cycles; occurrence of oligomenorrhea and amenorrhea
Endocrine abnormalities	Precocious or delayed puberty; abnormal female body habitus; evidence of masculinization
Pelvic abnormalities	Abnormal vaginal mucosa; evidence of cervical obstruction
Endometriosis	Pelvic or lower back pain exacerbated during premenstrual period and alleviated by menses
Pelvic infection	Inflammation and pelvic pain with positive culture results for pathogens

2   DIAGNOSE

NURSING DIAGNOSIS	SUBJECTIVE FINDINGS	OBJECTIVE FINDINGS
Sexual dysfunction related to female factor infertility	Individual or couple reports inability to conceive a child after a reasonable period of anticipatory (unprotected) sexual intercourse	Conception has not been achieved after 1 year of anticipatory (unprotected) intercourse
Knowledge deficit related to optimum techniques for attaining pregnancy	Couple expresses uncertainty about techniques for maximizing likelihood of conception	Couple uses ineffective or suboptimal techniques to promote conception
Low self-esteem, situational related to infertility	Couple expresses feelings of uncertainty about sexual compatibility or the stability of their relationship	Stated feelings or behaviors reveal feelings of self-degradation or worthlessness related to infertility

3   PLAN

Patient goals

1. Conception will be achieved.
2. The couple will learn effective techniques to maximize the likelihood of conception.
3. The couple will regain their feelings of self-worth.
4. The marital relationship will remain intact and positive.

4   IMPLEMENT

NURSING DIAGNOSIS	NURSING INTERVENTIONS	RATIONALE
Sexual dysfunction related to female factor infertility	Consult the physician about the fertility potential for the woman with a markedly elevated FSH level; help the couple obtain information about adoption, surrogate pregnancy, and embryo donation or egg donation.	A significantly elevated serum FSH indicates ovarian failure, with poor prognosis for fertility.
	Teach the patient to administer clomiphene citrate as directed.	Clomiphene citrate stimulates ovulation in as many as 95% of anovulatory women.[199]
	Advise the patient taking clomiphene citrate that follow-up evaluation and care are necessary.	The dosage often must be titrated to stimulate ovulation; combination therapy may be indicated.
	Administer HCG with clomiphene citrate as directed.	HCG may be administered with clomiphene to stimulate ovulation in individuals who do not respond to clomiphene alone; HCG is administered at midcycle, and ultrasonography typically is indicated to time the dosage of the drug accurately (Table 9-6, page 290).
	Administer HMG as directed.	HMG is administered to women who fail to respond to oral clomiphene therapy, to those who respond with ovulation but fail to conceive, and to women with pituitary or hypothalamic insufficiency; therapy usually is combined with HCG and clomiphene.
	Help the woman who is significantly obese or has other life-style factors leading to anovulation to change these habits or reduce body weight as indicated.	Life-style factors or significant obesity can predispose a woman to anovulation; eliminating these factors can significantly increase fertility potential.
	Administer GnRH or an analog as directed.	GnRH or an analog is used to restore ovulation in a woman who does not respond to nonpharmacologic measures to restore ovulation.
	If the patient has hyperprolactinemia in association with pituitary enlargement or hyperthyroidism, arrange for her to consult an endocrinologist.	Hyperprolactinemia can be caused by excessive thyroid secretion or pituitary adenoma; optimal care is delivered by a qualified expert.
	Administer or teach the patient to self-administer bromocriptine as directed.	Bromocriptine reduces idiopathic hyperprolactinemia and increases fertility potential.
	Administer or teach the patient to self-administer progestins as directed.	Progestins are administered as intramuscular injections or suppositories or in micronized capsule forms; progestins may enhance fertility potential in women with inadequate luteal phase function.

→ ❭ ❭

NURSING DIAGNOSIS	NURSING INTERVENTIONS	RATIONALE
	Help the woman with endometriosis to obtain care from a gynecologist as indicated.	Approximately 11% to 20% of women with endometriosis experience anovulation, and the disorder is found in 30% to 40% of infertile women, compared to 15% of fertile women; management of the condition by a qualified specialist may reverse anovulation and improve fertility potential.[201]
	Prepare the patient for myomectomy as directed.	Surgical myomectomy may be used for women with recurrent abortions.
	Prepare the patient for in vitro fertilization (IVF) and related procedures as directed.	IVF is used when more conservative measures to manage infertility prove unsuccessful (see In Vitro Fertilization).
	Prepare the patient for gamete intrafallopian tube transfer (GIFT) as directed.	GIFT is used when more conservative infertility treatment strategies prove unsuccessful (see Special Procedure: In Vitro Fertilization, page 295).
	Prepare the patient for surgical reconstruction of the fallopian tubes.	Obstruction of the tubes may respond to tubal reanastomosis; reanastomosis is most commonly performed to reverse tubal ligation.
Knowledge deficit related to optimum techniques for attaining pregnancy	Teach the couple the basic principles of reproduction, including the woman's menstrual cycle, events that accompany ovulation, and optimal frequency for intercourse.	The timing and frequency of intercourse may exacerbate or produce infertility in certain cases.
	Help the couple seek cultural solutions for culturally related habits that influence the frequency and timing of intercourse.	Typically, cultural remedies for infertility problems can be identified to resolve frequency and timing issues that reduce fertility potential.
Low self-esteem, situational related to infertility	Encourage both partners to express their feelings about infertility, individually and together; reassure them that these concerns are common and neither negative nor positive.	Expressing feelings allows the couple to identify issues related to low self-esteem and to cope with these feelings rather than blindly responding to them.
	Help the couple obtain medical care for infertility issues as indicated.	Seeking medical care for issues related to infertility provides an opportunity to aggressively and jointly pursue a positive solution to a legitimate health problem.
	Refer the couple with significant self-esteem disorders to a qualified counselor.	Significant self-esteem problems affecting the individual and couple are best managed by a specialist.

5 EVALUATE

PATIENT OUTCOME	DATA INDICATING THAT OUTCOME IS REACHED
Conception has been achieved.	Pregnancy has been attained and sustained, producing a viable infant.
The couple can describe effective techniques to maximize the likelihood of conception.	The couple accurately relates the events of the woman's menstrual cycle and the timing of ovulation; they can accurately state the basic principles of timing and frequency of intercourse.
The couple has regained their feelings of self-worth.	Individually and together, the couple expresses feelings of positive self-evaluation and identifies specific actions to resolve infertility problems.
The marital relationship has remained intact and positive.	Individually and together, the couple expresses resolve to remain within the relationship and to resolve infertility problems together.

PATIENT TEACHING

1. Teach the couple the basic principles of conception, including the menstrual cycle and the significance of ovulation.
2. Teach the patient the names, indications, actions, dosage, and scheduling of all medications.
3. Emphasize the significance of and provide written instructions about the dosage and scheduling of endocrine medications or clomiphene citrate. Help the patient determine her ovulatory cycle as indicated.
4. Teach the patient who measures basal body temperature about the biphasic temperature rise she can expect, the method to determine body temperature, and the significance of assessing the timing of ovulation.

IN VITRO FERTILIZATION

In vitro fertilization remains a relatively new technique for treating infertility.[199] The procedure requires removal of eggs from the ovary, fertilization in the laboratory, and reimplantation into the patient's uterus for impregnation. The procedure is performed after superovulation of the woman's ova. In some women clomiphene citrate may be administered alone or in combination with HMG and FSH to achieve superovulation; in others, luteinizing hormone–releasing hormone (LHRH), FSH, or HMG is administered alone to achieve superovulation. The process of ovulation is closely monitored by ultrasonic scans of the ovaries and serum estradiol and LH levels. The woman is deemed appropriate for IVF when two or three follicles are developing. Otherwise, the procedure is postponed until a more productive cycle is induced.

The aspiration of eggs from the woman's ovary occurs approximately 24 hours after a natural LH surge or 34 hours after administration of HCG. The eggs are retrieved by laparoscopic-guided aspiration or by transurethral, transvaginal, or percutaneous-transvesicular aspiration using ultrasonic guidance. Follicular fluid is aspirated, and the eggs are carefully identified. The man's sperm is capacitated (processed and incubated in a special medium) and allowed to fertilize the eggs in an in vitro setting; between 10,000 and 50,000 spermatozoa typically are placed with each mature egg.

After fertilization, the eggs are incubated in a special atmosphere (5% carbon dioxide and 5% or 20% oxygen) in various culture media. During incubation, the eggs are carefully examined for pronuclei to confirm fertilization and for blastomeres to confirm cleavage.

SURGICAL PROCEDURES TO ACHIEVE INFERTILITY

Although many couples seek to achieve fertility, others seek to attain infertility when they decide that their family is complete. In addition to pharmacologic and mechanical birth control methods, surgical procedures (tubal ligation in women, vasectomy in men) may be used to achieve infertility without compromising other sexual functions.

Vasectomy is the surgical resection of the vasa deferentia, which prevents sperm from entering the semen during ejaculation. Nursing management before surgery focuses on ensuring informed consent and teaching the patient that the procedure should be considered permanent. The surgery is performed with local anesthesia with one or two small surgical incisions. The vasa deferentia are identified by palpation and visual inspection, and then surgically cut and tied. A tissue sample may be sent to the pathology laboratory for identification. Cauterization may be used to increase the likelihood of complete obstruction. The skin may be reapproximated with several sutures or allowed to heal naturally. After surgery, the nurse emphasizes that infertility is not considered complete until one or more semen specimens are determined to be **aspermic** (without sperm). Pain after the procedure typically is minimal and managed with analgesics and by applying an ice pack to the scrotum.

Tubal ligation is the interruption of the fallopian tubes, which obstructs eggs seeking to enter the uterus for implantation and pregnancy. The procedure may be performed as part of more extensive surgery or as a laparoscopic procedure. After being cut the muscular tubes are tied and obstructed, and a tissue specimen may be sent to the pathology laboratory for identification. Preoperative nursing care centers on ensuring informed consent. The nurse may need to spend considerable time with the patient to ensure a full understanding of the procedure and its implications. Patients are advised that the procedure is not considered reversible. Advise the patient with preexisting menstrual disturbances that pain rarely occurs after tubal ligation. If a laparoscopic technique is used, some women may experience abdominal discomfort after the procedure. Other women may have more extensive incisions because of related surgical procedures. Analgesia and other pain-relieving strategies are employed as needed.

Even though vasectomy and tubal ligation are considered irreversible, pregnancy and reintroduction of sperm into the semen may be obtained in some cases by vasovasostomy and tubal reanastomosis.

After 2 to 3 days of laboratory culture, the eggs are placed in the patient's uterus, typically at the two- to eight-cell stage; they are introduced with a small catheter that is placed transcervically into the uterine cavity.

Special procedures may be used to enhance the fertility potential offered by IVF. In cases of severe oligospermia, sperm may be injected directly into the egg, or the egg may be treated by microscopic techniques to enhance fertility potential. Donation of embryos from one woman to another and implantation of frozen/thawed embryos have resulted in viable pregnancies.

A technique of gamete intrafallopian tube transfer (GIFT) has been developed as an alternative to IVF. Superovulation is achieved using techniques described for IVF. Then an injection of HCG is given, and the follicles are aspirated from the patient under laparoscopic guidance. Spermatozoa are mixed with the eggs,

and the resulting cells are drawn into a catheter and introduced into the uterine tubes. GIFT can be used only in women who are free of tubal disease.

INDICATIONS

Severe tubal disease or obstruction (except GIFT)
Antisperm antibodies
Oligospermia
Unexplained infertility

CONTRAINDICATIONS

None

COMPLICATIONS

Ectopic pregnancy

PREPROCEDURAL NURSING CARE

NURSING DIAGNOSIS	NURSING INTERVENTIONS	RATIONALE
Knowledge deficit related to procedure, its goals, and potential untoward effects	Reinforce preprocedural teaching provided by the urologist; discuss anticipated nursing care.	Anxiety before a medical procedure reduces the efficiency of learning and retention of knowledge; repeating teaching increases the efficiency of learning.
	Advise the patient that the timing of the procedure is crucial and that adhering to scheduled evaluations is crucial to the success of IVF.	IVF relies on the production of two or three follicles with mature eggs for successful fertilization and implantation into the uterus.
	Consult the physician about the method of egg retrieval to be used; instruct the patient about this method and the probable anesthesia.	Eggs are retrieved by laparotomy or by ultrasound-guided aspiration techniques; general or local anesthesia is required.
	Advise the patient that multiple births may occur with IVF.	IVF usually involves the transfer of three or four embryos to the uterus; several embryos may implant, leading to multiple births.

POSTPROCEDURAL NURSING CARE

NURSING DIAGNOSIS	NURSING INTERVENTIONS	RATIONALE
Altered tissue perfusion (potential) related to ectopic pregnancy	Teach the patient the signs and symptoms of ectopic pregnancy.	IVF may result in an ectopic pregnancy, although it significantly lowers this risk among women with tubal disease.
	Instruct the patient to seek medical care immediately if she experiences the signs of ectopic pregnancy.	An ectopic pregnancy may cause significant or life-threatening hemorrhage if not promptly treated.
Grieving (potential) related to unsuccessful IVF or GIFT procedure	Reinforce instruction on success rate of IVF or GIFT procedure.	Hope for successful pregnancy may affect the couple's perception of reality concerning the likelihood of pregnancy; prepare the couple for a possible unsuccessful attempt *before* the procedure.
	Encourage the patient and her spouse to discuss feelings of grief and loss after unsuccessful IVF or GIFT procedure.	Expressing feelings of loss encourages successful completion of the grieving process and provides opportunities for the couple to receive and provide support and reassurance.
	Teach the couple about the potential for *biochemical pregnancy* (laboratory tests indicating pregnancy without implantation of an embryo).	Signs of pregnancy may appear without successful implantation.

→ > >

NURSING DIAGNOSIS	NURSING INTERVENTIONS	RATIONALE
	Gently remind the couple that one unsuccessful IVF or GIFT procedure does not imply an inability to conceive using this method.	The chances for success are equal for couples undergoing repeated procedures.

PATIENT TEACHING

1. Teach the couple the significance of preparation for IVF or GIFT and the significance of strict compliance with all diagnostic and therapeutic procedures.
2. Instruct the couple that pregnancy is confirmed by the gynecologist and that home tests may not be accurate for women undergoing IVF or GIFT.
3. Instruct the man in the correct procedure for obtaining sperm. Remind the man with retrograde ejaculation or oligospermia that specialized procedures for sperm retrieval may be required (see Electroejaculation Stimulation, page 285).

CHAPTER 10

Patient Teaching Guides

Patient education has always been an important part of the nursing process. Nurses in charge of patients with genitourinary disorders are responsible for teaching these patients how to manage their bowel and urinary functions on a day-to-day basis. Because these functions usually are taken care of in private, many patients are embarrassed to even discuss catheter insertion or skin care for incontinence. It is the nurse's responsibility not only to educate these patients on how to manage their disorders, but also to protect patients' privacy and to provide them with the tools to maintain their dignity.

Written teaching guides can help reinforce patient teaching and encourage compliance. This chapter provides written handouts that can be photocopied and given to patients or their caregivers to take home and use for self-care. The handouts list step-by-step instructions for certain procedures. More than one guide may be needed for a particular patient.

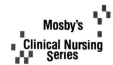

Choosing a Containment Device for Urinary Leakage

When urinary leakage is slight or temporary, a containment device such as a pad or diaper can be used to contain the leakage. There are basically five different types of containment devices for urinary leakage. Which one you choose should be based on these criteria:

- How much leakage you experience; the device should completely protect your clothing, bedding, and furniture
- How comfortable the device is; the smaller and thinner it is, the more comfortable it will be to wear
- How easy it is to use the device; ideally you should be able to put it on by yourself
- How inconspicuous the device is; it should not be bulky or make rustling noises when you walk
- How easy it is to clean or dispose of the device
- How affordable the device is

The containment devices

Diapers can hold large amounts of urinary leakage; however, they are large and bulky and can rustle when you walk. They are best used for people with severe incontinence or for those confined to a bed or wheelchair.

Adult undergarments can hold relatively large amounts of urinary leakage but may have trouble containing leakage when you are lying down.

Underpants with absorbent pads can hold relatively large amounts of urinary leakage. The device, which resembles a typical undergarment, has a space into which you insert a pad.

Sanitary pads can hold small amounts of urinary leakage. They are not ideal for urinary leakage, because they are constructed for menstrual flow. Instead, choose an incontinent pad with a wide front and back that is very absorbent (has a material capable of absorbing many times its weight in urine).

Male drip collectors can absorb small amounts of urine. The device fits comfortably over the penis and usually is used after a prostatectomy.

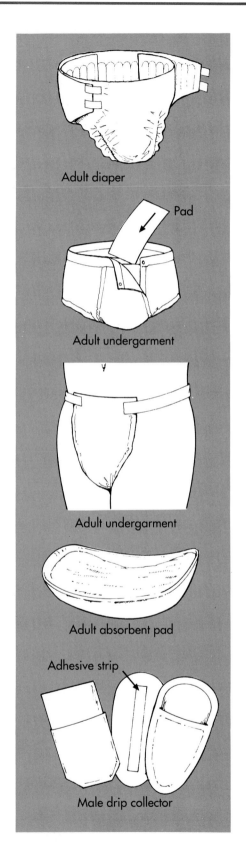

Adult diaper

Pad

Adult undergarment

Adult undergarment

Adult absorbent pad

Adhesive strip

Male drip collector

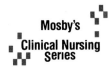

Skin Care for the Incontinent Patient

A patient who is incontinent cannot control the flow of urine. Incontinence may involve only a little urine leaking out when the person laughs, coughs, or lifts something, or may reflect total lack of bladder control.

Urine is very irritating to the skin. Skin that is continuously exposed to urine quickly becomes inflamed and irritated. If the condition continues, rashes and sores will appear.

It is important, therefore, that you follow a few simple procedures to help prevent this skin breakdown.

1. Keep the perineal area clean. Washing with soap and water is the best way to remove urine from your skin.
2. After washing, you may apply a skin barrier or moisture sealant to help moisturize and protect your skin. Ask your nurse to select the best barrier or sealant for you.
3. If your clothing or bedding gets wet, change them immediately.
4. If your skin becomes irritated or red, notify your nurse or doctor. There are prescription creams and sprays that your nurse or doctor can prescribe to relieve skin irritation.
5. Whenever possible, expose the perineal area to air.
6. If you use plastic sheets or pads on your bed, make sure you don't lie directly on the plastic. Put cotton sheets or pads over the plastic.
7. Wear adult briefs with pads, adult absorptive briefs, or an incontinent pad with superabsorbents to help absorb urine and keep it off your skin.

Skin care products

The following is a list of skin care products to help cleanse and protect your skin:

Cleansers are formulated to gently clean the skin without the irritation of soap. Because some cleansers contain fragrances, people who are allergic to fragrances should check the label or test a small amount of cleanser on a small area of skin to see if there is any skin irritation.

Wet wipes come in convenient containers and cleanse the skin without causing irritation.

Deodorizers are intended to cover up offensive odors. Deodorizers come in sprays or drops and are to be sprayed in the air or applied to ostomy pouches, leg bags, and bedside drainage systems. They are *not* to be applied to your skin.

Moisturizing creams and lotions help protect and soothe the skin of incontinent individuals.

Antifungal cream treats fungal infections of the skin.

Barrier films, creams, or salves are intended to protect skin from irritation and damage caused by urine and feces. These products can be used on skin that is already irritated and broken.

Powders, especially those with cornstarch, can help control moisture. Those who are allergic to fragrances should be aware that some powders contain fragrance.

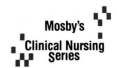

Mosby's
Clinical Nursing
Series

Keeping a Bladder Diary

You have been told to keep a bladder diary for 1 to 7 days, depending on the instructions from your nurse or doctor. The following is a guide on how to fill out the bladder diary sheet and how to measure your urine.

How to measure and record your urine

1. Your doctor or nurse will tell you what information they want you to include on the bladder diary sheet. You may be instructed to complete one or more of the columns on the sheet.
2. Record the time of day you urinated under the column labeled Time.
3. Always measure your urine with the plastic cup provided or with another measuring container marked in milliliters (ml) or ounces (oz).

4. Record the amount you urinated under the column labeled Amount Voided.
5. If you experience leakage, place a check in the Leakage column and write down the approximate time it occurred.
6. Record the amount you drink under the column labeled Amount Consumed; it is okay to use approximate volumes:
   - a cup of coffee or tea is 4 oz; a mug of coffee or tea is 8 oz
   - a glass of tea, water, or soda is 8 oz
   - a large tumbler is 12 oz
   - a can of soda is 12 oz
7. If you have any questions, call your doctor or nurse.

TIME	AMOUNT VOIDED	LEAKAGE	AMOUNT CONSUMED

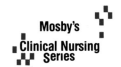

Fluid Intake: What, When, and How Much

If you have a problem with urinary infection, leakage of urine, or stones in the kidneys or bladder, your doctor may advise you to change the amount or type of fluids you drink or the time you drink them. The following guidelines will help you change your fluid intake.

Fluid intake when a urinary tract infection occurs

A urinary tract infection (cystitis, urinary tract infection) is an infection of your bladder that may involve your kidneys or urethra. When you have a urinary tract infection, your doctor or nurse will probably advise you to "force fluids"; this means to increase the amount of liquids you drink each day. The average-sized adult should drink 1,500 ml (1½ quarts) to 2,500 ml (2½ quarts) when forcing fluids.

The type of fluids you drink is important, also. Certain types of beverages may increase feelings of pain or urgency to urinate, and others are likely to lessen these feelings. It is best to avoid carbonated beverages or those containing caffeine. Citrus juices may irritate the bladder in some people. You may want to try eliminating these fluids one at a time to see how they affect your bladder. Clear liquids and water are excellent liquids when forcing fluids.

Fluid intake when urinary leakage (incontinence) occurs

Urinary leakage (incontinence) is the uncontrolled loss of urine. Often people with urinary leakage drink only very small amounts of liquids to lessen the leakage. However, cutting back on the amount of liquids you drink will not help your leakage; instead, it will concentrate your urine, making it more irritating to the bladder and increasing your chances for a urinary tract infection.

Even though you have urinary leakage, you should drink a normal amount of liquids each day. Drink about 1,500 ml (1½ quarts) each day.

The types of fluids you choose to drink may affect the likelihood of urinary leakage. Avoid drinking only carbonated beverages and those with caffeine. Some people with urinary leakage notice more bladder irritation when they drink citrus juices, and others do not notice any effect. You should try these fluids one at a time to see how they affect your bladder. When you drink fluids also affects your leakage. Many people drink several glasses of liquid with a meal and may go without drinking between meals. Others drink immediately before going to bed. These habits will make you more likely to leak urine. It is best to spread your intake of liquids throughout the day and to limit the amount you drink with meals to 8 ounces (240 ml). Sip water or a clear liquid from a squeeze bottle or tumbler. Limit fluids to sips (2 to 3 ounces) for 2 hours before going to bed at night. Be sure that you drink a total of 1,500 ml (1½ quarts) to 2,500 ml (2½ quarts) each day.

Fluid intake when urinary stones occur

Urinary stones are painful gravel or larger pebbles that grow from salts or other solid substances in the urine. These stones may block the passage of urine, causing pain and infection. Your doctor may recommend fluid intake to prevent stones to help you pass stones you already have.

Forcing fluids is advisable when you are trying to pass a urinary stone. You should drink at least 1,500 ml (1½ quarts) to 3,000 ml (3 quarts) of fluid each day according to your doctor's instructions.

The type of liquids you drink may affect the likelihood of developing a urinary stone. Different types of urinary stones are formed by different types of substances. Ask your doctor whether you should eliminate any type of liquids (or food) from your diet.

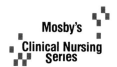

Pelvic Muscle Exercises

The pelvic floor is made up of muscles responsible for holding the body's lower organs, including the bladder. Because we walk upright, quite a bit of pressure is put on these organs as we walk, exercise, cough, or pick up something. When these muscles are weakened by childbirth or hormonal changes (such as those caused by menopause) or as a result of surgery or lower back injury, small amounts of urine may leak with physical activity. This condition is called stress incontinence, and it affects many women and some men.

Stress incontinence may be controlled without surgery in many cases. Exercising the pelvic muscles is a good way to strengthen them. Pelvic exercises (sometimes called Kegel exercises, after Dr. Arnold Kegel) are an excellent way to improve the fitness of the pelvic floor muscles.

Pelvic muscle exercises for women

First, it is important to locate and identify the correct muscles to exercise. The muscles you wish to exercise surround the urethra (the tube where urine leaves your body) and the vagina. You can find this muscle by practicing stopping your urine in midstream. Tighten (contract) the muscles to stop the urine; release the muscles to continue urination. Your nurse will help you locate the correct muscles. She may gently place a gloved finger in the vagina and ask you to contract the muscles around her finger, or she may use a special machine that helps you find and contract the correct muscles. The special machine uses sound or visual signals to help you understand how to contract and release the pelvic muscles. The nurse will also help you avoid tightening your abdominal or thigh muscles. Contracting these muscles will not help you strengthen the pelvic muscles.

As soon as you think you understand how to contract and release the pelvic muscles, you are ready to start your exercise program. Here's how to proceed:

- Choose a time and place to exercise. You will need about 15 minutes to do your exercises.

- You will find the best position to do your exercises with practice. Some women prefer to sit or stand; others lie on the back with the head elevated on a pillow.
- Tighten the pelvic muscles as hard as you can.
- Hold the muscle tight for 10 seconds—you may find it helpful to count to 10—then relax the muscle for 10 seconds.
- Repeat this exercise 10 times.
- Ask your nurse or doctor how many times a day (repetitions) you need to perform the exercise (generally, it is best to begin with 10 repetitions and work up to 35 to 50 repetitions every other day). Remember that one repetition consists of 10 seconds of tightening and 10 seconds of relaxation.

You may wish to try a variation of this exercise.

- While sitting, standing, or lying with your head elevated, tighten and release the pelvic muscles in rapid succession. Repeat this 15 times.
- In the same position, tighten the pelvic muscles while you exhale. Hold the muscle for a count of 30. Repeat this exercise 10 times.

Pelvic muscle exercises for men

First, it is important to locate and identify the correct muscles to exercise. The muscles you wish to exercise surround the urethra (the tube where urine leaves your body) and the anus (where stool leaves the body). You can find this muscle by practicing stopping your urine in midstream. Tighten (contract) the muscles to stop the urine; release the muscles to continue urination. Your nurse will help you locate the correct muscles. She may gently place a gloved finger in the lowest portion of your rectum. She will ask you to tighten the muscle around her gloved finger. She may also help you locate the pelvic muscles using a special machine. The special machine uses sound or visual signals to help you understand how to contract and release the pelvic muscles. The nurse will also help you avoid tightening your abdominal or thigh muscles. Contracting these muscles will not help you strengthen the pelvic muscles.

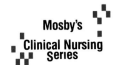

As soon as you think you understand how to contract and release the pelvic muscles, you are ready to start your exercise program. Here's how to proceed:

- Choose a time and place to exercise. You will need about 15 minutes to do your exercises.
- You will find the best position to do your exercises with practice. Some men prefer to sit or stand; others lie on the back with the head elevated on a pillow.
- Tighten the pelvic muscles as hard as you can.
- Hold the muscle tight for 10 seconds—you may find it helpful to count to 10—then relax the muscle for 10 seconds.
- Repeat this exercise 10 times.

- Ask your nurse or doctor how many times a day (repetitions) you need to perform the exercise (generally, it is best to begin with 10 repetitions and work up to 35 to 50 repetitions every other day). Remember that one repetition consists of 10 seconds of tightening and 10 seconds of relaxation.

You may wish to try a variation of this exercise.

- While sitting, standing, or lying with your head elevated, tighten and release the pelvic muscles in rapid succession. Repeat this 15 times.
- In the same position, tighten the pelvic muscles while you exhale. Hold the muscle for a count of 30. Repeat this exercise 10 times.

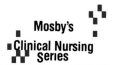
Intermittent Self-Catheterization for Men

When the bladder cannot empty itself completely (or at all), intermittent catheterization (IC) becomes necessary. This is a procedure that you do yourself, and to avoid introducing germs and possibly infection into the bladder, it is important that you carefully follow a clean procedure. Your doctor will tell you the maximum amount of fluid you should have in your bladder and how often you will need to catheterize yourself.

Equipment

Before you begin, make sure you have everything you need:
1. Catheter (and optional extension)
2. K-Y jelly (lubricant)
3. Basin for collecting urine
4. Plastic bag for storing the catheter
5. Handiwipes or a soapy washcloth and rinse cloth

Procedure

Catheterization may be performed while sitting on the toilet, in a wheelchair, in bed, or while standing.

1. Wash your hands thoroughly with soap and water.
2. Wash the penis and surrounding area with soap and water. Rinse with the rinse cloth.
3. Open the lubricant and squeeze a generous amount onto a paper towel.
4. Remove the catheter from its package, and roll the first 3 inches or so of the catheter in the lubricant.
5. Put one end of the catheter in the basin (or toilet). Hold your penis with one hand, and with the other gently insert the catheter through the urinary opening. As you push the catheter in, pull up on your penis to help the catheter slide in more easily.
6. Continue pushing the catheter in until urine begins to flow; then insert the catheter another 1 to 2 inches. Hold the catheter until all urine has been drained into a basin or toilet. To make sure your bladder is completely empty, take some deep breaths or press on your lower abdomen.
7. When the urine flow stops, pinch the catheter

closed and slowly remove it.
8. Empty the basin and rinse it.
9. Wash your hands.
10. Wash the catheter in warm, soapy water and rinse it, both inside and out. Dry it with a clean towel, and place it in a clean plastic bag until the next time you need it. If the catheter appears crusted, rinse or soak it in a solution of half distilled vinegar and half water. Catheters that show wear, become brittle, crack, or do not drain urine well need to be replaced.

When to call your doctor

1. If you have any problems inserting the catheter
2. If you have any symptoms of infection, such as the following:
   - Pain in the lower back and lower abdomen
   - Cloudy, foul-smelling urine
   - Bloody urine
   - Chills or fever
   - Lack of appetite or lack of energy, or both
   - Sandlike material (sediment) in the urine

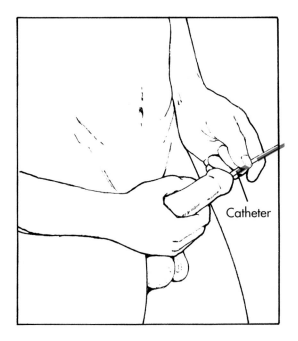

Catheter

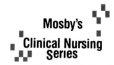

**Mosby's
Clinical Nursing
Series**

Intermittent Self-Catheterization for Women

When the bladder cannot empty itself completely (or at all) intermittent catheterization (IC) becomes necessary. This is a procedure that you do yourself, and to avoid introducing germs and possibly infection into the bladder, it is important that you carefully follow a clean procedure. Your doctor will tell you the maximum amount of fluid you should have in your bladder and how often you will need to catheterize yourself.

Equipment

Before you begin, make sure you have everything you need:

1. Catheter—use a short female catheter if you are doing catheterization on a toilet. Use a longer catheter if you are doing this procedure from a wheelchair.
2. K-Y jelly (lubricant)
3. Basin for collecting urine
4. Plastic bag
5. Handiwipes or a soapy washcloth and rinse cloth

Procedure

Catherization may be performed while sitting on the toilet, in a wheelchair, in bed, or while standing.

1. Wash your hands thoroughly with soap and water.
2. Wash your urinary area (urethral opening) and the surrounding area with soap and water. Use downward strokes and avoid the bowel area. Rinse with the rinse cloth.
3. Open the lubricant and squeeze a generous amount onto a paper towel.
4. Remove the catheter from its package, and roll the first 3 inches or so of the catheter in the lubricant.
5. Put one end of the catheter in the basin (or toilet). With the index finger and ring finger of one hand, spread the lips of the vulva, and with the middle finger locate the urethral opening. With the other hand, gently insert the catheter into the urethra.
6. Continue pushing the catheter in (about 2 to 3 inches) until urine begins to flow. Hold the catheter until all the urine has drained into a basin or toilet. To make sure your bladder is completely empty, take some deep breaths or press on your lower abdomen.
7. When the urine flow stops, pinch the catheter closed and slowly remove it.
8. Empty the basin and rinse it.
9. Wash your hands.
10. Wash the catheter in warm, soapy water and rinse it, both inside and out. Dry it with a clean towel, and

place it in a clean plastic bag until the next time you need it. If the catheter appears crusted, rinse or soak it in a solution of half distilled vinegar and half water. Catheters that show wear, become brittle, crack, or do not drain urine well need to be replaced.

When to call your doctor

1. If you have any problems inserting the catheter
2. If you have any symptoms of infection, such as the following:
   - Pain in the lower back and lower abdomen
   - Cloudy, foul-smelling urine
   - Bloody urine
   - Chills or fever
   - Lack of appetite or lack of energy, or both
   - Sandlike material (sediment) in the urine
   - Red or swollen urinary opening

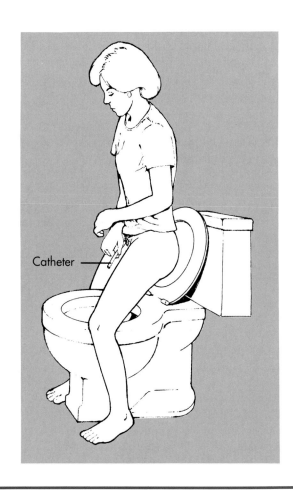

Catheter

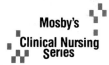
Care of an Indwelling Foley Catheter

An indwelling Foley catheter is a tube that empties urine from your bladder into a drainage bag. To prevent blockage of the catheter and contamination of the urine, it is important that you follow a few guidelines in caring for your catheter.

1. Empty your drainage bag once every 8 hours or as soon as it fills. Do not postpone emptying a full drainage bag, since this causes urine to back up in your bladder, making infection or leakage more likely.

2. Empty the bag by loosening the clamp on the end of the leg or bedside bag. Do not touch the the tip of the tube. After draining the urine into the toilet, you may clean the tip with a povidone-iodine (Betadine) solution.

3. Always keep the drainage bag lower than the catheter. Remember that urine will not drain uphill or against gravity. Check the tubing for kinks, since urine will not drain past a kink.

4. Regularly flush your bladder by drinking plenty of liquids. Clear liquids and water are ideal; remember to drink about 1½ to 2½ quarts each day. Ask your doctor for advice on the amount of liquids you need to drink.

5. Your catheter should be changed about every 4 weeks. Check your catheter regularly for encrustation and blockage. If these occur, you need to change your catheter at that time.

6. You may reuse your bedside and leg bags, but it is important to clean them carefully. First, rinse the inside of the bag with soapy water and then rinse very well with clear water. Then fill the bag with a solution that is one part vinegar to four parts water, and soak the inside for 30 minutes. Empty the bag and let it air dry.

7. Ask your doctor or nurse about bacteria and infection caused by indwelling catheters. People with an indwelling catheter will have some bacteria in the urine. A urinary tract infection occurs when enough bacteria get into the system to cause symptoms such as fever or blood in the urine. Because people who use catheters are at risk for urinary tract infection, you should know the following signs of infection:
   - Pain in the lower back or abdomen
   - Cloudy, foul-smelling urine
   - Bloody urine
   - Chills or fever
   - Poor appetite and lack of energy
   - Sandlike material (sediment) in the urine

Call your doctor or nurse if you have any of these symptoms.

Choosing a drainage bag

People who wear a catheter to empty the bladder use a drainage bag to hold the urine. These guidelines will help you choose the best drainage bag for your needs.

1. Usually it is best to wear a leg bag during the day. A leg bag empties urine from your catheter into a small bag that attaches to your thigh or calf. The leg bag should hold about 500 ml (½ quart) of urine.

2. The leg bag should be attached to your leg with cloth or Velcro straps or should fit into a cloth sleeve. Rubber straps are not the best choice, since they tend to irritate your skin.

3. You or the person who cares for you should be able to open and close the drainage valve of your leg bag easily.

4. The leg bag should not show under your clothing. Choose a leg bag that fills without bulging.

5. Usually it is best to wear a bedside bag while sleeping. The bag should hold at least 1,500 ml (1½ quarts) or more of urine.

6. The bedside bag should have plenty of tubing to allow you to move while in bed. You may wish to attach the bedside drainage bag to a stand while sleeping.

7. You or the person who cares for you should be able to open and close the drainage valve on your bedside bag easily.

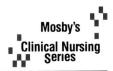

Preventing Urinary Tract Infections

A urinary tract infection (UTI) is any infection or inflammation located along the urinary tract. Most urinary tract infections occur in the bladder or urethra, the canal that carries the urine from the bladder to the urethral opening.

What causes urinary tract infections?

Urinary tract infections have a number of causes. Most are caused by bacteria from the bowel that invade the urinary tract. Because a woman's urethra is closer to the rectum than a man's is, women suffer many more urinary tract infections than men do. Other causes include overstretching of the bladder, urine left in the bladder (incomplete voiding), and lack of cleanliness when doing catheterization. Urethral inflammation can be caused by chemical irritants such as perfumed feminine hygiene products, sanitary napkins, spermicidal foams and jellies, and bubble bath.

What are the signs of a urinary tract infection?

Several signs indicate a urinary tract infection. You may have one or a combination of these symptoms:
1. A frequent and urgent need to urinate
2. Pain in the lower back and lower pelvic region
3. Cloudy, foul-smelling urine
4. Bloody urine
5. Chills or fever
6. Lack of appetite or lack of energy, or both
7. Sandlike material (sediment) in the urine

How to prevent a urinary tract infection or inflammation

The most important thing you can do to prevent a urinary tract infection is to practice good hygiene. Women should avoid wiping fecal matter into the urethral area. Wiping from front to back helps prevent germs and bacteria from entering the urethral opening. Showering or bathing daily also helps prevent the spread of germs, and drinking lots of fluids helps the bladder flush itself.

If you are catheterizing yourself, it is very important that you are careful to be very clean. It is very easy to insert germs along with the catheter into your urethra and bladder. Wash your hands frequently as you carry out the catheterization process. Wash the catheter in soapy water after each use and allow it to dry completely before using it again.

To prevent inflammation of the urinary tract, avoid perfumed feminine hygiene products, spermicidal jellies and foams, and bubble bath.

See your doctor if you think you might have a urinary tract infection. Such infections can lead to bladder and kidney damage, kidney stones, and urine retention.

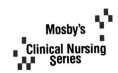

Mosby's
Clinical Nursing Series

Self-Irrigation for Reconstructed Bladders

Self-irrigation of a urinary continent pouch

Gather the following equipment before you begin:

- Normal saline (you may buy this or make your own: boil 1 quart of water, then add 2 teaspoons of salt and let cool; or, add 2 teaspoons of salt to 1 quart of distilled water)
- Irrigation kit containing an irrigation syringe and bottle
- Container for collecting urine

Irrigating your urinary pouch

1. Wash your hands.
2. Catheterize the stoma as usual.
3. Draw up 40 to 60 ml of normal saline into the syringe.
4. Hold the catheter upright, and place the tip of the syringe into the catheter.
5. Gently inject the normal saline into the pouch. *Do not force the liquid.*
6. Gently withdraw the saline from the pouch with the syringe. Watch for mucus.
7. Repeat steps 3 through 6 twice or until the drainage is clear.

Things to remember

1. Irrigate every _____day when at home.
2. Check the drainage tube for kinks and straighten them out.
3. To reduce mucus in your continent pouch:
   - Drink at least 1½ to 2 quarts of liquid every day. Water is particularly good.
   - Drink 8 ounces of cranberry juice, once in the morning and once at night. This will thin the mucus so that it is less likely to clog the catheter. You can drink pure cranberry juice or mix it with ginger ale or other beverages to improve the taste.

Notify your doctor if any of the following occur:

- No urine output from the pouch for 4 hours
- Blood in the urine
- Fever above 101° F (38.3° C)
- Sudden pain in your bladder
- Pain in your kidneys (flank pain)

Self-irrigation of an augmented bladder

Gather the following equipment before you begin:

- Normal saline (you may buy this or make your own: boil 1 quart of water, then add 2 teaspoons of salt and let cool; or, add 2 teaspoons of salt to 1 quart of distilled water)
- Irrigation kit containing an irrigation syringe and bottle
- Container for collecting urine

Irrigating your augmented bladder

1. Wash your hands.
2. Catheterize yourself as usual.
3. Draw up 40 to 60 ml of normal saline into the syringe.
4. Hold the catheter upright, and place the tip of the syringe into the catheter.
5. Gently inject the normal saline into the pouch. *Do not force the liquid.*
6. Gently withdraw the saline from the bladder with the syringe. Watch for mucus.
7. Repeat steps 3 through 6 twice or until the drainage is clear.

Things to remember

1. Irrigate every _____day when at home.
2. If the catheter is plugged, irrigate it immediately.
3. To reduce mucus in your augmented bladder:
   - Drink at least 1½ to 2 quarts of liquid every day. Water is particularly good.
   - Drink 8 ounces of cranberry juice, once in the morning and once at night. This will thin the mucus so that it is less likely to clog the catheter. You can drink pure cranberry juice or mix it with ginger ale or other beverages to improve the taste.

Notify your doctor if any of the following occur:

- No urine output from the pouch for 4 hours
- Blood in the urine
- Fever above 101° F (38.3° C)
- Sudden pain in your bladder
- Pain in your kidneys (flank pain)

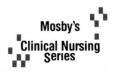

Self-Injection for a Pharmacologic Erection Program

If you cannot achieve or sustain an erection, you may be a candidate for penile injection therapy. An erection-producing drug is injected into the shaft of the penis. This drug works by expanding the blood vessels in the penis and allowing more blood to flow in. The penis swells and traps the blood, preventing it from escaping. The result is an erection that usually lasts 1 to 2 hours.

Guidelines for a pharmacologic erection

Your urologist will determine if you are a candidate for the pharmacologic erection program (PEP) and then choose the best drug and dosage for you. You must follow his or her instructions carefully. The nurse or doctor will show you how to inject the drug and how to adjust the dosage so that your erection lasts 1 to 2 hours. They also will advise you of possible side effects and tell you how often you can use the injections.

Instructions for self-injection

It is important that you inject the drug into the correct area of your penis. Take your penis and hold it tightly over either your left or right thigh. The erectile bodies of the penis lie on either side of the penis' shaft. This is the area into which you should inject the drug. Don't inject into the top or bottom of the penis.

Injection procedure

Before you begin, assemble your supplies. These include alcohol swabs, 1-ml syringes and needles, and the vial of injection drug.

Then:
1. Clean the top of the vial with an alcohol swab.
2. Remove the plastic cap from the needle on the syringe, and pull back on the barrel of the syringe to the point where you were instructed. Be careful not to touch the needle or let anything else touch the needle.
3. Stick the needle into the rubber top of the vial, and inject the air that is in the syringe into the vial.
4. Slowly withdraw the correct amount of medicine into the syringe. If there are air bubbles in the syringe, inject the medicine back into the vial and start again.
5. When the correct amount of medicine is in the syringe and has no air bubbles, remove the needle from the vial and cover it with the plastic cap. Lay the syringe down.
6. Holding only the tip, pull your penis straight out from your body. Then stretch it tightly across your left or right thigh; this is how you will position it for the injection.
7. Clean the area to be injected with an alcohol swab.
8. Pick up the needle and remove the cap.
9. Position your penis as in step 6 and, holding the syringe like a pencil, quickly "dart" the needle into the correct spot. Slowly inject the medication.
10. After the medicine has been injected, remove the nee-

dle, recap it, and throw away the syringe.
11. Press for 5 minutes on the injection site with an alcohol swab (this is to prevent bruising).

You should have no pain during the injection. If you do, remove the needle immediately and press down on the injection site for 5 minutes with an alcohol swab.

Things to remember

Your erection should last 1 to 2 hours, but it may last longer. However, any erection that lasts for more than 6 hours can be dangerous and should be reported to your urologist. The blood trapped in the penis can congeal and become unable to drain back out of the penis. This can lead to tissue damage. Your urologist may have to flush the penis, inject an antierection drug, or prescribe a medication to be taken by mouth. With a severe, prolonged erection, a shunt may be inserted to drain blood.

Make sure you keep your needles sterile. Don't let them touch anything before the injection.

You must see your urologist every 4 to 6 months to make sure that you are suffering no adverse reactions to this injection program.

Never inject yourself more than twice in a 24-hour period. If your first injection fails, you must wait another 24 hours before injecting again.

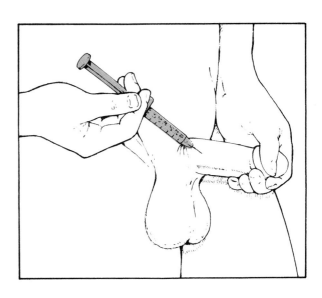

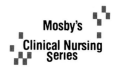
Testicular Self-Examination

Testicular cancer is a curable disease if it is discovered and treated early. Performing testicular self-examination (TSE) once a month greatly increases the chances that you will discover a cancerous lump or mass early enough for effective treatment.

When you do testicular self-examination you should be looking for hard nodules or lumps in the testes. Enlarged testes also may indicate a cancerous condition, and any enlargement or swelling that doesn't respond to medications should be investigated further.

How to do testicular self-examination

Boys should begin examining themselves at 15 years of age and should perform the examination once a month. Choose a day of the month that is significant to you, such as your birthday or the first or fifteenth of the month, to make it easier for you to remember to do the examination regularly.

It is best to examine the testicles in a warm place, such as the shower, because this promotes relaxation and descent of the scrotal contents. Soap your hands to increase your sensitivity to touch. Use both hands during the examination.

1. Examine each testicle separately; apply only gentle pressure while holding the scrotum in your palm. The testicles should be approximately equal in size and evenly round. No nodules should be present.

2. Examine your right testicle first. Lift your penis with your left hand, and with your right hand locate the epididymis, the cordlike structure at the back of your testicle. Feel along it with your thumb and first two fingers. The epididymis extends upward into the spermatic cord. Squeeze gently along the length of this cord, feeling for lumps and masses as you progress upward. It normally is tender to the touch.

3. Identify the vas deferens. It is a smooth, movable tube that can be traced up to the point where the scrotum joins the groin. It should be movable, nontender, and of equal size in the two testicles.

4. Repeat steps 2 and 3 to examine the left testicle, using your left hand.

Normal testicles should feel firm to the touch, but you should be able to move them. They should feel smooth and rubbery and should be free of lumps. If you notice any lumps or masses or anything unusual, call your doctor.

Know the signs of testicular cancer. They are:

- A change in the size or consistency of one testicle
- A lump or nodule on one testicle
- Pain or a sensation of testicular pressure or heaviness
- Enlargement of your nipples

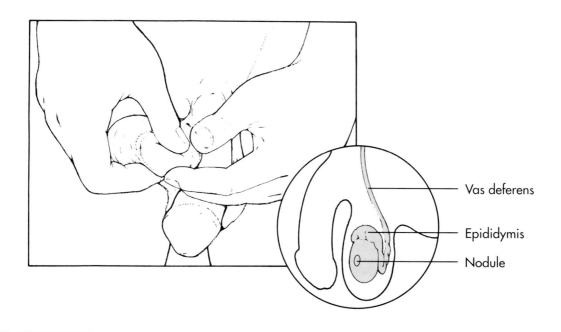

Vas deferens

Epididymis

Nodule

CHAPTER 11

Genitourinary Drugs

ANTIINFECTIVE MEDICATIONS

PENICILLINS

Penicillins comprise the most widely used family of antibiotics. They inhibit bacterial enzymes responsible for cell wall rigidity and enhance bacterial enzymes responsible for cell wall catabolism. Penicillins are categorized according to their structure and spectra of activity. Natural penicillins have a narrow spectrum of activity and are effective primarily against certain gram-positive bacteria. Aminopenicillins have a spectrum of activity that extends to many gram-negative bacteria. Extended-spectrum penicillins are effective against an even broader spectrum of organisms. Some penicillins are available in fixed combination with clavulanic acid or sulbactam sodium, forming drugs that are effective against bacteria resistant to single-agent penicillins.

Precautions/contraindications: Use during pregnancy should be limited to situations when clearly needed. Penicillins should be used cautiously in nursing mothers. Penicillins are contraindicated in patients with a history of hypersensitivity to penicillins, cephalosporins, cephamycins, or penicillamine. They are used cautiously in patients with impaired renal function, GI disease, infectious mononucleosis, or a history of asthma or allergies. *Carbenicillin, ticarcillin:* Platelet aggregation is inhibited; they must be used cautiously in patients with bleeding disorders.

Side effects/adverse reactions: *Allergic:* Rash, exfoliative dermatitis, erythema, contact dermatitis, hives, pruritus, wheezing, anaphylaxis, fever, blood dyscrasias, Stevens-Johnson syndrome, angioedema, serum sickness. *CNS:* Seizures, hallucinations, confusion, hyperreflexia, dysphasia, encephalopathy. *GI:* Nausea, vomiting, bloating, flatulence, diarrhea, cramps, thirst, bitter taste. *Hematologic:* Eosinophilia, hemolytic anemia, thrombocytopenia, leukopenia, neutropenia, agranulocytosis. *Hepatic:* Cholestatic jaundice. *Renal:* Acute interstitial nephritis (fever, hematuria, pyuria, albuminuria, oliguria), electrolyte imbalance following IV administration. *Skin:* Pain, induration at injection site.

Pharmacokinetics: Penicillins are distributed throughout the body and cross the placenta. Most if not all penicillins are excreted in breast milk. Penicillin G potassium and penicillin G sodium are readily absorbed systemically. Penicillin G benzathine and penicillin G procaine, however, are relatively insoluble and form tissue depots from which systemic absorption occurs slowly. Azlocillin, mezlocillin, piperacillin, and ticarcillin are not appreciably absorbed orally and must be given parenterally. Carbenicillin can be administered orally or parenterally.

Interactions: Penicillins have additive or synergistic effects when used concurrently with aminoglycosides; however, penicillins may inactivate aminoglycosides if the two are mixed in a syringe or IV bag. Probenecid increases serum concentration and prolongs penicillins' half-lives, an interaction exploited to therapeutic advantage in the treatment of gonorrhea and acute pelvic inflammatory disease. *Natural penicillins:* Hyperkalemia may occur with concurrent use of potassium-containing penicillins and other potassium-containing medications, angiotensin-converting enzyme (ACE) inhibitors, or po-

PENICILLINS

Natural penicillins

Penicillin G benzathine (Bicillin) 2.4 million U IM—Syphilis

Penicillin G potassium (Pfizerpen) 5-10 million U/day IM/IV—Gynecologic infections

Penicillin G procaine (Wycillin) 4.8 million U IM—Gonorrhea
  600,000 U/day IM—Syphilis

Penicillin G sodium (generic) 4.8 million U IM—Gonorrhea
  600,000 U/day IM—Syphilis

Aminopenicillins

Amoxicillin (Amoxil, Larotid, Polymox) 250-500 mg q 8 h PO—Gonorrhea, gynecologic infections, gonococcal urethritis

Amoxicillin/clavulanate (Augmentin) 250-500 mg/125 mg q 8 h PO—Urinary tract infections

Ampicillin (Omnipen, Principen) 250-500 mg q 6 h PO—Gynecologic infections, gonococcal urethritis
  200 mg/kg/day IV/IM

Ampicillin/sulbactam (Unasyn) 1-2/0.5-1 g q 6 h IM/IV—Gynecologic infections

Bacampicillin (Spectrobid) 1.6 g PO—Gonorrhea
  400-800 mg q 12 h PO—Urinary tract infections

Cyclacillin (Cyclapen) 250-500 mg q 6 h PO—Urinary tract infections

Broad-spectrum penicillins

Amdinocillin (Coactin) 10 mg/kg q 4-6 h IM/IV—Bacteremia, urinary tract infections

Azlocillin (Azlin) 100-300 mg/kg/day IV—Urinary tract infections

Carbenicillin (Geocillin) 382-764 mg q 6 h PO—Prostatitis, urinary tract infections
  (Geopen, Pyopen) 200 mg/kg/day IM/IV—Gynecologic infections, urinary tract infections
  4 g IM—Gonorrhea

Mezlocillin (Mezlin) 100-125 mg/kg/day IM/IV—Gynecologic infections, urinary tract infections

Piperacillin (Piperacil) 100-125 mg/kg/day IM—Gynecologic infections, gonococcal urethritis, urinary tract infections
  100-300 mg/kg/day IV

Ticarcillin (Ticar) 1 g q 6 h IM—Gynecologic infections, urinary tract infections
  150-300 mg/kg/day IV

Ticarcillin/clavulanate (Timentin) 3 g/100 mg q 4-8 h IV—Urinary tract infections

SUPERINFECTIONS

A potential sequela of antibiotic therapy is suppression of commensal flora that normally keep other organisms such as *Candida albicans*, *Proteus* sp., or *Pseudomonas* sp. from proliferating. Such suppression may enable one or more of these organisms to cause what is known as a superinfection. Superinfections commonly occur in the mouth, intestines, vagina, or urinary tract.

Oral candidiasis is characterized by creamy-white, cottage cheese–like patches on the tongue or elsewhere in the mouth. Scraping this exudate often reveals a raw, bleeding surface. Intestinal candidiasis causes rectal discharge, itching, and pain. Vaginal candidiasis is manifested by white or yellow discharge, itching, dryness, and dyspareunia. Signs and symptoms of urinary tract infections include frequency, urgency, dysuria, and incontinence.

If a superinfection develops, the physician must be notified and an alternate antibiotic may need to be selected. The organism involved must be treated with appropriate pharmacologic therapy. Good oral and vaginal hygiene may prevent or minimize the impact of candidiasis, and adequate fluid intake may do the same for urinary tract infections. Yogurt and buttermilk (if allowed) may help prevent intestinal superinfections by replenishing normal intestinal flora.

tassium-sparing diuretics. Chloramphenicol, erythromycins, sulfonamides, and tetracyclines may antagonize the bactericidal effect of natural penicillins. Sulfinpyrazone may decrease urinary secretion of penicillin G, resulting in a higher serum level. *Aminopenicillins:* Ampicillin rash is more likely to occur during concurrent use of ampicillin or bacampicillin and allopurinol, especially in hyperuricemic patients. Concurrent use of bacampicillin and disulfiram may cause a disulfiram-alcohol reaction. Ampicillin may decrease the efficacy of oral contraceptives. Tetracyclines may decrease the therapeutic efficacy of amoxicillin. *Broad-spectrum penicillins:* Concurrent use of other platelet-aggregation inhibitors, anticoagulants, heparin, or thrombolytic agents with high doses of carbenicillin or ticarcillin increases the risk of hemorrhage. The sodium content of carbenicillin disodium and ticarcillin disodium may alter lithium elimination. Additive hepatotoxicity may occur with concurrent use of azlocillin, mezlocillin, or piperacillin and other hepatotoxic agents.

Nursing considerations: Electrolyte imbalances may occur in patients receiving high doses of penicillins that contain sodium or potassium, as well as in patients receiving any penicillins intravenously. Patients with impaired renal or cardiac function require especially close monitoring. Penicillins interfere with urine glucose tests that employ cupric sulfate (e.g., Benedict's solution, Clinitest). Patients who normally use these methods should use an alternative (e.g., Diastix, Tes-Tape) during penicillin therapy. Penicillins may cause false-positive results in direct antiglobulin (Coombs') tests, interfering with hematologic studies and transfusion cross-matching procedures.

CEPHALOSPORINS

Cephalosporins and penicillins have similar mechanisms of action and pharmacologic properties. Like penicillins, they are classified into categories based on the spectrum of antibacterial activity.

Precautions/contraindications: Use during pregnancy should be limited to situations when clearly needed. Cautious use is required in nursing mothers. Cautious use is required in patients with a history of hypersensitivity reactions to cephalosporins or penicillins. Cautious use is required in patients with a history of GI disease or bleeding disorders and in patients with impaired hepatic or renal function.

Side effects/adverse reactions: *CNS:* Dizziness, headache, malaise, fatigue. With high doses or in patients with impaired renal function, seizures, encephalopathy, asterixis, and neuromuscular excitability may occur. *GI (most common):* Nausea, vomiting, diarrhea, abdominal pain, tenesmus, dyspepsia, glossitis. *Hematologic (rare):* Mild and transient neutropenia, thrombocytopenia, leukopenia, lymphocytosis, anemia, agranulocytosis, aplastic anemia, pancytopenia, hemolytic anemia, hypoprothrombinemia, hemorrhage. *Hepatic:* Hepatic dysfunction, including cholestasis. *Hypersensitivity:* Urticaria, pruritus, rash, fever, chills, reactions resembling serum sickness, eosinophilia, joint pain, edema, erythema, genital and anal pruritus, angioedema, Stevens-Johnson syndrome, erythema multiforme, toxic epidermal necrolysis, exfoliative dermatitis, and anaphylaxis. *Local:* IM injection: pain, tenderness, and induration. IV infusion: phlebitis and thrombophlebitis.

Pharmacokinetics: Cephalosporins readily cross the placenta and are excreted in breast milk. Except for cefuroxime, the presence of food delays absorption, resulting in later and lower peak levels, but does not affect the total amount absorbed. Cefuroxime's bioavailability is increased by administration with or shortly after food.

Interactions: A disulfiram-like reaction may occur if alcohol is ingested within 72 h after administration of cefamandole, cefoperazone, cefotetan, or moxalactam. The antibacterial activity of aminoglycosides, penicil-

---

CEPHALOSPORINS

First generation

Cefadroxil (Duracef, Ultracef) 1-2 g/day PO—Urinary tract infections

Cefazolin (Ancef, Kefzol) 250-1500 mg q 6 h IM/IV—Urinary tract infections

Cephalexin (Keflex, Keftab) 250-500 mg q 6-12 h PO—Prostatitis, urinary tract infections

Cephalothin (Keflin) 0.5-2 g q 4-6 h IM/IV—Urinary tract infections

Cephapirin (Cefadyl) 0.5-2 g q 4-6 h IM/IV—Urinary tract infections

Cephadrine (Anspor, Velosef) 250-1000 mg q 6-12 h PO—Urinary tract infections 0.5-1 g qid IM/IV

Second generation

Cefaclor (Ceclor) 250-500 mg q 8 h PO—Urinary tract infections

Cefamandole (Mandol) 0.5-1 g q 4-8 h IM/IV—Urinary tract infections

Cefmetazole (Zefazone) 2 g q 6-12 h IV—Urinary tract infections

Cefonicid (Monocid) 1 g/day IM/IV—Gonorrhea, urinary tract infections

Ceforanide (Precef) 0.5-1 g q 12 h IM/IV—Urinary tract infections

Cefotetan (Cefotan) 1-2 g q 12 h IM/IV—Gynecologic infections, urinary tract infections

Cefoxitin (Mefoxin) 1-2 g q 6-8 h IM/IV—Gynecologic infections, urinary tract infections

Cefuroxime (Ceftin, Kefurox, Zenacef) 125-500 mg q 12 h PO—Gonorrhea, urinary tract infections

Third generation

Cefixime (Suprax) 400 mg/day PO—Urinary tract infections

Cefoperazone (Cefobid) 2 g q 12 h IM/IV—Gynecologic infections, urinary tract infections

Cefotaxime (Claforan) 1-2 g q 6-8 h IM/IV—Gynecologic infections, urinary tract infections
1 g IM—Gonorrhea

Cefsulodin (Cefomondil) 0.5-3 g q 6 h IV—Urinary tract infections

Ceftazidime (Fortaz, Tazidime) 0.5-2 g q 8-12 h IM/IV—Gynecologic infections, urinary tract infections

Ceftizoxime (Cefizox) 0.5-2 g q 8-12 h IM/IV—Gonorrhea, gynecologic infections, urinary tract infections

Ceftriaxone (Rocephin) 1-2 g/day IM/IV—Gonorrhea, gynecologic infections, urinary tract infections

Moxalactam (Moxam) 2-6 g/day IM/IV—Gynecologic infections, urinary tract infections

PARENTERAL ADMINISTRATION OF ANTIINFECTIVES

Antiinfective agents tend to be very irritating. IM injection should be given deep into a large muscle. No more than 2 g of a medication should be injected into a single site. A record of injection sites should be kept to ensure maximal site rotation. Many agents can be reconstituted for intramuscular injection using a solution containing lidocaine or bacteriostatic water and benzyl alcohol to minimize pain; consult manufacturers' instructions.

Unintentional IV administration or injection too near a nerve should be carefully guarded against during IM injection. Always aspirate for blood; if any returns, withdraw the syringe. If a patient complains of immediate, severe pain upon injection, stop immediately; injection too near a nerve can cause permanent damage.

Assess IV sites daily; the risk of phlebitis is minimized by using a small needle in a large vein. Many antiinfectives should not be mixed with other medications; consult a compatibility chart.

lins, and chloramphenicol may be additive or synergistic with cephalosporins. Cephalosporins increase prothrombin time, altering anticoagulant requirements. Concurrent use of cephalosporins and nephrotoxic medications (e.g., aminoglycosides, bumetanide, colistin, ethacrynic acid, furosemide, polymyxin B, vancomycin) increases the risk of nephrotoxicity and should be avoided. Probenecid causes higher and prolonged serum levels.

Nursing considerations: Except for cefuroxime, which should be taken with food, oral cephalosporins should be taken on an empty stomach. They may be taken with meals, however, should GI upset occur. *Cefonicid, cefotaxime, ceftizoxime:* IM injection of 2 g should be split into two sites. Cephalosporins should not be mixed with aminoglycosides for IV infusion. Warn patients that dizziness may occur. They should avoid driving and other inherently hazardous activities until their specific response has been established. *Cefamandole, cefonicid, cefoperazone, cefotaxime, moxalactam:* Warn patients not to drink alcohol for 72 h after administration.

Cephalosporins interfere with urine glucose tests that use cupric sulfate (e.g., Benedict's solution, Clinitest). Patients who normally use these methods should use an alternative (e.g., Diastix, Tes-Tape) while taking cephalosporins. Cephalosporins may cause false-positive results in direct antiglobulin (Coombs') tests, interfering with hematologic studies and transfusion crossmatching.

SULFONAMIDES

Sulfonamides inhibit bacterial growth and reproduction and are effective against a wide range of gram-positive and gram-negative bacteria. They are commonly used to treat urinary tract infections and as alternatives to tetracyclines in the treatment of chlamydial infections. Some sulfonamides are available in fixed combination with the urinary analgesic phenazopyridine, as well as fixed in combination with trimethoprim, a bacteriostatic agent that acts synergistically to treat urinary tract infections.

Precautions/contraindications: Safe use during pregnancy has not been established, although sulfonamides are contraindicated during the third trimester. Use by nursing mothers is not recommended. Cautious use is required in patients with blood dyscrasias or G6PD deficiency, asthma, severe allergies, impaired hepatic or renal function, urinary obstruction, or a history of hypersensitity to sulfonamides, furosemide, thiazide diuretics, sulfonylureas, or carbonic anhydrase inhibitors.

Adverse effects: *Allergic:* Rash, pruritus, photosensitivity, fever, headache, joint pain, Stevens-Johnson syndrome, Lyell's syndrome, Behçet's syndrome. *CNS:* Ataxia, acute psychosis, confusion, depression, drowsiness, headache, dizziness, insomnia, and restlessness. *GI:* Nausea, vomiting (common), abdominal pain, anorexia, pharyngitis, glossitis, stomatitis, gastroenteritis, diarrhea, pancreatitis. *Hematologic:* Acute hemolytic anemia, agranulocytosis, aplastic anemia, eosinophilia, hypoprothrombinemia, leukopenia, methemoglobinemia. *Liver:* Jaundice, malaise, fever, right upper quadrant pain. *Renal:* Sulfonamide crystallization in urine (anuria, oliguria, hematuria, proteinuria, renal colic, urolithiasis). *Other:* Hypothyroidism, goiter, hypoglycemia, periorbital edema, scleral and conjunctival infection.

Pharmacokinetics: Sulfonamides readily cross the placenta and are excreted in breast milk.

Interactions: Aminobenzoates may antagonize the bacteriostatic effect of sulfonamides; concurrent use is not recommended. Antacids decrease absorption of oral sulfonamides, decreasing their therapeutic efficacy. Concurrent use with bone marrow depressants may increase leukopenic or thrombocytopenic effects, or both. Local parenteral anesthetics may decrease therapeutic efficacy. Some sulfonamides may form a precipitate with a by-product of methenamine metabolism; concurrent use is not recommended. Sulfonamides may increase the therapeutic or toxic effects of hydantoin anticonvulsants, methotrexate, oral anticoagulants, oral antidiabetic agents, phenylbutazone, and thiopental. Concurrent use with oral contraceptives may decrease the reliability of contraception and increase breakthrough bleeding. Sulfonamides may interfere with the thera-

---

SULFONAMIDES

Sulfacytine (Renoquid) 500 mg once, then 250 mg qid PO—Urinary tract infections

Sulfadiazine (Microsulfon) 2-4 g once, then 2-4 g/day PO—Urinary tract infections

Sulfamethizole (Proklar, Thiosulfil) 0.5-1 g tid or qid PO—Urinary tract infections

Sulfamethizole/phenazopyridine (Azo-Gamazole) 2-4 tabs bid or tid PO—Urinary tract infections (first 2 days)

Sulfamethizole/phenazopyridine/oxytetracycline (Urobiotic) 2-4 caps tid or qid PO—Urinary tract infections (first 2 days)

Sulfamethoxazole (Ganatol) 2 g once, then 1 g bid or tid PO—Chlamydial infections, gynecologic infections, urinary tract infections

Sulfamethoxazole/phenazopyridine (Azo-Ganantol) 4 tabs once, then 2 tabs q 12 h PO—Urinary tract infections (first 2 days)

Sulfamethoxazole/trimethoprim (co-trimoxazole) (Bactrim, Cotrim, Septra, Sulfamethoprim) 160 mg/800 mg q 12 h PO—Chlamydial infections, gonorrhea, gynecologic infections, urinary tract infections
8-12 mg/kg and 40-50 mg/kg daily IV

Sulfisoxazole (Gantrisin) 2-4 g once, then 4-8 g/day PO—Chlamydial infections, gynecologic infections, urinary tract infections
50 mg/kg once, then 100 mg/kg day IM/IV

Sulfisoxazole/phenazopyridine (Azo-Gantrisin) 4-6 tabs q 12 h PO—Urinary tract infections (first 2 days)

QUINOLONES

Cinoxacin (Cinobac) 1 g/day PO—Urinary tract infections

Ciprofloxacin (Cipro) 250-500 mg bid PO—Gonococcal urethritis, urinary tract infections, prostatitis

Nalidixic acid (NegGram) 1 g qid PO—Urinary tract infections

Norfloxacin (Noroxin) 400 mg bid PO—Urinary tract infections, prostatitis

---

peutic efficacy of penicillins. Probenecid decreases urinary excretion of sulfonamides. Concurrent use with other hemolytic or hepatotoxic agents may result in additive adverse effects.

Nursing considerations: Instruct patients to take oral sulfonamides with a full glass of water. Warn patients that drowsiness or dizziness may occur; they should avoid driving and other inherently hazardous activities until their specific response has been established. Warn patients that sulfonamides may turn urine rust colored or brown; combination agents that contain phenazopyridine may turn urine orange-red. These colors are clinically insignificant.

QUINOLONES

Quinolones are a group of antibiotics that act by inhibiting DNA replication, causing bacterial death. Four quinolones are useful in the treatment of urinary tract infections: cinoxacin, ciprofloxacin, nalidixic acid, and norfloxacin.

Precautions/contraindications: Quinolones have caused arthropathy in immature animals of various spe-

cies. Use during pregnancy, by nursing mothers, and in children is not recommended. Use is contraindicated in patients hypersensitive to quinolones. Quinolones should be used with caution in patients with CNS disorders or impaired renal or hepatic function.

Pharmacokinetics: All quinolones cross the placenta. Ciprofloxacin and nalidixic acid are excreted in breast milk; it is not known whether cinoxacin or norfloxacin is.

Nursing considerations: Quinolones may cause dizziness, drowsiness, or both. Patients should be warned not to drive or do other inherently hazardous activities until their specific response has been established. These effects may not occur until 30 minutes after the drug has been taken.

Cinoxacin

Side effects/adverse reactions: *Allergic:* Urticaria, pruritus, rash, edema. *CNS:* Headache, dizziness, insomnia, paresthesias, agitation, anxiety. *Eye:* Photophobia, vision problems. *GI:* Nausea, vomiting, anorexia, constipation, metallic taste, rectal itching, sore gums, abdominal cramps, diarrhea. *Other:* Swelling of extremities, arthropathy, palpitation, perineal burning, tinnitus.

Pharmacokinetics: *Peak level:* 2-3 h. *Half-life:* 1½ h. *Protein binding:* 60%-80%. *Duration of effect:* 6-8 h. *Route of elimination:* Urine.

Interactions: Probenecid decreases tubular excretion of cinoxacin, resulting in decreased concentration in the urine.

Nursing considerations: Cinoxacin may be taken with food.

Ciprofloxacin

Side effects/adverse reactions: *Allergic:* Rash, erythema, angioedema, edema of the face and hands, fever, flushing, photosensitivity, pruritus. *CNS:* Headache, restlessness, anorexia, ataxia, blurred vision, convulsive seizures, depression, dizziness, drowsiness, hallucinations, insomnia, irritability, lethargy, malaise, paresthesia, tinnitus, tremors, weakness. *CV:* Hypertension, syncope, angina pectoris, palpitations, atrial flutter, myocardial infarction, cerebral thrombosis, ventricular ectopy. *Eye:* Vision problems, eye pain. *GI:* Nausea, diarrhea, vomiting, abdominal pain. *Hematologic:* Eosinophilia, pancytopenia, leukopenia, anemia, leukocytosis, bleeding, diathesis. *Musculoskeletal:* Back pain, joint pain, or stiffness. *Renal:* Crystalluria, cylindruria, hematuria, nephritis, renal failure, urinary retention, polyuria, vaginitis, urethral bleeding. *Respiratory:* Dyspnea, bronchospasm, pulmonary embolism, edema of larynx or lungs, hemoptysis, hiccoughs.

Pharmacokinetics: *Peak level:* 1-2 h. *Half-life:* 4 h. *Protein binding:* 20%-40%. *Metabolism:* Liver. *Route of elimination:* Urine, feces, bile.

Interactions: Antacids, ferrous sulfate, and sucralfate may reduce absorption of ciprofloxacin by chelation; concurrent use is not recommended. Ciprofloxacin reduces the hepatic metabolism and clearance of caffeine, increasing the risk of CNS stimulation. Ciprofloxacin also reduces the hepatic metabolism and clearance of theophylline, increasing the risk of theophylline toxicity. Probenecid decreases tubular secretion of ciprofloxacin, decreasing urine concentration and increasing the risk of toxicity. Urinary alkalinizers reduce the solubility of ciprofloxacin in urine, increasing the risk of crystalluria and nephrotoxicity.

Nursing considerations: Instruct patients to take ciprofloxacin on an empty stomach. Warn patients against taking antacids within 2 hours of the time they take ciprofloxacin.

Nalidixic acid

Side effects/adverse reactions: *Allergic:* Rash, urticaria, eosinophilia, pruritus, photosensitivity, arthritis, arthralgia, anaphylaxis. *CNS:* Confusion, depression, dizziness, drowsiness, excitement, hallucinations, headache, insomnia, malaise, myalgia, peripheral neuritis, sensory abnormalities, syncope, increased intracranial pressure, seizures, sixth cranial nerve palsy, and acute toxic psychoses. *Eye:* Vision problems, nystagmus. *GI:* Nausea, vomiting, diarrhea, abdominal pain. *Hematologic:* Leukopenia, thrombocytopenia, hemolytic anemia. *Metabolic:* Metabolic acidosis, especially in premature infants.

Pharmacokinetics: *Peak urine level:* 3-4 h. *Half-life:* 6 h. *Protein binding:* 93%-97%. *Metabolism:* Liver. *Route of elimination:* Urine, feces.

Interactions: Antacids may interfere with absorption of nalidixic acid; space doses of each as far apart as possible. Concurrent use with nitrofurantoin decreases the therapeutic efficacy of nalidixic acid. Nalidixic acid may displace oral anticoagulants from protein-binding sites, causing increased anticoagulation.

Nursing considerations: Remain with patients for

several minutes after giving the first few doses; assess for adverse allergic or CNS effects. CNS effects tend to occur 30 min after initial administration, as well as after the second and third doses. Monitor hematology, as well as renal and liver function if therapy exceeds 2 wk. Nalidixic acid interferes with urine glucose tests that use cupric sulfate (e.g., Benedict's solution, Clinitest). Patients who normally use these methods should use an alternative (e.g., Diastix, Tes-Tape) while taking nalidixic acid.

Norfloxacin

Side effects/adverse reactions: *CNS:* Headache, dizziness, insomnia, depression, visual disturbances. *GI:* Nausea, vomiting, anorexia, abdominal cramps, diarrhea, dry mouth. *Allergic:* Rash, erythema. *Hematologic:* Eosinophilia, lowered WBC. *Hepatic:* Jaundice, fever, malaise, right upper quadrant pain, change in color or consistency of stools.

Pharmacokinetics: *Peak level:* 1-2 h. *Half-life:* 3-4 h. *Protein binding:* 10%-15%. *Route of elimination:* Urine, bile, feces.

Interactions: Antacids interfere with the absorption of norfloxacin. Nitrofurantoin antagonizes the antibacterial action of norfloxacin. Probenecid decreases urinary excretion of norfloxacin. Norfloxacin reduces the clearance of theophylline, increasing the risk of theophylline toxicity. Urinary alkalinizers reduce the solubility of norfloxacin in urine, increasing the risk of crystalluria and nephrotoxicity.

Nursing considerations: Norfloxacin should be taken on an empty stomach, with a full glass of water. Norfloxacin may cause dry mouth.

AMINOGLYCOSIDES

Aminoglycosides are broad-spectrum antibiotics used to treat serious infections in which less toxic agents are ineffective or contraindicated. Aminoglycosides act by interfering with bacterial protein synthesis. They have a high incidence of toxic reactions, which limits their clinical usefulness.

Precautions/contraindications: During pregnancy aminoglycosides should be used only in life-threatening situations or for severe infections in which less toxic drugs cannot be used. They should be used with caution and in reduced dosages in neonates. Ototoxicity and nephrotoxicity, the most serious adverse effects, are most likely to occur when these drugs are administered in high doses, for prolonged periods, or in conjunction with other ototoxic or nephrotoxic medications. Geriatric and dehydrated patients, as well as patients with impaired renal function, are at greatest risk. Aminoglycosides should be used with caution in patients with tinnitus, vertigo, or subclinical, high-frequency hearing impairment. Aminoglycosides should

PSEUDOMEMBRANOUS COLITIS

Pseudomembranous colitis is a potentially lethal consequence of antibiotic therapy that occurs while the drug is being taken or up to 2 wk after it is discontinued. Although this disorder is most often associated with clindamycin, ampicillin, and the cephalosporins, almost all antibiotics can cause it.

Pseudomembranous colitis is characterized by profuse watery and sometimes bloody diarrhea with cramps, tenesmus, and low-grade fever. Diarrhea occurs as a result of selective overgrowth of *Clostridium difficile*, which produces a toxin that causes the "summit lesion" characteristic of the disease. Sequelae of pseudomembranous colitis include dehydration, electrolyte imbalance, perforation, toxic megacolon, and death.

Patients should be instructed to report promptly diarrhea that occurs during and after antibiotic therapy. Such a report warrants immediate assessment to rule out pseudomembranous colitis. Physician notification is required, accompanied by a description of the onset and duration of the problem, character of stools, associated symptoms, and the patient's temperature and weight. A stool sample may be required. Patients should be told not to take anything for the diarrhea until receiving instructions from the physician, since antidiarrheals may delay removal of the toxin from the colon.

Once pseudomembranous colitis has been confirmed, antibiotics should be withdrawn, and treatment begun with metronidazole. Cases refractory to metronidazole usually respond to vancomycin. A similar colitis without pseudomembrane formation may occur and may even be more common. If *C. difficile* toxin is detected, it should be treated in the same manner as pseudomembranous colitis.

AMINOGLYCOSIDES

Amikacin (Amikin) 15 mg/kg/day IM/IV—Urinary tract infections

Gentamicin (Garamycin) 3-5 mg/kg/day IM/IV—Urinary tract infections

Netilmicin (Netromycin) 3-6.5 mg/kg/day IM/IV—Urinary tract infections

Tobramycin (Mebcin, Tobrex) 3-5 mg/kg/day IM/IV—Urinary tract infections

arachnoiditis, acute organic brain syndrome, visual disturbances, scotomas, eighth cranial nerve damage. *Other:* Arthralgia, hepatomegaly, splenomegaly, hepatic necrosis, increased salivation, alopecia, pseudotumor cerebri, pulmonary fibrosis, laryngeal edema.

Pharmacokinetics: Aminoglycosides cross the placenta, and small amounts are excreted in breast milk. Because aminoglycosides are not appreciably absorbed by the GI tract, parenteral administration is required. Following IM administration, aminoglycosides attain peak plasma level in ½-2 h and can be detected for 8-12 h. They are widely distributed into body fluids, with minimal protein binding. A small amount of each dose accumulates in body tissues. The plasma half-lives of aminoglycosides usually are 2-4 h; they are excreted unchanged in urine.

Interactions: Additive or synergistic activity occurs with beta-lactam antibiotics and vancomycin, although antagonism has also been reported. Penicillins, chloramphenicol, clindamycin, and tetracycline can inactivate aminoglycosides in vitro. Antivertigo agents (e.g., dimenhydrinate) may mask signs of aminoglycoside ototoxicity. Concurrent use of general anesthetics or neuromuscular blocking agents may cause additive neuromuscular blockade and subsequent respiratory paralysis. Indomethacin may increase serum aminoglycosides. The serum glycoside level and renal function should be monitored during concurrent use with nonsteroidal antiinflammatory agents. Other neurotoxic, nephrotoxic, or ototoxic medications may have additive effects with aminoglycosides.

Nursing considerations: The risk of toxicity and the narrow therapeutic range dictate dosage based on peak and trough levels during therapy.

TETRACYCLINES

Tetracyclines are broad-spectrum antibiotics useful against gram-positive bacteria, gram-negative bacteria, rickettsia, and spirochetes. Tetracyclines inhibit protein synthesis in bacteria, limiting growth and reproduction.

Precautions/contraindications: Tetracyclines are contraindicated during pregnancy unless alternate drugs

also be used with caution in patients with impaired renal function, neuromuscular disorders, or a history of hypersensitivity to aminoglycosides.

Side effects/adverse reactions: *Allergic:* Rash, urticaria, stomatitis, pruritus, generalized burning, fever, eosinophilia, transient agranulocytosis, anaphylaxis. *CV:* Tachycardia, myocarditis, hypotension, hypertension. *GI:* Nausea, vomiting, anorexia. *Hematologic:* Anemia, leukopenia, granulocytopenia, thrombocytopenia. *Local:* Irritation, pain, sterile abscess, subcutaneous atrophy, fat necrosis, thrombophlebitis. *Renal:* Tubular necrosis, renal function changes, proteinuria, cells or casts in urine, nonoliguric azotemia, aminoaciduria, metabolic acidosis, hypocalcemia, hypomagnesemia, hypokalemia. **Nervous system:** Peripheral neuropathy, encephalopathy, seizures, weakness, headache, tremor, lethargy, paresthesia, peripheral neuritis,

NEOMYCIN/POLYMYXIN B (NEOSPORIN G.U. IRRIGANT)

The neomycin sulfate and polymyxin B sulfate combination is used to provide continuous irrigation in urinary bladders to help prevent bacteriuria and septicemia associated with the use of indwelling catheters. Systemic absorption, with resultant toxicity, is the primary risk of this therapy. The drug should not be administered if there is any chance of inadvertent absorption, as could occur or in body spaces other than urinary bladders. The duration of therapy is also limited to 10 days to minimize the risk of systemic absorption.

Usual dosage: See manufacturer's instructions.

Precautions/contraindications: Use is contraindicated in pregnant women.

Nursing considerations: Irrigation should be continuous; flow should not be interrupted for more than a few minutes at a time. A superinfection of resistant organisms may occur. Urine specimens should be collected and cultured during irrigation to assess for resistant organisms. If any are found, the physician should be notified and appropriate steps taken to treat these organisms. If signs and symptoms of aminoglycoside toxicity develop, the physician is notified immediately.

TETRACYCLINES

Demeclocycline (Declomycin) 600 mg/day PO—Gonorrhea, gynecologic infections, urinary tract infections

Doxycycline (Vibramycin) 50-100 mg q 12 h PO/IV—Gonorrhea, gynecologic infections, prostatitis, syphilis, urinary tract infections

Methacycline (Rondomycin) 600 mg/day PO—Gonorrhea, gynecologic infections, syphilis, urinary tract infections

Minocycline (Minocin) 200 mg/day PO/IV—Gonorrhea, gynecologic infections, urinary tract infections, prostatitis

Oxytetracycline (Terramycin) 1-2 g/day PO—Gonorrhea, gynecologic infections, syphilis, urinary tract infections
  250-300 mg/day IM
  0.5-1 g/day IV

Tetracycline (Achromycin, Sumycin, Tetracyn) 1-2 g/day PO—Gonorrhea, gynecologic infections, syphilis, urinary tract infections
  250-300 mg/day IM
  250-500 mg q 12 h IV

---

are ineffective or cannot be used. Use by nursing mothers is not recommended. Tetracyclines can cause permanent tooth discoloration, enamel hypoplasia, and a decrease in the linear skeletal growth rate in children under 8 yr of age.

Tetracyclines should be used with caution, and at a reduced dosage, in patients with impaired renal function. Doxycycline and minocycline, which are less affected by renal function than hepatic function, should be used cautiously in patients with impaired hepatic function. Cautious use is also required in patients with a history of hypersensitivity to tetracyclines.

Side effects/adverse reactions: *CNS:* Dizziness, drowsiness, fatigue, ataxia. *Hematologic:* Hemolytic anemia, thrombocytopenia, leukocytosis, leukopenia, neutropenia, atypical lymphocytes. *GI:* Anorexia, thirst, nausea, vomiting, diarrhea, flatulence, abdominal discomfort, epigastric distress. *Liver:* Hepatotoxicity. *Skin:* Paresthesia, photosensitivity, discoloration of nails. *Local:* Pain with IM injection; thrombophlebitis with IV administration. *Allergic:* Dermatoses, rashes, pruritus, urticaria, eosinophilia, angioedema, pericarditis, anaphylaxis, serum sickness.

Pharmacokinetics: Tetracyclines are well absorbed in the stomach and upper small intestine and are distributed throughout all tissues and fluids, including across the placenta and into breast milk. They are deposited in the fetal skeleton and calcifying teeth.

Interactions: Aluminum, calcium, iron, magnesium, manganese, and zinc salts interfere with GI absorption of tetracyclines, decreasing their therapeutic efficacy. Kaolin, pectin, bismuth subsalicylate, cimetidine, cholestyramine, colestipol, and sodium bicarbonate also impair absorption of tetracyclines. Barbiturates, phenytoin, and carbamazepine speed the elimination of doxycycline; other tetracyclines are unaffected.

Tetracyclines enhance the effect of oral anticoagulants, either by causing hypoprothrombinemia or by interfering with vitamin K production by normal intestinal flora. Tetracyclines increase the bioavailability of digoxin but impair the therapeutic efficacy of penicillins, other beta-lactam antibiotics, and oral contraceptives. Concurrent use with methoxyflurane, bumetanide, thiazide diuretics, ethacrynic acid, and furosemide causes additive renal toxicity. Tetracycline hydrochloride may increase serum lithium.

Nursing considerations: Oral tetracyclines should be taken on an empty stomach with a full glass of water; patients should remain upright for 10 min to ensure esophageal passage. Tetracyclines should not be taken with milk, antacids, laxatives, iron, vitamins, or antidiarrheal preparations. They should not be given to patients with esophageal obstruction or compression. Observe patients carefully during the first 30 min after parenteral administration. Assess renal, hepatic, and hematologic systems periodically during prolonged tetracycline therapy. *Doxycycline, minocycline:* May be taken without regard to meals.

Warn patients that dizziness may occur. They should avoid driving and other inherently hazardous activities until their specific response has been established. Warn patients to avoid direct sun or ultraviolet light and to report erythema promptly. Tetracyclines interfere with urine glucose tests that use cupric sulfate (e.g., Benedict's solution, Clinitest). Patients who normally use these methods should use an alternative (e.g., Diastix, Tes-Tape) while taking tetracycline.

URINARY ANTIINFECTIVE DRUGS
Methenamine (Hiprex, Mandelamine, Urex)

Methenamine is a bactericidal agent that relies on its own catabolism to achieve its desired effect. Readily absorbed in the GI tract, methenamine is excreted intact into urine, where it is hydrolyzed into formaldehyde and ammonia. The formaldehyde metabolite is a nonspecific antibacterial agent effective against both grampositive and gram-negative bacteria. Hydrolysis depends on urine acidity of pH 5.5 or less.

Indications: Prophylaxis or suppression of recurrent urinary tract infections.

Usual dosage: *Methenamine, methenamine mandelate:* 1 g qid PO; *methenamine hippurate:* 1 g bid PO.

Precautions/contraindications: Safe use during pregnancy or by nursing mothers has not been established. Methenamine is contraindicated in patients with renal insufficiency, severe hepatic impairment, severe dehydration, or a history of hypersensitivity to methenamine. Cautious use is required in patients with gout.

Side effects/adverse reactions: *GI:* Abdominal cramps, anorexia, diarrhea, nausea, vomiting. *Renal:* Albuminuria, bladder irritation, hematuria, crystalluria, dysuria, urinary frequency or urgency. *Allergic:* Rash, pruritus, stomatitis, and urticaria. *Other:* Dyspnea, edema, headache, muscle cramps, lipoid pneumonitis (oral suspension form only), tinnitus.

Pharmacokinetics: Methenamine crosses the placenta and is excreted in breast milk. *Peak level:* 2 h (3-8 h with enteric-coated tablets). *Half-life:* 4 h. *Route of elimination:* Urine.

Interactions: Sulfamethizole forms an insoluble precipitate with formaldehyde in acidic urine; concurrent use is contraindicated. Urinary alkalinizers impair the therapeutic effect of methenamine.

Nursing considerations: Methenamine should be taken with food or a full glass of water, or enteric-coated tablets should be used to decrease gastric irritation. Instruct patients about the need to maintain acid urine. Teach them how to monitor urine pH and how foods affect urine pH. Meat, fish, fowl, shellfish, eggs, cheese, peanut butter, corn, lentils, cranberries, plums, prunes, the juices of these fruits, breads, and pasta tend to increase urine acidity. Milk, cream, buttermilk, vegetables (except corn and lentils), and fruit (except cranberries, plums, and prunes) tend to decrease urine acidity. Warn patients not to take over-the-counter medications that contain sodium carbonate or sodium bicarbonate.

Nitrofurantoin (Furadantin, Macrodantin)

Nitrofurantoin acts by inhibiting several bacterial enzyme systems. Although it usually inhibits only bacterial growth and reproduction, nitrofurantoin destroys bacteria in sufficient concentration and a sufficiently acid urine.

Indications: Treatment and prevention of urinary tract infections.

Usual dosage: 50-100 mg qid PO (acute infection); 50-100 mg/day PO (suppression of chronic infections).

Precautions/contraindications: Nitrofurantoin is contraindicated in pregnant women at term and in infants younger than 1 mo of age because of the risk of hemolytic anemia. Its safe use during pregnancy or by nursing mothers has not been established. Nitrofurantoin is contraindicated in patients with a history of hypersensitivity to nitrofurantoin, as well as in patients with anuria, oliguria, or significant renal impairment. Cautious use is required in patients with G6PD deficiency because of the risk of hemolysis, as well as in patients with anemia, diabetes mellitus, electrolyte imbalances, vitamin B deficiency, or debilitating disease.

Side effects/adverse reactions: *CNS:* Cerebellar dysfunction, dizziness, drowsiness, headache, intracranial hypertension, nystagmus, retrobulbar neuritis, peripheral neuropathy, trigeminal neuralgia. *Hematologic:* Hemolytic anemia, granulocytopenia, thrombocytopenia, eosinophilia, agranulocytosis, leukopenia, megaloblastic anemia. *GI:* Anorexia, nausea, vomiting, diarrhea, abdominal pain, parotitis, pancreatitis. *Renal:* Crystalluria. *Allergic:* Anaphylaxis, drug fever, rashes, pruritus, urticaria, angioedema, exfoliative dermatitis, erythema multiforme, Stevens-Johnson syndrome, arthralgia, cholestatic jaundice, asthmatic symptoms. *Respiratory:* Dyspnea, cough, chest pain, permanent impairment of pulmonary function. *Hepatic:* Hepatitis and cholestatic jaundice. *Other:* Photosensitivity, alopecia, hypotension.

Pharmacokinetics: Nitrofurantoin is rapidly absorbed in the GI tract. It crosses the placenta and is excreted in breast milk. *Peak urine level:* 30 min. *Half-life:* 20 min. *Protein binding:* 20%-60%. *Route of elimination:* Urine, bile.

Interactions: Urinary alkalinizers may decrease the drug's therapeutic efficacy. Antacids containing magnesium trisilicate decrease GI absorption, thereby decreasing therapeutic efficacy. Anticholinergic medications increase GI absorption, thereby increasing therapeutic efficacy. Nitrofurantoin antagonizes the effect of nalidixic acid. Probenecid decreases nitrofurantoin tubular secretion, lowering urine levels but raising serum levels and the risk of adverse effects.

Nursing considerations: Warn patients that urine may turn dark yellow or brown—an expected and harmless phenomenon. Monitor the patient's pulmonary status closely, especially during the first week of therapy. Liver function and peripheral neurologic status should also be monitored. Nitrofurantoin should be taken with food or milk to minimize gastric irritation. Nausea occurs commonly with microcrystals, less commonly with macrocrystals (Macrodantin). Nitrofurantoin can stain the teeth if direct contact occurs: tablets should not be crushed, and the oral suspension should be diluted in milk, water, infant formula, or fruit juice; patients should rinse their mouths after taking the drug.

Trimethoprim (Proloprim, Trimpex)

Trimethoprim destroys bacteria by inhibiting bacterial metabolism of folic acid. It is commonly used in combination form with sulfamethoxazole but is also effective alone against most common urinary tract pathogens.

Indications: Urinary tract infections.

Usual dosage: 200 mg/day PO.

Precautions/contraindications: Trimethoprim may interfere with folic acid metabolism; it should be used during pregnancy only if the benefits outweigh potential risk. It should be used with caution in children with the fragile X chromosome associated with mental retardation. Trimethoprim is contraindicated in patients with a history of hypersensitivity to it or who have megaloblastic anemia secondary to folate deficiency. Cautious use is required in patients with impaired renal or hepatic function or with possible folate deficiency.

Side effects/adverse reactions: *Hematologic:* Megaloblastic anemia, neutropenia, thrombocytopenia, methemoglobinemia, leukopenia. *GI:* Epigastric discomfort, glossitis, nausea, vomiting, abnormal taste sensation. *Skin:* Rashes, pruritus, exfoliative dermatitis, phototoxicity. *Other:* Fever.

Pharmacokinetics: Trimethoprim crosses the placenta and is excreted in breast milk. It is readily absorbed from the GI tract. *Peak level:* 1-4 h. *Half-life:* 8-11 h. *Protein binding:* 42%-46%. *Metabolism:* Liver. *Route of elimination:* Urine.

Interactions: Trimethoprim inhibits phenytoin metabolism, increasing the risk of phenytoin toxicity. Concurrent use with phenytoin also increases the incidence of folate deficiency.

Nursing considerations: Monitor hematologic status.

MEDICATIONS THAT ALTER BLADDER FUNCTION

ANTICHOLINERGICS/ANTISPASMODICS/SPASMOLYTICS

A group of medications known as anticholinergics/antispasmodics/spasmolytics is the mainstay of pharmacologic therapy of instability incontinence. These agents relax smooth muscle in the bladder, increasing the volume that stimulates involuntary contraction, decreasing the amplitude of involuntary contractions, and increasing the total bladder capacity.

Precautions/contraindications: These agents should be used during pregnancy only when clearly needed. Anticholinergic agents may inhibit lactation; use by nursing mothers is not recommended. Cautious use is required in children and geriatric patients. Geriatric patients may respond to usual doses of anticholinergic agents with excitement, agitation, drowsiness, or confusion. Cautious use is required in patients with a history of sensitivity to belladonna alkaloids or derivatives, as well as in those with impaired hepatic or renal function. Medication-related tachycardia may affect individuals with hyperthyroidism, existing tachycardia, cardiac disease, and acute hemorrhage. GI hypomotility may exacerbate reflux esophagitis, gastric ulcers, GI infections, intestinal atony, ulcerative colitis, and pyloric obstruction; paralytic ileus may result in some of these conditions. Esophageal sphincter relaxation may also exacerbate reflux esophagitis. Anticholinergic effects may exacerbate benign prostatic hyperplasia, hypertension, myasthenia, urinary retention, toxemia of pregnancy, xerostomia (dry mouth), brain damage in children, glaucoma, and autonomic neuropathy. An abnormal increase in pupillary dilation and tachycardia may occur in patients with Down's syndrome. A decrease in bronchial secretions may cause inspissation and formation of bronchial plugs in patients with chronic lung disease.

Side effects/adverse reactions: Although these medications share basic pharmacologic properties, antispasmodics and spasmolytics generally have fewer adverse effects than anticholinergics. Differences also exist among primarily anticholinergic agents. *Allergic:* Anaphylaxis, urticaria, rash. *CNS:* Confusion, drowsiness, euphoria, amnesia, fatigue, dreamless sleep, headache, nervousness, weakness, dizziness. Toxicity: paradoxical excitement (restlessness, hallucinations, delirium). *CV:* Bradycardia, tachycardia, dysrhythmias, AV dissociation, cutaneous vasodilation (causing a flushing of the skin). *GI:* Xerostomia, reduced gastric acid secretion, hypomotility, prolonged GI transit time, constipation, relaxation of lower esophageal sphincter, nausea, vomiting. *GU:* Urinary hesitancy and retention, impotence. *Ophthalmic:* Mydriasis, cycloplegia, increased intraocular pressure, blurred vision, photophobia (especially with scopolamine). *Respiratory:* Reduced bronchial secretions, bronchodilation. *Other:* Anhidrosis.

Interactions: Antacids and adsorbent antidiarrheals reduce GI absorption of these agents, with subsequent loss of efficacy. Doses should be spaced at least 1 h apart. These agents decrease GI absorption of ketoconazole; if used, ketoconazole should be administered at least 2 h before one of these agents. Concurrent use with potassium chloride increases the risk of GI lesions. Concurrent use with monoamine oxidase (MAO) inhibitors or other medications with anticholinergic activity may result in intensified anticholinergic effects. Urinary alkalinizers delay excretion of these agents, increasing the therapeutic and adverse effects. Concurrent use with antimyasthenic agents or opioid analgesics increases the risk of GI hypomotility. Concurrent use with glucocorticoids, corticotropin, or haloperidol may increase intraocular pressure; these agents can also decrease haloperidol's efficacy. Concurrent use with guanadrel, guanethidine, or reserpine may antagonize the inhibitory action of anticholinergic agents on gastric acid secretion. Metoclopramide's effects on GI motility may be antagonized by these agents. *Scopolamine:* Scopolamine may decrease the emetic effect of apomorphine in the treatment of poisoning; concurrent use can also cause additive CNS depressant effects. Concurrent use with CNS depression-producing agents can cause additive CNS depressant effects.

Nursing considerations: Unless otherwise indicated, anticholinergic agents should be administered ½-1 h before a meal. Anticholinergic agents may antagonize the effect of pentagastrin and histamine; they should be held for 24 h before conducting gastric acid secretion tests. Warn patients not to drive or do other hazardous activities until their response to their medication has been established. Instruct patients about orthostatic hypotension and how to minimize its effects. Instruct patients about dry mouth. Warn patients to use caution during hot weather, since anticholinergic agents inhibit sweating. Paralytic ileus is a special risk for patients with GI problems or who are taking other medications that predispose them to GI hypomotility. These patients should be warned of this risk and told to notify their physician promptly should any GI problems occur. *Transdermal scopolamine:* Patients should wash and dry their hands thoroughly before and after applying the patches; the patches should be applied to hairless, intact skin behind the ear. Warn patients that alcohol's effects may be enhanced while using the patch. Residual cycloplegia and mydriasis may interfere with neuroradiologic tests for intracranial neoplasm, subdural hematoma, or aneurysm.

Dicyclomine (Bentyl)

Dicyclomine is an antispasmodic agent with little anticholinergic activity. It has few adverse effects at the usual dosage.

Indications: Instability (urge or reflex) incontinence.
Usual dosage: 10-20 mg tid or qid PO.
Pharmacokinetics: *Onset of action:* 1-2 h. *Peak level:* 60-90 min. *Duration of effect:* 4 h. *Metabolism:* Liver. *Route of elimination:* Urine (80%), feces (8%).

Flavoxate (Urispas)

Flavoxate has a direct spasmolytic effect on smooth muscle, as well as anticholinergic, local anesthetic, and analgesic properties. Adverse effects are relatively uncommon.

Indications: Instability incontinence, bladder spasm, dysuria.
Usual dosage: 100-200 mg tid or qid PO.
Pharmacokinetics: *Onset of action:* 1 h. *Peak level:* 2 h. *Route of elimination:* Urine.

Hyoscyamine (Cystospaz, Levsin)

Hyoscyamine is an anticholinergic agent with typical anticholinergic side effects.

Indications: Cystitis, neurogenic bladder, renal colic, and bladder spasm associated with infection, inflammation, or use of an indwelling catheter.
Usual dosage: *Hyoscyamine:* 0.15-0.3 mg qid PO; *hyoscyamine sulfate:* 0.125-0.25 mg qid PO, or extended-release: 0.375 mg q 12 h.
Pharmacokinetics: *Onset of action:* 20-30 min. *Duration of effect:* 4-6 h. *Half-life:* 3½ h. *Metabolism:* Liver. *Route of elimination:* Urine.

Hyoscyamine/scopolamine (Bellafoline)

Indications: Instability incontinence, bladder spasms.
Usual dosage: 0.25-0.5 mg tid PO.

Methantheline (Banthine)

Methantheline is an anticholinergic agent that has fewer CNS and ocular effects than other anticholinergic agents but greater orthostatic hypotension.

Indications: Instability incontinence, bladder spasm.
Usual dosage: 50-100 mg qid PO.
Pharmacokinetics: *Onset of action:* 30 min. *Duration of effect:* 6 h.

Oxybutynin (Ditropan)

Oxybutynin is an antispasmodic agent with anticholinergic and local anesthetic activity. Its adverse reactions reflect its anticholinergic nature.

Indications: Instability incontinence, bladder spasms.
Usual dosage: 5 mg bid or tid PO.

Pharmacokinetics: *Onset of action:* 30-60 min. *Peak effect:* 3-6 h. *Duration of effect:* 6-10 h. *Metabolism:* Liver. *Route of elimination:* Urine.

Propantheline bromide (Pro-Banthine)

Propantheline is an anticholinergic agent with fewer CNS and ocular effects than other anticholinergic agents but greater orthostatic hypotension.

Indications: Instability incontinence, bladder spasm.

Usual dosage: 15-30 mg before meals, then 30 mg at HS, up to 120 mg/day PO.

Pharmacokinetics: Food decreases absorption of propantheline. *Onset of action:* 30-45 min. *Duration of effect:* 4-6 h. *Half-life:* 1.6 h. *Metabolism:* GI tract, liver. *Route of elimination:* All body fluids.

Scopolamine (Transderm-Scop)

Scopolamine is an anticholinergic agent with more pronounced CNS effects than other agents. Although primarily used as an antiemetic or antivertigo agent, it occasionally is used to treat unstable bladder contractions.

Indications: Instability incontinence, bladder spasms.

Usual dosage: 1 patch to postauricular skin q 3 days.

Pharmacokinetics: *Onset of action:* 4 h; 0.5 mg released at a constant rate over 72 h. *Duration of effect:* Up to 72 h. *Route of elimination:* Urine.

Terolidine

Terolidine is an investigational agent with calcium channel–blocking and anticholinergic properties that has been marketed in Europe since 1986. Side effects common to other calcium antagonist are rare.

Indications: Instability incontinence, bladder spasms.

Usual dosage: 25 mg bid PO.

Pharmacokinetics: *Half-life:* 60 h; steady-state achieved in 10 days.

TRICYCLIC ANTIDEPRESSANT

Imipramine (Tofranil)

Imipramine is a tricyclic antidepressant that is structurally related to the phenothiazines. Like other tricyclic antidepressants, it blocks reuptake of norepinephrine and serotonin by presynaptic neurons in the CNS. It has anticholinergic, antihistaminic, hypotensive, sedative, mild analgesic, and peripheral vasodilator effects. Its use in urge incontinence and enuresis is thought to be related to its anticholinergic activity. Although primarily used to treat urge incontinence and nocturnal enuresis in children, imipramine has also been used to treat neurogenic disorders of urine storage. It reportedly is useful in conjunction with propantheline or oxybutynin to treat hyperreflexia.

XEROSTOMIA (DRY MOUTH)

Xerostomia is a common side effect of anticholinergic agents, caused by decreased salivation. An annoyance in the short term, chronic xerostomia hinders mechanisms that normally ensure oral health, possibly resulting in caries, oral infections, and periodontal disease.

Patients taking medications that cause xerostomia should be warned of these sequelae and instructed in how to prevent and recognize them. Patients need to practice strict oral hygiene and receive dental care regularly. Patients should be instructed to brush with a soft toothbrush after every meal and floss daily before brushing. If they note painful or bleeding gums, they should see their dentist promptly. Other signs of problems are halitosis (bad breath) and teeth that are sensitive to heat or cold.

Patients should be instructed to drink plenty of water (unless restricted) and to rinse the mouth frequently with tepid water. They should avoid commercial mouthwashes because these often contain alcohol, which exacerbates the problem. Sugarless gum, sugarless sourballs, lemon drops, and bits of ice can also provide relief. However, if these measures fail, saliva substitutes are available.

Indications: Instability incontinence, enuresis.

Usual dosage: 75-100 mg/day PO.

Precautions/contraindications: Safe use during pregnancy has not been established. Serious adverse reactions may occur to nursing infants. Adolescent and elderly patients are especially sensitive to dosage changes and side effects. Cautious use is required in patients with a history of hypersensitivity to tricyclic medications, cardiovascular disorders, defects in bundle-branch conduction, asthma, GI disorders, urinary retention, glaucoma or increased intraocular pressure, hepatic or renal function impairment, hyperthyroidism, prostate hypertrophy, seizure disorders, active alcoholism, bipolar disorder, schizophrenia, and blood disorders and during the acute post-MI recovery period.

Side effects/adverse reactions: *Anticholinergic:* Dry mouth, nose, and throat, blurred vision, increased intraocular pressure, hyperthermia, constipation, adynamic ileus, urinary retention, delayed micturition, dilation of the urinary tract, esophageal reflux, hiatal hernia. *CNS:* Drowsiness (most frequent), weakness, lethargy, fatigue, agitation, excitement, nightmares, restlessness, insomnia, confusion, disturbed coordination, disorientation, headache, delusions, hallucinations, anxiety, emotional instability, exacerbation of depression, hypomania, panic, hostility, euphoria, exacerbation of psychosis, EEG changes, seizures, coma. *Other nervous system:* Peripheral neuropathy, dizziness, tinnitus, dysarthria, numbness, tingling, paresthesia, ataxia. *Allergic:* Rash, erythema, petechiae, urticaria, pruritus, eosinophilia, edema, drug fever, photosensitivity. Some brands contain tartrazine, which causes an allergic reaction in some people, especially those hypersensitive to aspirin. *Blood:* Agranulocytosis, thrombocytopenia, eosinophilia, leukopenia, purpura. *CV:* Orthostatic hypotension, ECG changes, conduction disturbances, dysrhythmias, tachycardia, bradycardia, ventricular fibrillation, ventricular ectopy, syncope, hypertension, thrombosis, thrombophlebitis, stroke, CHF, peripheral vasospasm, collapse, sudden death. *Endocrine:* Increased or decreased libido, impotence, testicular swelling, painful ejaculation, breast engorgement, galactorrhea, gynecomastia, SIADH, elevation or reduction of serum glucose. *GI:* Anorexia, nausea, vomiting, diarrhea, abdominal cramps, epigastric distress, stomatitis, peculiar taste, black tongue. *Hepatic:* Jaundice, hepatitis. *Other:* Alopecia, flushing, chills, diaphoresis, interstitial pneumonitis, parotid swelling, increased appetite, weight gain or loss.

Pharmacokinetics: Imipramine is excreted in breast milk. *Peak level:* 1-2 h. *Half-life:* 8-16 h.

Interactions: Enhanced CNS depression, anticholinergic effects, or both can occur with concurrent use of other CNS depression-producing agents (including alcohol), anticholinergic agents, and medications with anticholinergic activity. Concurrent use with MAO inhibitors may cause hyperpyretic episodes, severe convulsions, hypertensive crisis, and death. Concurrent use with cocaine or pimozide can result in cardiac dysrhythmias. Sympathomimetic agents may enhance cardiovascular effects. Imipramine may decrease the therapeutic efficacy of anticonvulsants, methylphenidate, clonidine, guanadrel, and guanethidine. Concurrent use with glucocorticoids may exacerbate mental depression. Concurrent use with antithyroid agents increases the risk of agranulocytosis. Barbiturates and carbamazepine decrease plasma imipramine. Imipramine enhances the therapeutic effect of oral anticoagulants and increases the hazards of electroconvulsive therapy. Concurrent use with disulfiram may cause transient delirium. Concurrent use with intrathecal metrizamide may cause additive seizure threshold–lowering effects; withhold imipramine for at least 48 h before and 24 h after myelography.

Nursing considerations: Imipramine should be taken with or immediately after food to minimize gastric irritation. Tell patients that positive results usually take 1-2 wk to occur. Instruct patients that prompt reporting of their response to imipramine is required to prevent serious adverse effects. Warn patients that many over-the-counter medications contain agents that interact with imipramine and that they should not take medications of any kind without first consulting their physician. Warn patients to avoid driving or other hazardous activities until their response to imipramine has been established. Warn patients about orthostatic hypotension and how to minimize its effects. Instruct patients about dry mouth.

CHOLINERGIC AGENT

Bethanechol (Urecholine)

Bethanechol is a cholinergic (parasympathomimetic) medication that directly stimulates muscarinic receptors, primarily in the urinary and GI tracts. Its principal actions are to increase esophageal and ureteral peristalsis, contract the detrusor muscle of the urinary bladder, increase maximal voluntary voiding pressure, and decrease the capacity of the urinary bladder. Bethanechol induces the strongest contractions in denervated smooth muscle; when injected SC it is used to diagnose neurogenic bladder.

Indications: Urinary retention caused by deficient detrusor contractility.

Usual dosage: 10-50 mg bid-qid PO; 2.5-5 mg tid or qid SC.

Precautions/contraindications: The safe use of bethanechol during pregnancy, while nursing, or in children under 8 yr of age has not been established. Never administer bethanechol by IM or IV routes; a severe cholinergic reaction is likely. Bethanechol is contraindicated when the strength or integrity of the GI or bladder wall is in question or when increased muscular activity of the GI tract or urinary bladder may cause harm. Cautious use is required in patients with a history of hypersensitivity to bethanechol, hyperthyroidism, peptic ulcer, obstructive pulmonary disease, latent or active bronchial asthma, pronounced bradycardia or hypotension, hypertension, vasomotor instability, coronary artery disease, AV conduction defects, epilepsy, parkinsonism, marked vagotonia, cystitis, or bacteriuria.

Side effects/adverse reactions: Adverse effects are dose related and rare with oral administration. *CV:* Hypotension with reflex tachycardia, orthostatic hypotension, vasomotor response, heart block, atrial fibrillation (hyperthyroid patients), chest pain. *Eyes:* Lacrimation, miosis. *GI:* Abdominal cramps, diarrhea, salivation, nausea, vomiting, substernal pressure, involuntary defecation, colic, belching, borborygmus. *GU:* Urgency. *Other:* General malaise. *Respiratory:* Bronchial constriction, asthmatic attack, dyspnea. *Skin:* Flushing, sweating, sensation of heat about the face.

Pharmacokinetics: Bethanechol does not cross the blood-brain barrier. *Onset of action:* 30 min (PO); 5-15 min (SC). *Peak effect:* 60-90 min (PO); 15-30 min (SC). *Duration of effect:* 1 h (PO); 2 h (SC).

Interactions: Concurrent use with ganglionic blocking agents (e.g., mecamylamine) may cause a critical hypotensive response. Cholinesterase inhibitors (e.g., ambenonium, neostigmine) produce additive cholinergic effects. Procainamide and quinidine antagonize the effects of bethanechol.

Nursing considerations: Oral doses should be taken on an empty stomach. Inadvertent IM or IV administration must not occur; aspirate carefully for blood before parenteral administration. Assess vital signs q 5 min until stable after SC injection. Atropine should be immediately available to treat overdose or a cholinergic reaction. Teach patients how to recognize and manage orthostatic hypotension. Warn patients that dizziness may occur. They should avoid driving and other inherently hazardous activities until their specific response has been established. A bed pan or urinal should be immediately available to the patient; supervise ambulation.

ALPHA-SYMPATHOMIMETIC AGENTS
Ephedrine, pseudoephedrine, phenylpropanolamine

Alpha-sympathomimetic medications stimulate alpha-adrenergic receptors in the bladder neck and proximal urethra and are commonly used to treat stress incontinence. These agents are common ingredients in over-the-counter cough and cold medications. Phenylpropanolamine also depresses the appetite center in the CNS and is used as a diet aid in prescription and over-the-counter medications.

Indications: Stress incontinence, enuresis, retrograde ejaculation.

Usual dosage: *Ephedrine:* 25-50 mg qid PO; *pseudoephedrine:* 30-60 mg qid PO; *phenylpropanolamine:* 25 mg tid PO.

Precautions/contraindications: Safe use of these agents during pregnancy or by nursing mothers has not been established. Cautious use is required in patients with a history of hypersensitivity to sympathomimetic agents, glaucoma, coronary artery disease, angina, cardiac dysrhythmias, hypertension, hyperthyroidism, prostate hypertrophy, or diabetes mellitus.

Side effects/adverse reactions: Adverse effects are generally less pronounced and occur less often with pseudoephedrine and phenylpropanolamine. *CNS:* Insomnia, headache, nervousness, confusion, restlessness, anxiety, dizziness (with toxicity: euphoria, delirium, hallucinations, irritability, suicidal behavior, personality changes, convulsions, respiratory depression, somnolence, coma, paranoid psychosis). *CV:* Palpitation, tachycardia, precordial pain, dysrhythmias. *GI:* Nausea, vomiting, anorexia. *GU:* Dysuria, urinary retention. *Other:* Sweating, thirst, hyperglycemia.

Pharmacokinetics: These agents are excreted in breast milk. *Ephedrine:* Onset of action: 15-60 min. Duration of effect: 2-5 h. *Metabolism:* Liver. *Route of*

elimination: Urine; acid urine increases excretion. **Pseudoephedrine:** *Onset:* 30 min. *Duration:* 4-6 h. **Phenylpropanolamine:** *Onset:* 15-30 min. *Duration:* 3 h (extended-release form: 12-16 h).

Interactions: These agents decrease the therapeutic efficacy of antihypertensive agents (including diuretics). Concurrent use with beta-adrenergic blocking agents may result in unopposed alpha-adrenergic activity: hypertension, bradycardia, and heart block may occur. Concurrent use with CNS stimulation–producing agents (including caffeine and cocaine) or other sympathomimetic agents may cause additive CNS stimulation. Digitalis glycosides sensitize the heart to sympathomimetic agents; dysrhythmias may result. Diuretics decrease the therapeutic efficacy of sympathomimetic agents. Concurrent use with hydrocarbon inhalation anesthetics may cause severe ventricular dysrhythmias. Concurrent use with levodopa may also cause cardiac dysrhythmias; decreased sympathomimetic dosage is recommended.

Concurrent use of these agents with MAO inhibitors causes prolonged and intensified cardiostimulation and vasopressor effects. Concurrent use within 14 days of one another is contraindicated. These agents decrease the antianginal effects of nitrates. Concurrent use of one of these agents and thyroid hormones may cause enhanced effects of either. Concurrent use with tricyclic antidepressants may cause hypertension as a result of enhanced sympathomimetic vasopressor effects. *Ephedrine:* Ephedrine alters the metabolism of glucocorticoids and corticotropin. Alpha-adrenergic blocking agents decrease the pressor response to ephedrine. Dihydroergotamine, ergoloid mesylates, ergonovine, ergotamine, methylergonovine, methysergide, and oxytocin enhance vasoconstriction caused by ephedrine, resulting in peripheral vascular ischemia and gangrene or severe hypertension. Methyldopa decreases the therapeutic efficacy of ephedrine. Concurrent use of ephedrine and ritodrine may cause enhanced effects of either agent. Urinary alkalinizers decrease excretion of ephedrine and pseudoephedrine, with subsequent prolongation of effects. *Pseudoephedrine:* Rauwolfia alkaloids decrease the therapeutic efficacy of pseudoephedrine.

Nursing considerations: Avoid administration at night, when stress incontinence is not provoked. Warn patients that many over-the-counter medications— especially cough and cold remedies and diet pills— contain agents that add to the effect of these medications, increasing the likelihood and severity of side effects. Tell them to check with their physician before taking any over-the-counter medications. *Ephedrine:* Warn patients that dizziness may occur. They should avoid driving and other inherently hazardous activities until their specific response has been established.

Teach patients how to check their pulse; tell them to report an increase in rate or inception of an irregular rhythm. *Pseudoephedrine:* Tablets may be crushed and taken with a fluid of the patient's choice.

ALPHA-BLOCKERS

Benign prostatic hyperplasia (BPH) causes symptoms in two ways: (1) anatomic obstruction, and (2) increased bladder outlet resistance resulting from sympathetic stimulation of alpha-adrenoceptors in the prostate, prostatic capsule, and bladder neck. Since 1978, alpha-adrenergic antagonists have been used to relieve symptoms of BPH by decreasing bladder outlet resistance. Phenoxybenzamine was the first such agent used. It blocks both alpha$_1$ and alpha$_2$ receptors and has been used with considerable success. However, phenoxybenzamine's adverse effects, as well as concerns that it could cause cancer, have prompted researchers to seek alternatives. Two that have come into favor are prazosin and terazosin—alpha$_1$ antagonists that have fewer adverse effects and have proved useful in treating hypertension.

Phenoxybenzamine (Dibenzyline)

Indications: Benign prostatic hyperplasia, bladder neck dyssynergia, detrusor, striated sphincter dyssynergia.

Usual dosage: 20-60 mg/day PO.

Precautions/contraindications: Elderly patients may be especially sensitive to hypotensive and hypothermic effects. Cautious use is required in patients with a history of hypersensitivity to phenoxybenzamine, cerebrovascular insufficiency, congestive heart failure, coronary artery disease, renal function impairment, or respiratory infection.

Side effects/adverse reactions: *CNS:* Lethargy and shock (overdose only), drowsiness, fatigue, dizziness, confusion, headache, dry mouth. *CV:* Orthostatic hypotension, tachycardia, palpitation. *GI:* GI irritation, vomiting. *Ophthalmic:* Miosis, drooping of eyelids. *Respiratory:* Nasal congestion. *Other:* Inhibition of ejaculation, allergic contact dermatitis.

Pharmacokinetics: *Peak effect:* 4-6 h. *Half-life:* 5-12 h. *Metabolism:* Liver. *Route of elimination:* Urine.

Interactions: Vasodilation is exaggerated when phenoxybenzamine is used with alcohol. Phenoxybenzamine decreases the therapeutic efficacy of diazoxide. Concurrent use with guanadrel or guanethidine increases the risk of orthostatic hypotension and bradycardia. Sympathomimetic agents decrease the therapeutic efficacy of phenoxybenzamine. With agents that stimulate both alpha- and beta-adrenergic receptors (e.g., epinephrine), vasodilation, severe hypotension, and tachycardia may result.

Nursing considerations: Taking the drug with milk may reduce GI irritation. While the optimal dosage is being determined, monitor vital signs in both recumbent and standing positions; patients should be observed for at least 4 days between dose increases. Instruct patients about the risk of orthostatic hypotension and how to minimize its effects. Tell patients that adverse effects generally decrease with continued use, but orthostatic hypotension and palpitation may reappear under conditions that cause vasodilation (e.g., exercise, eating a large meal). Tell patients that beneficial effects may not appear for several weeks and that effects may last several days after therapy has stopped. Warn patients that many over-the-counter medications contain agents that interact with phenoxybenzamine and that they should not take any without first consulting their physician.

Prazosin (Minipress)

Indications: Benign prostatic hypertrophy, bladder neck dyssynergia, detrusor, striated sphincter dyssynergia.

Usual dosage: 1-2 mg daily, up to 8 mg daily in 2-3 divided doses PO.

Precautions/contraindications: Cautious use is required in patients with a history of hypersensitivity to prazosin, renal function impairment, and in men with sickle-cell trait.

Side effects/adverse reactions: Side effects usually disappear with continued therapy. *CNS:* Dizziness, drowsiness, headache, fatigue, paresthesias, depression, vertigo, nervousness, hallucinations, nightmares, lethargy. *CV:* Palpitations, syncope, tachycardia, orthostatic hypotension, exacerbation of angina, edema. *GI:* Nausea, vomiting, diarrhea, constipation, abdominal pain, pancreatitis. *GU:* Urinary frequency, incontinence, impotence, priapism (especially in men with sickle-cell anemia). *Respiratory:* Dyspnea, nasal congestion. *First-dose effect:* Marked orthostatic hypotension and syncope ½-2 hours after initial dose, increase in dosage, or addition of a hypotensive agent. Patients remain at risk for this effect for several days. *Other:* Asthenia, sweating, blurred vision, tinnitus, epistaxis, reddening of sclera, rash, alopecia, pruritus, fever.

Pharmacokinetics: *Onset of action:* 2 h. *Peak effect:* 2-3 h. *Duration of effect:* 6-12 h. *Metabolism:* Liver. *Route of elimination:* Bile, feces, urine.

Interactions: Concurrent use with calcium channel blockers or other hypotension-causing agents may cause additive hypotensive effects. Nonsteroidal antiinflammatory agents decrease the antihypertensive effects of prazosin. Sympathomimetic agents decrease its therapeutic efficacy. With agents that stimulate both alpha- and beta-adrenergic receptors (e.g., epinephrine), vasodilation, severe hypotension, and tachycardia may result.

Nursing considerations: Advise patients to take prazosin at night to minimize postural hypotension. Monitor vital signs closely after the first dose; supervise ambulation until the risk of a first-dose effect has passed. Warn patients about the first-dose effect and the possibility of dizziness or syncope. Instruct them not to drive or do other hazardous activities until their response to prazosin has been established. Instruct patients to lie down at the first signs of lightheadedness, dizziness, or blurred vision. Warn patients that many over-the-counter medications contain agents that interact with prazosin and that they should not take any without first consulting their physician.

Terazosin (Hytrin)

Indications: Benign prostatic hypertrophy, bladder neck dyssynergia, detrusor, striated sphincter dyssynergia.

Usual dosage: Data are not available for this use.

Precautions/contraindications: Cautious use is required in patients with a history of hypersensitivity to terazosin.

Side effects/adverse reactions: See prazosin.

Pharmacokinetics: *Peak effect (antihypertensive):* 2-3 h. *Half-life:* 12 h. *Route of elimination:* Urine, feces.

Interactions: See prazosin.

Nursing considerations: See prazosin.

SKELETAL MUSCLE RELAXANTS

Normal emptying of the bladder depends on detrusor contraction occurring in coordination with relaxation of the internal and external sphincters. Spinal cord injury or disease disrupts this process. Detrusor-sphincter dyssynergia refers to a condition in which detrusor contraction does not occur in concert with external sphincter relaxation; obstruction of the urinary tract results. Nonspecific antispasmodic medications such as diazepam and baclofen have been used to treat this problem, but the adverse effects of these drugs at the levels required for treatment limit their acceptability.

HORMONAL AGENTS

ESTROGENS

The primary treatment of advanced metastatic prostate cancer is endocrine therapy to decrease circulating androgens. This causes tumor cells to atrophy. One strategy used for this purpose is administering large doses of estrogen. Estrogens are also used to treat atrophic vaginitis, a condition in postmenopausal women characterized by dry, thin vaginal walls that lack rugal folds.

Precautions/contraindications: Estrogens are contraindicated during pregnancy. Use by nursing mothers is not recommended. Women undergoing unopposed estrogen replacement therapy have a higher risk of endometrial cancer than women undergoing cyclic therapy. Systemic estrogens increase the risk of breast cancer in men; this risk is unproved in women. Estrogens are contraindicated in patients with breast cancer (because of the risk of promoting tumor growth) and women with vaginal bleeding. Estrogen therapy can exacerbate gallbladder disease, hypercalcemia, hepatic porphyria, thrombophlebitis, endometriosis, and uterine fibroids. Estrogens should be used with caution in patients with hepatic dysfunction, jaundice, or hypersensitivity to estrogens. Cautious use is required in men with cardiovascular disease, because the large doses needed to treat prostate cancer are associated with an increased risk of myocardial infarction, pulmonary embolism, and thrombophlebitis.

Side effects/adverse reactions: *Breast:* Pain, tenderness, enlargement, tumors. *CV:* Hypertension, peripheral edema (with prostate cancer therapy only: thromboembolism, thrombus formation). *GI:* Abdominal cramping or bloating, anorexia, nausea, vomiting, diarrhea, cholestatic jaundice, gallbladder disease. *Nervous system:* Chorea, dizziness, headaches. *Skin:* Chloasma, melasma, erythema multiforme, erythema nodosum, hemorrhagic eruption, hirsutism, alopecia, porphyria cutanea, skin irritation or redness (with transdermal patches only). *Other:* Decreased libido (men), increased libido (women), intolerance to contact lenses.

Pharmacokinetics: Estrogens are readily absorbed through the skin and mucous membranes and are distributed through most body tissues, including breast milk. *Protein binding:* 50%-80%. *Metabolism:* Liver, muscle, kidneys, gonads. *Route of elimination:* Urine.

Interactions: Estrogens alter the metabolism and elimination of glucocorticoids, resulting in increased therapeutic and adverse effects. Concurrent use with corticotropin enhances the antiinflammatory effects of endogenous cortisol. Carbamazepine, phenylbutazone, phenytoin, primidone, rifampin, and barbiturates enhance the metabolism of estrogens, thereby decreasing their therapeutic efficacy. Estrogens increase absorption of calcium. Estrogens decrease metabolism of cyclosporine, increasing the risks of hepatotoxicity and nephrotoxicity. Concurrent use with hepatotoxic medications increases the risk of hepatotoxicity. Smoking and tobacco increase the risk of serious cardiovascular effects resulting from estrogen use; a decreased therapeutic efficacy also results. Estrogens decrease the therapeutic efficacy of oral anticoagulants and tamoxifen. Estrogens increase the effects of succinylcholine and tricyclic antidepressants.

Nursing considerations: Oral estrogens for atrophic vaginitis can be administered continuously or cyclically

---

ESTROGENS

Chlorotrianisene (TACE) 12-25 mg/day PO—Atrophic vaginitis, prostate cancer

Conjugated estrogens (Premarin) 0.3-1.25 mg/day PO—Atrophic vaginitis
    1.25-2.5 mg/day topical
    1.25-2.5 mg tid PO—Prostate cancer

Dienestrol (DV, Ortho Dienestrol) Cyclic topical application (See manufacturer's instructions)—Atrophic vaginitis

Diethylstilbestrol (DES) 1-3 mg/day PO—Prostate cancer

Diethylstilbestrol diphosphate (Stilphostrol) 50-200 mg tid PO—Prostate cancer
    IV (See manufacturer's instructions)

Esterified estrogens (Estratab, Menest) 0.3-1.25 mg/day PO—Atrophic vaginitis
    1.25-2.5 mg tid PO—Prostate cancer

Estradiol (Estrace) Cyclic topical application (See manufacturer's instructions)—Atrophic vaginitis
    1-2 mg tid—Prostate cancer

Estradiol transdermal (Estraderm) 1 patch 2 times/wk topical—Atrophic vaginitis

Estradiol valerate (Delestrogen) 10-20 mg q 4 wk IM—Atrophic vaginitis
    30 mg q 1-2 wk IM—Prostate cancer

Estrone (Estroject, Estrone-A) 0.1-0.5 mg 2 or 3 times/wk IM—Atrophic vaginitis
    2-4 mg 2 or 3 times/wk IM—Prostate cancer

Estropipate (Ogen) 0.75-6 mg/day PO—Atrophic vaginitis

Ethinyl estradiol (Estinyl) 0.15-3 mg/day PO—Prostate cancer

Polyestradiol (Estradurin) 40 mg q 2-4 wk IM—Prostate cancer

(periods of treatment alternating with periods without treatment, or alternating with a progestin). Topical estrogens are administered cyclically. Estrogen (both oral and parenteral forms) should be given immediately after food if nausea is a problem. Monitor hepatic function and blood pressure at regular intervals. Men should have regular breast examinations. Women should have annual serum lipid profile determinations, mammograms, and Pap tests. Women with an intact uterus may require periodic endometrial biopsy. Withdrawal bleeding can occur in women with an intact uterus who are receiving cyclic estrogen therapy with a progestin.

Warn patients (especially men on higher dosages) about the possibility of dizziness. Tell them not to drive or do other hazardous activities until their response to estrogens has been established. Estrogens may cause gingival hyperplasia and other problems such as gingivitis or irritation and bleeding of gingival tissues. Instruct patients to brush with a soft toothbrush after every meal and to floss daily before brushing. Patients also need close dental management during estrogen therapy. Warn patients about the risks of smoking during estrogen therapy. Warn men of the risk of cardiovascular effects and the signs and symptoms of thromboembolism or thrombus formation (leg pain, chest pain, shortness of breath, hemoptysis, dizziness, changes in vision or speech, numbness or weakness in the extremities).

ANTIANDROGENIC AGENTS

An alternative to estrogen therapy for prostate cancer uses a group of medications called antiandrogens, because they block either the action of androgens in androgen-sensitive tissues or the production of androgens; both actions provide palliation. Flutamide (Eulexin) is an example of a "pure" antiandrogen that blocks androgens at the androgen-receptor site. Goserelin (Zoladex) and leuprolide (Lupron) are examples of luteinizing hormone–releasing hormone (LHRH) analogs that suppress the release of luteinizing hormone—the hormone responsible for stimulating testes to produce androgens. Often an LHRH analog is used in conjunction with a "pure" antiandrogen. Aminoglutethimide is an agent that achieves a medical adrenalectomy, thereby blocking adrenal production of androgens. Ketoconazole, a synthetic imidazole-derivative antifungal agent, blocks adrenal and testicular androgen production; its efficacy in prostate cancer is under investigation.

Antiandrogenic agents are also used to treat benign prostatic hyperplasia. Megestrol acetate (Megace) is a progestin that binds to androgen receptors, preventing stimulation and subsequent growth. Proscar is an agent (currently undergoing clinical trials) that inhibits conversion of testosterone to dihydrotestosterone, a more potent androgen; it reportedly has fewer side effects than other antiandrogenic agents.

ANDROGENS

Androgens are steroid hormones that promote male characteristics. They are produced primarily by the testes and mediated by hormones released from the pituitary gland. A deficiency of circulating testosterone, the most important androgen, results from either a problem with the pituitary-hypothalamus mechanism of hormone regulation or direct testicular failure. Replacement therapy with the androgens fluoxymesterone, methyltestosterone, and testosterone effectively treats such deficiency.

Vasodilators for Pharmocologic Erection Therapy

For the past 10 years the vasodilators papaverine hydrochloride, phentolamine mesylate, and alprostadil (prostaglandin E_1) have been used to treat impotence. When injected into the corpora carvernosa, they cause relaxation of the trabecular cavernous smooth muscle and vasodilation of the penile arteries. Subsequent blood flow into the corpora cavernosa causes swelling and elongation of the penis. Alprostadil also causes the glans and corpus spongiosum to swell. These agents also reduce venous outflow, possibly by increasing venous resistance.

Indications: Diagnosis and treatment of impotence.

Precautions/contraindications: These agents are contraindicated for enhancing erections in men who are not impotent; priapism and permanent damage to penile tissues may occur. Cautious use is required in patients with severe coagulation defects, a history of priapism, sickle cell disease, and allergy or intolerance to a specific agent. Systemic use of papaverine may cause hepatotoxicity; although systemic absorption is slow following intracavernosal injection, use in patients with impaired hepatic function must be weighed against the risks.

Interactions: The vasodilating effect of these agents is reversed by alpha-adrenergic sympathomimetics, especially metaraminol, epinephrine, and phenylephrine.

Nursing Considerations: Patients must be closely supervised by a physician experienced in the use of these agents and familiar with proper management of sustained erection and priapism. Intracavernosal administration of phenylephrine is used to treat sustained erection and priapism. These agents should not be self-administered by patients without thorough training and understanding of the need for strict adherence to instructions. Regular palpation of the penis by the patient and physician should be done to assess for developing fibrosis or curvature.

Alprostadil (Prostaglandin E_1)

Usual dosage: 2.5-20 µg intracavernosal. Alprostadil should not be administered more than 2 times/wk or 2 days in succession.

Side effects/adverse reactions: Priapism, bruising, bleeding, or pain at the injection site. If inadvertent subcutaneous injection occurs, bruising, bleeding, and swelling at the injection site can occur.

Pharmacokinetics: *Peak effect:* 20 min. *Duration of effect:* 1-3 h.

Papaverine

Usual dosage: 30 mg.

Side effects/adverse reactions: Dizziness, fibrosis, burning along the penis, difficulty ejaculating, tingling at the tip of the penis, priapism, bruising, bleeding, or pain at the injection site.

Pharmacokinetics: Papaverine is slowly released into the venous circulation; few if any systemic effects occur. *Peak effect:* 10 min. *Duration of effect:* 1-6 h; prolonged with concurrent use of phentolamine.

Phentolamine (Regitine)

Usual dosage: 0.5-1 mg mixed with papaverine hydrochloride (30 mg). This mixture should not be administered more often than 2 times/wk or 2 days in succession.

Side effects/adverse reactions: Dizziness, fibrosis, burning along the penis, difficulty ejaculating, tingling at the tip of the penis, priapism, bruising, bleeding, or pain at the injection site.

Pharmacokinetics: Phentolamine is slowly released into the venous circulation; few if any systemic effects result. *Peak effect:* 10 min. *Duration of effect:* 1-6 h.

Urinary Analgesics

Phenazopyridine (Pyridium)

Phenazopyridine is an azo dye with local anesthetic effect on urinary tract mucosa. Although it shows slight antibacterial action in vitro, it has little if any antibacterial effect in vivo. In the treatment of urinary tract infections, it must be administered in conjunction with an antibacterial agent. Phenazopyridine is used for the first 2 days of treatment to provide symptomatic relief.

Indications: Symptomatic relief of urinary tract irritation resulting from infection, catheterization, surgery, endoscopy, and other procedures.

Usual dosage: 200 mg tid, after meals.

Precautions/contraindications: Phenazopyridine is contraindicated in patients with glomerulonephritis, pyelonephritis, uremia, significant renal impairment or disease, and in patients with severe hepatitis. It should be used with caution in patients with GI disturbance or G6PD deficiency.

Side effects/adverse reactions: Adverse effects caused by phenazopyridine occur infrequently, except in patients with impaired renal function, with high dosage, or after prolonged use. *GI:* Nausea. *Hematologic:* Methemoglobinemia, hemolytic anemia. *Dermatologic:* Yellowish tinge of skin or sclera. *CNS:* Headache, vertigo. *Renal:* Renal stones, acute renal failure. *Allergic:* Jaundice, hepatitis.

Pharmacokinetics: Phenazopyridine appears to cross the placenta.

Interactions: None established.

Nursing considerations: This drug should be taken with food or immediately after meals to prevent GI upset. Warn patients that vertigo may occur. They should avoid driving and other inherently hazardous activities until their specific response to therapy has been established. Phenazopyridine interferes with urine tests based on color reactions or spectrometry. Phenazopyridine turns urine orange-red and can stain fabrics. Fluid intake should be maintained at 2500-3000 ml/day.

Atropine/hyoscyamine/methenamine/methylene blue/phenyl salicylate/benzoic acid (Urised)

This is a combination agent used to relieve local symptoms of urinary tract infections and diagnostic procedures that irritate urinary tract mucosa. Atropine and hyoscyamine possess anticholinergic properties, relaxing smooth muscle spasms along the urinary tract. Phenyl salicylate possesses analgesic properties. Methenamine, methylene blue, and benzoic acid are antibacterial agents.

Indications: Urinary tract infections and for relief of symptoms resultant from diagnostic procedures that cause urinary tract irritation.

Usual dosage: 1-2 tablets qid PO.

Precautions/contraindications: Cautious use is required in children with brain damage and patients with cardiac disease, severe dehydration, GI obstructive disease, glaucoma, G6PD deficiency, impaired hepatic function, hyperthyroidism, myasthenia gravis, nonobstructive prostatic hypertrophy, urinary retention, obstructive uropathy, impaired renal function, and intolerance to individual constituents of this medication. Cautious use is also required in patients over 40 yr of age because of the risk of precipitating undiagnosed glaucoma.

Side effects/adverse reactions: *Allergic:* Skin rash, hives. *Anticholinergic:* Drowsiness, dizziness, tachycardia, flushing, shortness of breath, dyspnea, dysuria, vision changes, increased intraocular pressure, dry mouth, nose, or throat. *GI:* Nausea, vomiting, stomach upset or pain. *GU:* Hematuria, pain or burning while urinating. *Salicylate effects:* Bloody stools, diarrhea, headache, dizziness, tinnitus, sweating, unusual tiredness or weakness.

Pharmacokinetics: This agent is well absorbed from the GI tract. *Route of elimination:* Urine.

Interactions: Drug interactions with each constituent should be considered (see sections on anticholinergic agents and methenamine).

Nursing considerations (see also sections on anticholinergic agents and methenamine): Methylene blue may turn urine or feces blue or bluish green; this is clinically insignificant.

MEDICATIONS USED TO TREAT OR PREVENT URINARY CALCULI

Urinary calculi arise from a variety of causes. Pharmacologic prevention and treatment are based on assess-

---

MEDICATIONS USED TO TREAT OR PREVENT URINARY CALCULI

Orthophosphates

Monobasic potassium phosphate (K-Phos) 228 mg qid PO—Calcium calculi

Potassium/sodium phosphates (Neutra-Phos) 225 mg qid PO—Calcium calculi

Thiazide diuretics

Hydrochlorothiazide (Hydrodiuril) 25-50 mg bid PO (or equivalent in other agents)—Calcium calculi

Urinary alkalinizers

Acetazolamide (Diamox) 250 mg HS PO—Cystine calculi, uric acid calculi IV (See manufacturer's instruction)

Potassium citrate (Urocit-K) up to 100 mEq/day PO—Calcium calculi, cystine calculi, renal tubular acidosis, uric acid calculi

Sodium bicarbonate (baking soda) up to 16 g/day PO—Cystine calculi, renal tubular acidosis, uric acid calculi

Sodium citrate (generic) 1-2 g q 2-4 h PO—Cystine calculi, renal tubular acidosis, uric acid calculi

Miscellaneous agents

Allopurinol (Zyloprim) 200-300 mg/day PO—Calcium calculi, uric acid calculi

Cellulose sodium phosphate (Calcibind) 5 g bid or tid PO—Calcium calculi

Pyridoxine (Vitamin B_6) 100-400 mg/day—Calcium calculi

---

ment of risk factors present and diagnosis of the cause of calculi. Medications presented herein are selected agents used to prevent the formation of calculi or to dissolve stones already formed. Hydration is one of the most effective interventions.

Orthophosphates acidify urine, increasing the solubility of calcium. Thiazide diuretics decrease calcium excretion in the distal tubule, reducing urine calcium. Urinary alkalinizers increase the solubility of uric acid and cystine. Potassium citrate also increases urine citrate, which binds with calcium, preventing calcification. Allopurinol prevents the formation of uric acid. Cellulose sodium phosphate binds with calcium ions, reducing calcium available for calcification. Pyridoxine acts as a coenzyme involved in the metabolism of protein, carbohydrates, and fat. It prevents and treats calcium oxalate calculi caused by primary hyperoxaluria.

References

CHAPTER 1: COLOR ATLAS OF ANATOMY AND PHYSIOLOGY

1. Boyarsky S, Labay P: Principles of ureteral physiology. In Bergman H, editor: *The ureter*, New York, 1981, Springer-Verlag.
2. Bradley WE: Physiology of the urinary bladder. In Walsh PC, Gittes RF, Perlmutter AD, and Stamey TA, editors: *Campbell's urology*, ed 5, Philadelphia, 1986, WB Saunders.
3. Crouch JE: *Functional human anatomy*, Philadelphia, 1982, Lea & Febiger.
4. de Tajada IS, Goldstein I, and Krane RJ: Local control of penile erection: nerves, smooth muscle, and endothelium, *Urologic Clinics of North America* 15, 9-16, 1988.
5. Dixon J, Gosling J: Structure and innervation in the human. In Torrens M, Morrison JFB, editors: *The physiology of the lower urinary tract*, London, 1987, Springer-Verlag.
6. Gosling J, Chilton C: The anatomy of the bladder, urethra and pelvic floor. In Mundy AR, Stephenson TP, and Wein AJ, editors: *Urodynamics: principles, practice and application*, London, 1984, Churchill Livingstone.
7. Gray DP, Heuther SE: Structure and function of the reproductive systems. In McCance KL, Heuther SE, editors: *Pathophysiology*, St Louis, 1990, Mosby–Year Book.
8. Griffiths D, Holstege G, Dalm E, and de Wall H: Control and coordination of bladder and urethral function in the brainstem of the cat, *Neurology and Urodynamics* 9:63-82, 1990.
9. Holstege G, Griffiths DJ, Dewall H, and Dalm E: Anatomic and physiologic observations on supraspinal control of bladder and urethral sphincter muscle contractions in the cat, *Journal of Comparative Neurology* 250:449-461, 1986.
10. Leeson CR, Leeson TS: *Histology*, Philadelphia, 1986, WB Saunders.
11. Lipschultz LI, Howards SS: *Infertility in the male*, New York, 1983, Churchill Livingstone.
12. Mann T, Lutwick-Mann C: *Male reproductive function and semen*, Berlin, 1981, Springer-Verlag.
13. Olsson CA: Anatomy of the upper urinary tract. In Walsh PC, Gittes RF, Perlmutter AD, and Stamey TA, editors: *Campbell's urology*, ed 5, Philadelphia, 1986, WB Saunders.
14. Sarma KP: *Tumors of the urinary bladder*, New York, 1969, Appleton-Century-Crofts.
15. Seeley RR, Stephens TD, and Tate P: *Anatomy and physiology*, ed 2, St Louis, 1986, Mosby–Year Book.
16. Siroky MB, Krane RJ: Neurophysiology of erection. In Krane RJ, Siroky MB, and Goldstein I, editors: *Male sexual dysfunction*, Boston, 1983, Little, Brown.
17. Staskin DR et al: Pathophysiology of stress incontinence, *Clinics in Obstetrics and Gynecology* 12:357, 1985.
18. Tanagho EA: Anatomy of the genitourinary tract. In Tanagho EA, McAninch JW, editors: *Smith's general urology*, Philadelphia, 1992, WB Saunders.
19. Tucker S: Female reproductive system. In Thompson J et al, editors: *Clinical nursing*, St Louis, 1989, Mosby–Year Book.
20. Williams P, Warwick R: *Gray's anatomy*, Philadelphia, 1980, WB Saunders.

CHAPTER 2: ASSESSMENT

21. Gray ML: Assessment of patients with urinary incontinence. In Doughty D, editor: *Nursing management of urinary and fecal incontinence*, St Louis, 1991, Mosby–Year Book.
22. Malasanos L, Barkauskas V, Moss M, and Stoltenberg-Allen K: *Health assessment*, St Louis, 1986, Mosby–Year Book.
23. Seidel HM, Ball JW, Dains JE, and Benedict WE: *Mosby's guide to physical examination*, St Louis, 1991, Mosby–Year Book.

CHAPTER 3: DIAGNOSTIC STUDIES

24. Friedenberg, RM: Excretory urography. In Pollack HM, editor: *Clinical urography*, Philadelphia, 1990, WB Saunders.
25. Marshall VF: Methods in urologic diagnosis. In Emmett JL, Witten DM, editors: *Clinical urography*, Philadelphia, 1971, WB Saunders.
26. Novick A: Renovascular hypertension. In Kendall AR, Karafin R, editors: *Urology: Goldsmith's practice of surgery*, Philadelphia, 1983, Harper & Row.
27. Tumeh SS, Treves S, and Adelstein SJ: Radionuclides in genitourinary disorders. In Walsh PC, Gittes RF, Perlmutter AD, and Stamey TA, editors: *Campbell's urology*, ed 5, Philadelphia, 1986, WB Saunders.
28. Whitaker R: Clinical application of upper tract urodynamics, *Urologic Clinics of North America* 6:137, 1979.
29. Williams RD: Magnetic resonance imaging. In Gillenwater JY, Grayhack JT, Howards SS, and Duckett JW, editors: *Adult and pediatric urology*, Chicago, 1991, Mosby–Year Book.

CHAPTER 4: INFLAMMATIONS OF THE GENITOURINARY SYSTEM

30. Andriole VT: Urinary tract infections in pregnancy, *Urologic Clinics of North America* 2:485, 1975.
31. Barrett DM, Wein AJ: Voiding dysfunction: diagnosis, classification, and management. In Gillenwater JY, Grayhack, JT, Howards SS, and Duckett JW, editors: *Adult and pediatric urology*, Chicago, 1991, Mosby–Year Book.
32. Carson CC: Urinary tract infections. In Resnick MI, Older RA, editors: *Diagnosis of genitourinary disease*, New York, 1982, Thieme Medical Publishers.
33. Davies G, Castro JE: Cystitis glandularis, *Urology* 10:128, 1977.
34. Dejuana CP, Everett JC: Interstitial cystitis: experience and review of recent literature, *Urology* 10:325, 1977.
35. Drach GW: Prostatitis: man's hidden infection, *Urologic Clinics of North America* 2:499, 1975.
36. Farrar WE: Infections of the urinary tract, *Medical Clinics of North America* 67:187, 1983.
37. Farnell B, Thomas P: Tuberculosis at the epididymis, *Canadian Medical Association Journal* 128:1296, 1983.
38. Hope-Stone HF: Radiotherapy in the management of invasive bladder cancer. In Smith PH, Prout GR, editors: *Bladder cancer*, London, 1984, Butterworth Publishers.
39. Ireton RC, Berger RE: Prostatitis and epididymitis, *Urologic Clinics of North America* 11:83, 1984.
40. Iselbacher KJ et al, editors: *Harrison's principles of internal medicine*, New York, 1980, McGraw-Hill.
41. Jensen H, Nielsen K, and Frimodt-Moller C: Interstitial cystitis: review of the literature, *Urologia Internationalis* 44:189, 1989.
42. Kay D: Host defense mechanisms in the urinary tract, *Urologic Clinics of North America* 2:407, 1975.
43. Klauber GT, Sant GR: Disorders of the male external genitalia. In Kerlalis PP, King LR, and Belman AB, editors: *Clinical pediatric urology*, Philadelphia, 1985, WB Saunders.
44. McCormick NB, Vinson RK: Interstitial cystitis: how women cope, *Urologic Nursing* 9:11, 1989.
45. Meares EM: Prostatitis, *Annual Review of Medicine* 30:279, 1979.
46. Michigan S: Genitourinary fungal infections, *Journal of Urology* 116:390, 1976.
47. Nistal M, Paniagua R: *Testicular epididymal pathology*, New York, 1984, Thieme Medical Publishers.
48. Oesterling JE: Scrotal surgery. In Glen JF, editor: *Urologic surgery*, Philadelphia, 1991, JB Lippincott.
49. Parsons CL, Schmidt JP, and Pollen JJ: Successful treatment of interstitial cystitis with sodium pentosonpolysulfate, *Journal of Urology* 130:51, 1983.
50. Rowland RG, Donogue JP: Scrotum and testis. In Gillenwater JY, Grayhack JT, Howards SS, and Duckett JW, editors: *Adult and pediatric urology*, Chicago, 1991, Mosby–Year Book.
51. Schaeffer AJ: Catheter-associated bacteriuria, *Urologic Clinics of North America* 13:735, 1986.
52. Slade DKA: Interstitial cystitis: a challenge to urology, *Urologic Nursing* 9:5, 1989.

53. Smith DR, editor: *General urology*, Los Altos, Calif, 1981, Lange Medical Books.

54. Soebel J, Kaye D: Urinary tract infections. In Gillenwater JY, Grayhack JT, Howards SS, and Duckett JW, editors: *Adult and pediatric urology*, Chicago, 1991, Mosby–Year Book.

55. Stamey TA: *Pathogenesis and treatment of urinary tract infections*, Baltimore, 1980, Williams & Wilkins.

56. Stamey TA: Urinary tract infections in women. In Harrison J et al, editors: *Campbell's urology*, Philadelphia, 1978, WB Saunders.

57. Walton KN: Urinary tract infections. In Hurst JW, editor: *Medicine for the practicing physician*, Boston, 1983, Butterworth Publishers.

CHAPTER 5: URINARY INCONTINENCE/ VOIDING DYSFUNCTION

58. Anson C, Gray ML, Bennett JK, and Green BG: Secondary complications following spinal injury, *Journal of the American Paraplegia Society* 14:106, 1991.

59. Barrett DM, Furlow W: Implantation of a new semiautomatic artificial genitourinary sphincter: experience with patients utilizing a new concept of primary and secondary activation, *Progress in Clinical and Biological Research* 78:375, 1981.

60. Barrett DM, Wein AJ: Voiding dysfunction: diagnosis, classification and management. In Gillenwater JY, Grayhack JT, Howards SS, and Duckett JW, editors: *Adult and pediatric urology*, ed 2, Chicago, 1991, Mosby–Year Book.

61. Barrett DM, Wein AJ: *Controversies in neurology*, New York, 1984, Churchill Livingstone.

62. Bates CP, Rowen D, Bradley WE, Sterling AM Glen E, Zinner N, Griffiths D, Hald T, and Melchior H: Standardization of terminology of lower urinary tract function, *Urology*, 9, 237-9.

63. Bradley WE, Scott FB: Physiology of the urinary bladder. In Walsh PC, et al, editors: *Campbell's urology*, ed 5, Philadelphia, 1986, WB Saunders.

64. Benness C, Abbott D, Cardozo L, Savvas M, and Studd J: Lower urinary tract dysfunction in postmenopausal women: the role of estrogen deficiency, *Neurology and Urodynamics* 10:315, 1991.

65. Cella M: The nursing costs of urinary incontinence in a nursing home population, *Nursing Clinics of North America* 23:159, 1988.

66. Chapell CR, Gilpin SA, Moss H, Milner T, Burnstock G, Gosling J, Miroy EJ, and Turner-Warwick RT: The role of neural factors in the etiology of detrusor instability associated with prostatic obstruction, *Journal of Urology* 141:290, 1989.

67. Chilton CP: The distal urethral sphincter mechanism and the pelvic floor. In Mundy AR, Stephenson TP, and Wein AJ, editors: *Urodynamics: principles, practice and application*, Edinburgh, 1984, Churchill Livingstone.

68. Colling J, Ouslander J, Hadley BJ, Campbell EB, and Eisch J: Patterned urge-response toileting for urinary incontinence. In key aspects of elder care (conference proceedings), April 11-13, 1991, Chapel Hill, NC.

69. Cucci A: Detrusor instability in prostatic outlet obstruction in relation to urethral opening pressure, *Neurology and Urodynamics* 9:17-24, 1990.

70. Diokno AC, Hollander JB, and Bennett CJ: Bladder neck obstruction in women: a real entity, *Journal of Urology* 132:294, 1984.

71. Dougherty MC et al: The effect of exercise on the circumvaginal muscles in postpartum women, *Journal of Nurse-Midwifery* 34:8, 1989.

72. Faller N: Toilet training people with mental retardation. In Jeter KF, Faller N, and Notron C: *Nursing for continence*, Philadelphia, 1990, WB Saunders.

73. Fantl JA, Wyman JF, McClish DK, Harkins SW, Elswick RK, Taylor JR, and Hadley EC: Efficacy of bladder training in older women with urinary incontinence, *Journal of the American Medical Association* 265:609-613, 1991.

74. Gray ML: Assessment and investigation of urinary incontinence. In Jeter KF, Faller NA, and Norton C, editors: *Nursing for continence*, Philadelphia, 1990, WB Saunders.

75. Gray ML: Assessment of the incontinent individual. In Doughty DB, editor: *Nursing management of urinary and fecal incontinence*, St Louis, 1991, Mosby–Year Book.

76. Gray ML, Siegel SW, Troy R, Faller N, Bakst A, and Hocevar B: Management of urinary incontinence. In Doughty DB, editor: *Nursing management of urinary and fecal incontinence*, St Louis, 1991, Mosby–Year Book.

77. Gray ML, Bennett JK, Green BG, and Killorin W: Urethral pressure gradient in the prediction of upper urinary tract distress following spinal injury in males, *Journal of the American Paraplegia Society* 14:105-106, 1991.

78. Gray ML, Dobkin K: Genitourinary system. In Thompson J et al: *Mosby's clinical nursing*, St Louis, 1989, Mosby–Year Book.

79. Gray ML, Dougherty MC: Urinary incontinence: pathophysiology and treatment, *Journal of Enterostomal Therapy* 14:152-162, 1987.

79a. Hessee U, Schussler B, Frimberger J, Obernitz NV, and Senn E: Effectiveness of a three-step pelvic floor reeducation in the treatment of stress urinary incontinence: a clinical assessment, *Neurology and Urodynamics* 9:397-398, 1990.

80. Kim MJ, McFarlane GH, and McLane AM: *Pocket guide to nursing diagnosis*, St Louis, 1991, Mosby–Year Book.

81. Kandel ER, Schwartz JH: *Principles of neural science*, New York, 1981, Elsevier North Holland.

82. Lose G, Colstrup H: Measurement of urethral power generation during contraction of the pelvic floor, *Neurology and Urodynamics* 10:397-398, 1991.

83. Malizia AA: Intravescial/suburetic injection of polytef: serial radiologic imaging, *Journal of Urology* 139:185a, 1988 (abstract 92).

84. Madersbacher H, Knoll M, and Kiss G: Intravesical application of oxybutynin: mode of action in controlling detrusor hyperreflexia, *Neurology and Urodynamics* 10:375-376, 1975.

84a. McGuire EJ, Appell RA: Collagen injection for the dysfunctional urethra, *Contemporary Urology* 3(9):11-20, 1991.

85. McGuire EJ, Savastano JA: Stress incontinence and detrusor instability/urge incontinence, *Neurology and Urodynamics* 4:313-316, 1985.

86. McGuire TJ, Kramer VN: Autonomic dysreflexia in the spinal cord injured: what the physician should know about this medical emergency, *Postgraduate Medicine* 80:81-89, 1986.

87. Mundy AR: The unstable bladder, *Clinics in Obstetrics and Gynecology* 12:15, 1985.

87a. National Institutes of Health: Consensus Development Conference statement: urinary incontinence in adults, vol 7, no 5, Bethesda, Md, 1988, Department of Health and Human Services.

88. Oesterling JE: The obstructive prostate and the intraurethral stent, *Contemporary Urology* 3(10):60-69, 1991.

89. Roberts JA, Sussel E, and Kaack M: Bacterial adherence to urethral catheters, *Journal of Urology* 144:264, 1990.

90. Rosenbaum TP, Shah PJR, Rose GA, and Lloyd Davies RW: Cranberry juice helps the problem of mucus production in enterocystoplasties, *Neurology and Urodynamics* 8:344, 1989.

91. Schaefer W, Lengen PH, and Thorner M: The real pressure/flow relationship during obstructed voiding, *Neurology and Urodynamics* 9:423-424, 1990.

92. Symmonds RE: Incontinence: vesical and urethral fistulae, *Clinics in Obstetrics and Gynecology* 27:499-514, 1984.

93. Wheatley JK: Causes and treatment of bladder incontinence, *Comprehensive Therapy* 9:27, 1983.

94. Williams P, Warwick R: *Gray's anatomy*, Philadelphia, 1980, WB Saunders.

95. Worth PHL: Postprostatectomy incontinence. In Mundy AR, Stephenson TP, and Wein AJ: *Urodynamics: principles, practice and application*, Edinburgh, 1984, Churchill Livingstone.

CHAPTER 6: OBSTRUCTIVE UROPATHIES

96. Andersen JT: Prostatism: clinical, radiologic and urodynamic aspects, *Neurology and Urodynamics* 1:241, 1982.

97. Andriana RT, Carson CC: Urolithiasis, *Clinical Symposia* 38:3, 1986.

98. Birkhoff JD: Natural history of benign prostatic hypertrophy. In Hinman JF Jr: *Benign prostatic hypertrophy*, New York, 1983, Springer-Verlag.

99. Boyarsky S: Ureteral surgery. In Glenn JF, editor: *Urologic surgery*, ed 2, New York, 1975, Harper & Row.

100. Boyce WH: Renal calculi. In Glenn JF, editor: *Urologic surgery*, ed 2, New York, 1975, Harper & Row.

101. Chaussy C, Brendel W, and Schmiedt E: Extracorporeally induced destruction of kidney stones by shock waves, *Lancet* 1:1265-1268, 1980.

102. Cucci A: Detrusor instability in prostatic outlet obstruction in relation to urethral opening pressure, *Neurology and Urodynamics* 9:17-24, 1990.

103. Drach GW: Urinary lithiasis. In Harrison JH et al, editors: *Campbell's urology*, Philadelphia, 1978, WB Saunders.

103a. Finkbiner AE, Bissada NK: For BPH, drugs hold promise, *Contemporary Urology* 4(2):49-54, 1992.

104. Finlayson B: Renal lithiasis in review, *Urologic Clinics of North America* 1:181, 1974.

105. Gillenwater JY: Hydronephrosis. In Gillenwater JY, Grayhack JT, Howards SS, and Duckett JW, editors: *Adult and pediatric urology*, Chicago, 1991, Mosby-Year Book.

106. Gillenwater JY: Extracorporeal shockwave lithotripsy for the treatment of urinary calculi. In Gillenwater JY, Grayhack JT, Howards SS, and Duckett JW, editors: *Adult and pediatric urology*, Chicago, 1991, Mosby-Year Book.

107. Grayhack JT, Kozlwoski JM: Benign prostatic hyperplasia. In Gillenwater JY, Grayhack JT, Howards SS, and Duckett JW, editors: *Adult and pediatric urology*, Chicago, 1991, Mosby-Year Book.

108. Jenkins AD: Calculus formation. In Gillenwater JY, Grayhack JT, Howards SS, Duckett JW, editors: *Adult and pediatric urology*, Chicago, 1991, Mosby-Year Book.

109. Jenkins AD: Upgrading extracorporeal shockwave lithotripsy, *Contemporary Urology* 3(10):11-22, 1991.

110. Kelalis PP: Obstructive uropathy: ureteropelvic junction. In Kelalis PP, King LR, and Belman AB, editors: *Clinical pediatric urology*, Philadelphia, 1985, WB Saunders.

111. King LR: Obstructive uropathy: posterior urethra. In Kelalis PP, King LR, and Belman AB, editors: *Clinical pediatric urology*, Philadelphia, 1985, WB Saunders.

112. Lapides J: Tips on self-catheterization, *Urology Digest* 6:11, 1977.

113. Lawson RK: Smaller means safer intraureteral electrohydraulic lithotripsis, *Contemporary Urology* 3:51-58, 1991.

113a. Lepor H: What will replace TURP? *Contemporary Urology* 4(2):30-41, 1992.

114. Malek RS: Obstructive uropathy: calyx. In Kelalis PP, King LR, and Belman AB, editors: *Clinical pediatric urology*, Philadelphia, 1985, WB Saunders.

115. Paulson DF: Renal calculi in children. In Glenn JF, editor: *Urologic surgery*, ed 2, New York, 1975, Harper & Row.

116. Resnick MI: Surgery of renal calculi, *AUA Update Series* 2(lesson 29):2, 1983.

117. Rose BD: Pathophysiology of renal disease, New York, 1981, McGraw-Hill.

118. Ruano-Gil D, Coca-Payeras A, and Tejedo-Maten A: Obstruction and normal recanalization of the ureter in the human embryo: its relation to congenital ureteric obstruction, *European Urology* 1:287, 1975.

119. Spirnak JP, Resnick MI: Kidney and ureteral stone surgery. In Gillenwater JY, Grayhack JT, Howards SS, and Duckett JW, editors: *Adult and pediatric urology*, Chicago, 1991, Mosby-Year Book.

120. Stamey TA: *Pathogenesis and treatment of urinary tract infection*, Baltimore, 1980, Williams & Wilkins.

121. Walker III DR: Obstructive uropathy: bladder and bladder neck. In Kelalis PP, King LR, and Belman AB, editors: *Clinical pediatric urology*, Philadelphia, 1985, WB Saunders.

122. Walsh PC, Lepor H, and Eggelston JC: Radical prostatectomy and preservation of sexual function: anatomical and pathological considerations, *Prostate* 4:473-485, 1983.

123. Walsh PC, Wilson JD: The induction of prostatic hypertrophy in the dog with androstanediol, *Journal of Clinical Investigation* 57:1093, 1976.

124. Weiss RM: Obstructive uropathy: pathophysiology and diagnosis. In Kelalis PP, King LR, and Belman AB, editors. *Clinical pediatric urology*, Philadelphia, 1985, WB Saunders.

125. Wilson JD: The pathogenesis of benign prostatic hypertrophy, *American Journal of Medicine* 68:745, 1980.

126. Weiss RM, Coolsaet BRLA: The ureter. In Gillenwater JY, Grayhack JT, Howards SS, and Duckett JW, editors: *Adult and pediatric urology*, Chicago, 1991, Mosby-Year Book.

CHAPTER 7: GENITOURINARY CANCER

127. Baker LH, Mebust WK, Chin TDY, et al: The relationship of herpes virus to carcinoma of the prostate, *Journal of Urology* 125:370-374, 1981.

128. Beahrs OH, Myers MH, editors: *American Joint Committee on Cancer: Manual for staging of cancer*, ed 2, Philadelphia, 1983, JB Lippincott.

129. Benson RC Jr, Hasan SM, Jones AG, et al: External beam radiotherapy for palliation of pain from metastatic carcinoma of the prostate, *Journal of Urology* 127:69-71, 1982.

130. Benson RC Jr, Gill GM, and Cummings KB: A randomized, double-blind crossover trial of diethylstilbestrol (DES) and estramustine phosphate (Emcyt) for stage D prostatic carcinoma, *Seminars in Oncology* 121:452-454, 1983.

131. Blair A, Fraumeni JF Jr: Geographic patterns of prostate cancer in the United States, *JNCI* 61:1379-1384, 1978.

132. Boyd SD: Kock pouch urinary diversion. In Glenn JF, editor: *Urologic surgery*, Philadelphia, 1991, JB Lippincott.

133. Bracken RB: Secondary renal neoplasms: an autopsy study, *Southern Medical Journal* 72:806, 1979.

134. Carroll PR: Urothelial carcinoma: cancers of the bladder, ureter and renal pelvis. In Tanagho EA, McAninch JW, editors: *Smith's general urology*, Norwalk, Conn, 1992, Lange Medical Publishers.

135. Catalona WJ: Bladder cancer. In Gillenwater JY, Grayhack JT, Howards SS, and Duckett JW, editors: *Adult and pediatric urology*, Chicago, 1991, Mosby-Year Book.

136. Clayman RV: Symposium: laparoscopy: new yet familiar, *Contemporary Urology* 3(10):34-50, 1991.

137. Cohen AJ, Li FP, Berg S, et al: Hereditary RCC associated with chromosomal translocation, *New England Journal of Medicine* 301:592-595, 1979.

138. Cole P, Hoover R, and Friedell GH: Occupation and cancer of the lower urinary tract, *Cancer* 29:1250, 1972.

139. deKernion JB, Berry D: The diagnosis and treatment of renal cell carcinoma, *Cancer* 44(suppl):1947, 1980.

140. de Vere-White RW: Pelvic lymph node dissection. In Glenn JF, editor: *Urologic surgery*, Philadelphia, 1991, JB Lippincott.

141. Driecer R, Williams RD: Renal parenchymal neoplasms. In Tanagho EA, McAninch JW, editors: *Smith's general urology*, Norwalk, Conn, 1992, Lange Medical Publishers.

142. Fallon B: Parenchymal tumors: clinical and diagnostic features. In Culp DA, Loening SA, editors: *Genitourinary oncology*, Philadelphia, 1985, Lea & Febiger.

143. Fossa SD, Kjosleth I, and Lund G: Radiotherapy of metastasis from renal cancer, *European Urology* 8:340, 1982.

144. Glashan RW, Robinson MRG: Cardiovascular complications in the treatment of prostatic carcinoma, *British Journal of Urology* 53:624-627, 1981.

145. Graham SD: Radical transcoccygeal prostatectomy. In Glenn JF, editor: *Urologic surgery*, Philadelphia, 1991, JB Lippincott.

146. Gray ML: Treatment modalities for bladder cancer, *Seminars in Oncology Nursing* 2:260-264, 1986.

147. Gray ML, Dobkin K: Genitourinary system. In Thompson J et al: *Mosby's clinical nursing*, St Louis, 1989, Mosby-Year Book.

148. Hermausen DK: Techniques of orchiectomy. In Glenn JF, editor: *Urologic surgery*, Philadelphia, 1991, JB Lippincott.

149. Karcioglu ZA, Sorper RM, van Reinsvelt HA, et al: Trace element concentrations in RCC, *Cancer* 42:1330, 1978.

150. Katz SA, Davis JE: Prognosis and treatment reflected by survival, *Urology* 10:10-11, 1977.

151. Kipling MD, Waterhouse JAH: Cadmium and prostatic carcinoma, *Lancet* 1:730-731, 1967.

152. Kozlowski JM, Grayhack JT: Carcinoma of the prostate. In Gillenwater JY, Grayhack JT, Howards SS, and Duckett JW, editors: *Adult and pediatric urology*, Chicago, 1991, Mosby-Year Book.

153. Kramer SA, Kelalis PP: Pediatric urologic oncology. In Gillenwater JY, Grayhack JT, Howards SS, and Duckett JW, editors: *Adult and pediatric urology*, Chicago, 1991, Mosby-Year Book.

154. Lang DJ, Kummer JF, and Hartley DP: Cytomegalovirus in semen: persistence and demonstration in extracellular fluid, *New England Journal of Medicine* 291:121, 1974.

155. Leionen A: Embolization of renal carcinoma, *Annals of Clinical Research* 17:299-305, 1985.

156. Lornoy W et al: Renal cell carcinoma: a new complication of analgesic nephropathy, *Lancet* 1:271, 1986.

157. Malizia AA, Banks DW, Walton KN, Walton GR, Ambrose AA, and Newton NC: Modified radical prostatectomy: preservation of bladder neck and proximal prostatic urethra, *Journal of Urology* 139:462A, 1988 (abstract 1194).

158. Morrison AS: Advances in the etiology of urothelial cancer, *Urologic Clinics of North America*, 11:557, 1984.

159. Narayan P: Neoplasms of the prostate gland. In Tanagho EA, McAninch JW, editors: *Smith's general urology*, Norwalk, Conn, 1992, Lange Medical Publishers.

160. Okabe T, Urobe A, Kato T: Production of erythropoietin-like activity by human renal and hepatic carcinomas in cell culture, *Cancer* 55:1918, 1985.

161. Paganinni-Hill A, Ross RK, and Henderson BE: Epidemiology of renal cancer. In Skinner DG, Lieskovsky G, editors: *Diagnosis and management of genitourinary cancer*, Philadelphia, 1988, WB Saunders.

162. Paulson DF, Rabson AS, and Fraley EE: Viral neoplastic transformation of hamster prostate tissue in vitro, *Science* 159:200-201, 1968.

163. Paulson DF: Radical cystectomy. In Glenn JF, editor: *Urologic surgery*, Philadelphia, 1991, JB Lippincott.

164. Presti JC Jr, Herr HW: Genital tumors. In Tanagho EA, McAninch JW, editors: *Smith's general urology*, Norwalk, Conn, 1992, Lange Medical Publishers.

165. Prout GR: Classification and staging of bladder carcinoma, *Seminars in Oncology* 6:189-197, 1979.

166. Richie JP: Retroperitoneal lymphadenectomy. In Glenn JF, editor: *Urologic surgery*, Philadelphia, 1991, JB Lippincott.

167. Robson CJ, Churchill BM, and Anderson W: The results of radical nephrectomy for renal cell carcinoma, *Journal of Urology* 101:297, 1969.

168. Rost A and Brosig W: Preoperative irradiation of renal cell carcinoma, *Urology* 10:414, 1977.

169. Rowland RG, Donohue JP: Scrotum and testis. In Gillenwater JY, Grayhack JT, Howards SS, and Duckett JW, editors: *Adult and pediatric urology*, Chicago, 1991, Mosby–Year Book.

170. Sander S, Biesland HO: Laser in the treatment of localized prostatic carcinoma, *Journal of Urology* 132:280-281, 1984.

171. Schumann LM, Mandel J, Blackard C, et al: Epidemiologic study of prostatic cancer: preliminary report, *Cancer Treatment Reports* 61:181-186, 1977.

172. Smith JA, Middleton RG: Bladder cancer. In Smith JA Jr: *Lasers in urologic surgery*, Chicago, 1985, Year Book Medical Publishers.

173. Soloway MS: How I follow patients with bladder cancer, *Contemporary Urology* 3(9):42-49, 1991.

174. Srinivas V et al: Sarcomas of the kidney, *Journal of Urology* 32:13, 1984.

175. Sueppel C: Men need education about prostate cancer, *Innovations in Urology Nursing* 3:1, 1991.

176. Wagle DG, Moore RH, and Murphy GP: Secondary carcinomas of the kidney, *Journal of Urology* 114:30, 1975.

177. Walsh PC: Radical retropubic prostatectomy. In Walsh PC, Gittes RF, Perlmutter AD, and Stamey TA, editors: *Campbell's urology*, Philadelphia, 1986, WB Saunders.

178. Walther PJ: Radical perineal prostatectomy. In Glenn JF, editor: *Urologic surgery*, Philadelphia, 1991, JB Lippincott.

179. Watt R: Bladder cancer: etiology and pathophysiology, *Seminars in Oncology Nursing* 2:256-259, 1986.

179a. Wilkinson GB and Retzer A: Prostate awareness week: how we did it! *Urologic Nursing* 11:19, 1991.

180. Williams RD: Renal, perirenal and ureteral neoplasms. In Gillenwater JY, Grayhack JT, Howards SS, and Duckett JW, editors: *Adult and pediatric urology*, Chicago, 1991, Mosby–Year Book.

CHAPTER 8: ERECTILE DYSFUNCTION/ IMPOTENCE

181. Abosief SR, Lue TF: Hemodynamics of penile erection, *Urologic Clinics of North America* 15:1-8, 1988.

182. Bennett AH: Venous arterialization for erectile dysfunction, *Urologic Clinics of North America* 15:111-114, 1988.

183. Benson GS, Boileau MA: The penis: sexual function and dysfunction. In Gillenwater JY, Grayhack JT, Howards SS, and Duckett JW, editors: *Adult and pediatric urology*, Chicago, 1991, Mosby–Year Book.

184. Kass I, Updegraff K, and Muffly RB: Sex in chronic obstructive pulmonary disease, *Medical Aspects of Human Sexuality* 6:33, 1972.

185. Kaufman JJ, Lindner A, and Rax S: Complications of penile prosthesis surgery for impotence, *Journal of Urology* 128:1192, 1982.

186. Kedia KR: Vascular disorders and male erectile dysfunction, *Urologic Clinics of North America* 8:153, 1981.

187. Krane RJ: Penile prosthesis, *Urologic Clinics of North America* 15:103, 1988.

188. Lewis RW: Venous surgery for impotence, *Urologic Clinics of North America* 15:115-122, 1988.

189. Lue TF: Male sexual dysfunction. In Tanagho EA, McAninch JW, editors: *Smith's general urology*, Norwalk, Conn, 1992, Lange Medical Publishers.

190. Michal V, Kramar R, and Psopichal J: External iliac steal syndrome, *Journal of Cardiovascular Surgery* 19:255, 1978.

191. Morales A, Condra MS, Owen JE, Fenemore J, and Surridge DH: Oral and transcutaneous pharmacologic agents in the treatment of impotence, *Urologic Clinics of North America* 15:87-94, 1988.

192. Smith AD: Causes and classification of impotence, *Urologic Clinics of North America* 8:79, 1981.

193. Wagner G, Green R: *Impotence*, New York, 1981, Plenum Press.

194. Wiedman CL, Northcutt RC: Endocrine aspects of impotence, *Urologic Clinics of North America* 8:143, 1981.

195. Witherington RF: Suction device therapy in the management of erectile impotence, *Urologic Clinics of North America* 15:123-128, 1988.

CHAPTER 9: INFERTILITY

196. Belker AM: Surgery for male infertility. In Glenn JF, editor: *Urologic surgery*, Philadelphia, 1991, JB Lippincott.

197. Belman AB: The dilemma of the adolescent varicocele, *Contemporary Urology* 3(9):21-29, 1991.

198. Lipshultz LI, Howards SS, and Buch JP: Male infertility. In Gillenwater JY, Grayhack JT, Howards SS, and Duckett JW, editors: *Adult and pediatric urology*, Chicago, 1991, Mosby–Year Book.

199. Martin M: Infertility. In Pernoll M, editor: *Current obstetric and gynecologic diagnosis and treatment*, Norwalk, Conn, 1991, Appleton & Lange.

200. McClure RD: Male infertility. In Tanagho EA, McAninch JW, editors: *Smith's general urology*, Norwalk, Conn, 1992, Lange Medical Publishers.

201. Muse KN Jr, Wilson EA: Endometriosis. In Pernoll M, editor: *Current obstetric and gynecologic diagnosis and treatment*, Norwalk, Conn, 1991, Appleton & Lange.

202. Thorneycroft IH: Amenorrhea. In Pernoll M, editor: *Current obstetric and gynecologic diagnosis and treatment*, Norwalk, Conn, 1991, Appleton & Lange.

203. Urban ND: Adult height and fertility in men with congenital virilizing adrenal hyperplasia, *New England Journal of Medicine* 299:1392, 1978.

CHAPTER 11: GENITOURINARY DRUGS

204. Goodman AG, Goodman LS, and Gilman A, editors: *Goodman and Gilman's the pharmacologic basis of therapeutics*, New York, 1980, Macmillan.

205. Govoni LE, Hayes JE: *Drugs and nursing implications*, Norwalk, Conn, 1988, Appleton-Century-Crofts.

Index